Inflammatory Bowel Disease: From Diagnosis to Treatment

Inflammatory Bowel Disease: From Diagnosis to Treatment

Guest Editors

Laura Maria Minordi
Daniela Pugliese

MDPI

Basel • Beijing • Wuhan • Barcelona • Belgrade • Novi Sad • Cluj • Manchester

Guest Editors
Laura Maria Minordi
Dipartimento di Diagnostica per Immagini, Radioterapia Oncologica ed Ematologia
Fondazione Policlinico Universitario "A. Gemelli" IRCCS
Rome
Italy

Daniela Pugliese
Dipartimento di Medicina e Chirurgia Traslazionale
Università Cattolica del Sacro Cuore
Rome
Italy

Editorial Office
MDPI AG
Grosspeteranlage 5
4052 Basel, Switzerland

This is a reprint of the Special Issue, published open access by the journal *Journal of Clinical Medicine* (ISSN 2077-0383), freely accessible at: https://www.mdpi.com/journal/jcm/special_issues/JLXWJH20J4.

For citation purposes, cite each article independently as indicated on the article page online and as indicated below:

Lastname, A.A.; Lastname, B.B. Article Title. *Journal Name* **Year**, *Volume Number*, Page Range.

ISBN 978-3-7258-4819-5 (Hbk)
ISBN 978-3-7258-4820-1 (PDF)
https://doi.org/10.3390/books978-3-7258-4820-1

Contents

Preface

Inflammatory bowel diseases (IBDs) are a group of chronic inflammatory intestinal conditions with unknown etiologies; Crohn's disease (CD) and ulcerative colitis (UC) represent the two main types. Diagnosis of both conditions is usually performed using a combination of clinical symptoms, laboratory tests, and endoscopic features. Moreover, the use of radiological exams, such as magnetic resonance imaging (MRI) or computed tomography (CT) enterography, is crucial in clinical practice for both the diagnosis and staging of CD, since the inflammation transmurally involves the bowel wall. CT has been proven to enable the precise evaluation of disease activity and complications, such as fistulas and strictures, especially when presenting acutely. However, MRI has replaced CT in recent years, because it offers comparable sensitivity, specificity, and accuracy in the diagnosis and evaluation of CD, especially concerning disease activity, without exposure to radiation. IBDs require continuous medical therapy to control inflammation and avoid disease progression. Over time, the therapeutic armamentarium for IBDs has significantly increased with the advent of several different advanced therapies (including both biological therapies and small molecules). However, surgery still remains a valid option in cases with complications, such as abscesses, fistulas, perforation, and strictures (the frequency of which ranges from 48% to 52% at 5 years after the diagnosis of CD) or for medically refractory diseases. The monitoring and adjustment of therapy based on those assessments is important in evaluating patients' responses to medical therapy and identifying those who require surgery. This reprint aims to provide information on clinical, diagnostic, and treatment methods for IBDs.

Laura Maria Minordi and Daniela Pugliese
Guest Editors

Journal of
Clinical Medicine

MDPI

Systematic Review

Small Intestinal Contrast Ultrasonography (SICUS) in Crohn's Disease: Systematic Review and Meta-Analysis

Giuseppe Losurdo [1,*], Margherita De Bellis [1], Raffaella Rima [1], Chiara Maria Palmisano [2], Paola Dell'Aquila [1], Andrea Iannone [1], Enzo Ierardi [1], Alfredo Di Leo [1] and Mariabeatrice Principi [1]

1 Section of Gastroenterology, Department of Precision and Regenerative Medicine and Ionian Area, University of Bari, 70124 Bari, Italy; margideb@gmail.com (M.D.B.); paoladellaquila@tiscali.it (P.D.); ianan@hotmail.it (A.I.); ierardi.enzo@gmail.com (E.I.); alfredo.dileo@uniba.it (A.D.L.); b.principi@gmail.com (M.P.)

2 Internal Medicine Unit "C. Frugoni", Department of Interdisciplinary Medicine, University of Bari "Aldo Moro", Piazza Giulio Cesare 11, 70124 Bari, Italy; chiarapalmi8@gmail.com

* Correspondence: giuseppelos@alice.it; Tel.: +39-0805594430; Fax: +39-0805593088

Abstract: The diagnosis of Crohn's Disease (CD) is based on a combination of clinical symptoms, laboratory tests, endoscopy, and imaging data. In Small Intestine Contrast Ultrasonography (SICUS), the ingestion of a macrogol solution as an oral contrast medium may optimize image quality. We performed a meta-analysis to evaluate the diagnostic performance of SICUS for CD. A literature search was performed in August 2023. We selected only studies where SICUS was compared to a technique that allows the assessment of the whole gastrointestinal tract, such as an MRE, a CT scan, or a surgical evaluation. We estimated pooled weighted sensitivity, specificity, and likelihood ratio for positive and negative tests (PLR/NLR) of SICUS. Summary receiver operating characteristic curves (SROC) were drawn, and pooled areas under the curve (AUC) were calculated. Five studies with 325 CD patients were included. SICUS showed a pooled sensitivity for the diagnosis of 95% (95% confidence interval CI 89–99%), a specificity = 77% (95% CI 60–90%), and the AUC was 0.94. SICUS demonstrated a pooled sensitivity for strictures of 78% (95% CI 63–88%) and a specificity = 96% (95% CI 85–99%), with AUC = 0.93. For abscesses, SICUS demonstrated a pooled sensitivity of 100% (95% CI 59–100%) and a specificity of 90% (95% CI 74–98%). Fistulae were detected with a pooled sensitivity of 77% (95% CI 46–95%) and a specificity of 92% (95% CI 75–99%). SICUS demonstrated excellent diagnostic performance compared to the gold standard despite some clinical scenarios (stenosis/fistulae) showing suboptimal diagnostic effectiveness.

Keywords: Crohn's disease; diagnosis; ultrasound; magnetic resonance enterography; oral contrast; SICUS

1. Introduction

Crohn's disease (CD) is a chronic condition with immunological pathogenesis, which can affect any site of the gastrointestinal tract in a segmental and transmural way, from the mouth to the anus. A total of 50% of patients have an involvement of the terminal ileum and colon, while 30% have an isolated small bowel involvement, while the remaining 20% of cases are confined to the colon. Among patients with small bowel disease, the terminal ileum is affected in 90% of cases [1].

CD is characterized by periods of remission alternated with phases of a flare-up. The inflammatory process can evolve towards either a fibrostenotic-obstructive picture or a penetrating-fistulizing one [1]. Symptoms can be insidious or nonspecific and depend on the site and severity of the disease. The development of adhesions leads to the formation of fistulas, as CD induces transmural damage. Abdominal and pelvic abscesses develop in 10 to 30% of patients. Other complications include intestinal obstruction, occurring in 40% of cases, massive hemorrhage, malabsorption, and severe perianal disease [1].

The diagnosis of CD relies on a combination of clinical symptoms, laboratory tests, and imaging data [2]. Ileopancolonoscopy is the first technique involved in diagnosis, management, and monitoring; however, endoscopy is not always a thorough investigation and is limited by invasiveness, poor patient compliance, and a risk of bowel perforation. Ileopancolonoscopy also fails to evaluate the extent of ileal disease, transmural damage, and lesions in the perineal region, such as fistulas and abscesses. Therefore, other imaging techniques, including ultrasonography, computed tomography (CT), and magnetic resonance enterography (MRE), have been more frequently used recently. Indeed, transabdominal ultrasound is non-invasive, does not use ionizing radiation, and is easily accepted by patients. Nowadays, intestinal ultrasound use is increasing as a clinically important first-line technique both in patients with suspected CD and disorder follow-up [3].

In particular, in small intestinal contrast ultrasonography (SICUS), introducing an oral contrast medium may optimize image quality and increase sensitivity and diagnostic accuracy in detecting small intestine lesions [3]. This method, therefore, has become relevant for investigating patients with CD for the classification of disease activity, the analysis of small bowel stenosis/mural fibrosis, and the evaluation of specific therapy responses [3]. In SICUS, patients are examined in the fasting state and after ingestion of an oral macrogol contrast solution consisting of polyethylene glycol (PEG) in powder at a dose ranging from 125 to 800 mL (usually 375 mL), dissolved in 250 mL of water [3]. The introduction of an oral contrast medium allows for distension of the intestinal lumen, with better visualization of the intestinal wall and accuracy in detecting complications related to CD, including strictures, abscesses, and fistulas [3]. Furthermore, its use has been proposed in the preoperative evaluation of CD, offering precision in detecting the presence of dilatation upstream of the stenosis [4,5]. Thus, SICUS has emerged as a valuable, well accepted, and radiation-free technique in the detection of intestinal damage in CD.

Therefore, we aimed to perform a systematic review and meta-analysis in order to evaluate the pooled diagnostic performance of SICUS in patients with CD in comparison to gold-standard techniques able to assess the transmural activity of the disease.

2. Materials and Methods

2.1. Eligibility Criteria and Study Selection

Methods of analysis and inclusion criteria were based on "Preferred Reporting Items for Systematic Reviews and Meta-Analyses" (PRISMA) recommendations [6], and its extension for diagnostic test accuracy (PRISMA-DTA) was taken into account [7]. A PRISMA-DTA checklist is provided in Supplementary Material S1. We excluded review articles, experimental in vitro studies, and single case reports. In cases of studies analyzing overlapping periods from the same registry/database, we considered only the study that examined the longest period and the largest number of patients.

2.2. Data Collection Process

A literature search was performed and updated in August 2023. Relevant publications were identified through research in PubMed, Web of Science, and Scopus. Only in extenso papers were selected; therefore, abstracts or conference proceedings were excluded. The search terms were Crohn's Disease, ultrasound, oral contrast, and SICUS. We used the following string, using Boolean operators AND/OR: Crohn's Disease AND (ultrasound OR small bowel OR oral contrast OR SICUS). We selected only studies in which SICUS was compared to a technique that allowed assessment of the whole gastrointestinal tract, such as magnetic resonance enterography (MRE), computed tomography (CT), or surgical evaluation. Therefore, in the case of comparison with colonoscopy, the study was excluded. In our search strategy, we included only papers in which the gold standard was able to assess all the bowel walls; therefore, if SICUS was compared only to enteroclysis or capsule endoscopy, it could not be included. Titles and abstracts of papers were screened by two reviewers (MDB and RR). Successively, data were extracted from the relevant studies by one reviewer and checked by a second reviewer, and thus inserted into dedicated tables. A third reviewer (GL) came to a decision on any disagreements.

Reviewers independently extracted from each paper the following data: (i) publication year, (ii) country, (iii) single- or multi-center study, (iv) study design, (v) number of patients included, (vi) oral contrast agent, (vii) ultrasound device, and (viii) number of true positive/negative and false positive/negative results. If the study did not provide sufficient data to extract true positive/negative and false positive/negative outcomes, it was excluded from the final analysis.

2.3. *Summary Measures and Planned Methods of Analysis*

The end-point was to estimate the pooled weighted sensitivity, specificity, and likelihood ratio for positive and negative tests (PLR and NLR, respectively) and the diagnostic odd ratio (DOR) of SICUS. Summary receiver operating characteristic curves (SROC) were drawn, and pooled areas under the curve (AUC) were calculated. A random effect model was followed in all analyses. We assessed heterogeneity using the χ^2 test, and if it was statistically significant, the I^2 statistic was computed. If necessary, a subgroup analysis was performed. The data were expressed as proportions/percentages, and 95% confidence intervals (CI) were calculated. A p-value < 0.05 was considered statistically significant. All analyses were performed according to the general principles of meta-analysis [8]. The MetaDisc software version 1.4 was used [9].

Two reviewers (GL and PD) independently assessed the quality of the included studies using the Quality Assessment of Diagnostic Accuracy Studies version 2 (QUADAS-2) instrument [10]. This tool is designed to assess the quality of primary diagnostic accuracy studies for inclusion in the systematic review (Supplementary Material S2).

3. Results

3.1. *Study Selection*

After a bibliography search, five studies were included in the analysis [11–15]. Such studies are reported in Table 1. The process of study selection is summarized in Figure 1. All studies but one [12] were performed in the adult population. Three studies were performed in the UK [11–13] and two in Italy [14,15]. All studies used PEG as an oral contrast agent, with final volume ranging from 250 mL to 1000 mL. Overall, 325 patients with CD were recruited.

3.2. *Final Diagnosis*

The term "final diagnosis" in the selected papers was defined as "the final judgement of the physician after performing all diagnostic tests and referred only to CD". For this analysis, four studies provided sufficient data [11–13,15]. One hundred and twenty-one patients were recruited. SICUS showed a pooled sensitivity of 95% (95% CI 89–99%), a specificity of 77% (95% CI 60–90%), a positive LR of 2.73 (0.93–8.05), a negative LR of 0.15 (0.06–0.41) and a DOR = 24.94 (5.90–105.47). The AUC of the SROC curve was 0.94. Further details are shown in Figure 2.

Table 1. Summary of main characteristics of included studies.

Article, Year	Country	Age Population	Type of Study	Study Population and Indication	N Male/Female	US Device	Contrast Agent	Amount of Contrast Agent	Ultrasound Diagnostic Criteria for CD	Gold Standard
Chatu, 2012 [11]	UK	36 (SD ± 15)	Retrospective	Suspected or already diagnosed CD. Performed for first diagnosis or detection of complications	64/79	Toshiba Medical Systems, Tochigi, Japan/GE Healthcare, Milwaukee, WI, USA	PEG Klean® Prep (Norgine)	1 sachet in 1000 mL	(1) distended bowel wall thickness >3 mm; (2) absence of peristalsis; (3) stiffened bowel loop; (4) presence of a stricture, fistula, abscess; (5) absence of wall stratification; (6) increased power Doppler activity; (7) mesenteric lymph node hypertrophy; (8) mesenteric fat hypertrophy	Final diagnosis, enclosing CT
Hakim, 2019 [12]	UK	15 (2–17)	Retrospective	Suspected or already diagnosed CD. Performed for first diagnosis or detection of complications	49/44	Toshiba Medical Systems, Tochigi, Japan/GE Healthcare, Milwaukee, WI, USA	Pediatric PEG (Movicol)	1 sachet/250 mL 250–1000 mL (body weight-ba sed)	Same as [11]	Magnetic Resonance Enterography (MRE)
Kumar, 2015 [13]	UK	29.6 (SD ± 10.7)	Prospective	Patients with suspicion of CD. Performed for first diagnosis or detection of complications	12/13	Toshiba Medical Systems, Tochigi, Japan/GE Healthcare, Milwaukee, WI, USA	PEG Klean® Prep (Norgine)	1 sachet in 1000 mL	Same as [11]	Magnetic Resonance Enterography (MRE)
Onali, 2012 [14]	Italy	44 (19–73)	Prospective	Patients with CD who needed surgery	8/7	Hitachi, EUB 6500, Japan	PEG (Promefarm, Milano, Italy)	375 mL (250–500 mL)	Same as [11], except lymphnodes enlargement (defined as >1 cm);	Surgical and pathological findings
Pallotta, 2012 [15]	Italy	37.7 (12–78)	Prospective	Patients with CD who needed surgery	28/21	Toshiba Tosbee (Tokyo, Japan)	PEG 4000 (Promefarm, Milan, Italy)	375 mL (250–500 mL)	Increased wall thickness (>3 mm). Bowel stenosis was defined as lumen diameter < 1. Bowel dilatation was defined as lumen diameter > 2.5 cm. Hypoechoic peri-intestinal lesions were defined fistulas when duct-like Abscesses in case of round-like mass with a diameter > 2 cm	Surgical and pathological findings

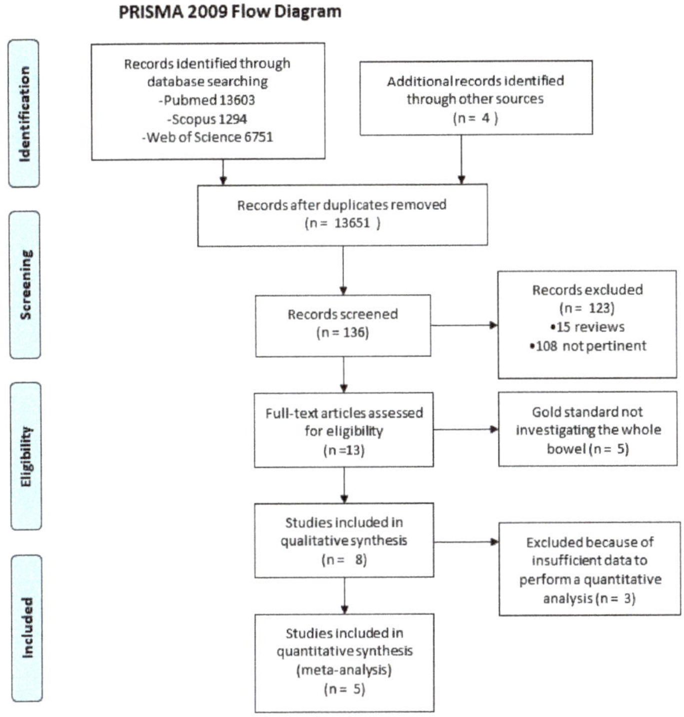

Figure 1. Flowchart summarizing the process of figure selection.

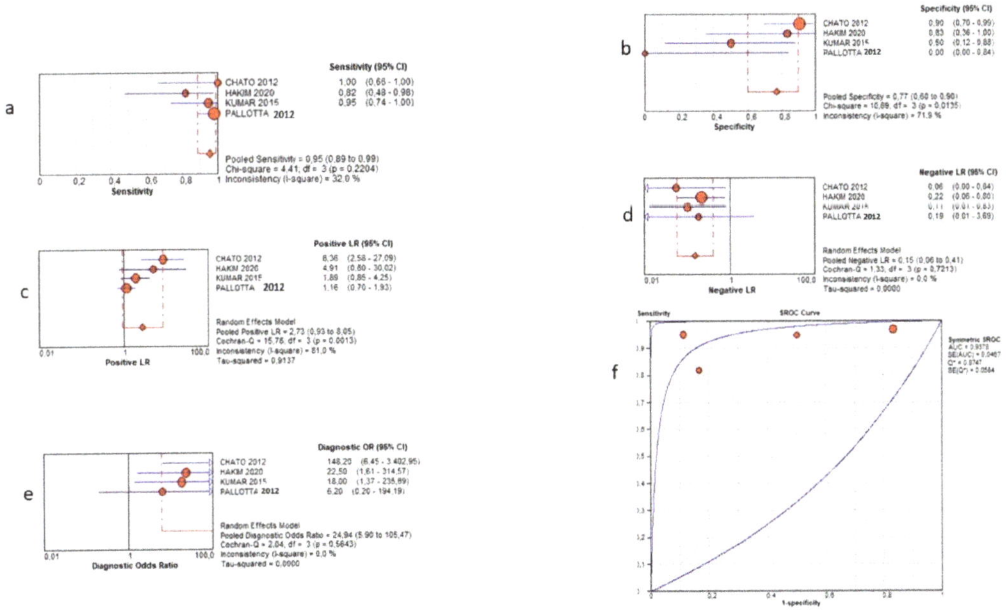

Figure 2. Sensitivity (**a**), specificity (**b**), positive likelihood ratio (**c**), negative likelihood ratio (**d**), diagnostic odd ratio (**e**), and AUC (**f**) for diagnosis of CD.

3.3. Strictures

The presence of strictures was examined in 94 patients within all studies. SICUS demonstrated a pooled sensitivity of 78% (95% CI 63–88%), a specificity of 96% (95% CI 85–99%), a positive LR of 6.37 (0.93–8.05), a negative LR of 0.23 (0.05–1.15), and a DOR = 30.99 (7.07–135.82). The AUC of the SROC curve was 0.93. Such results are summarized in the plots in Figure 3.

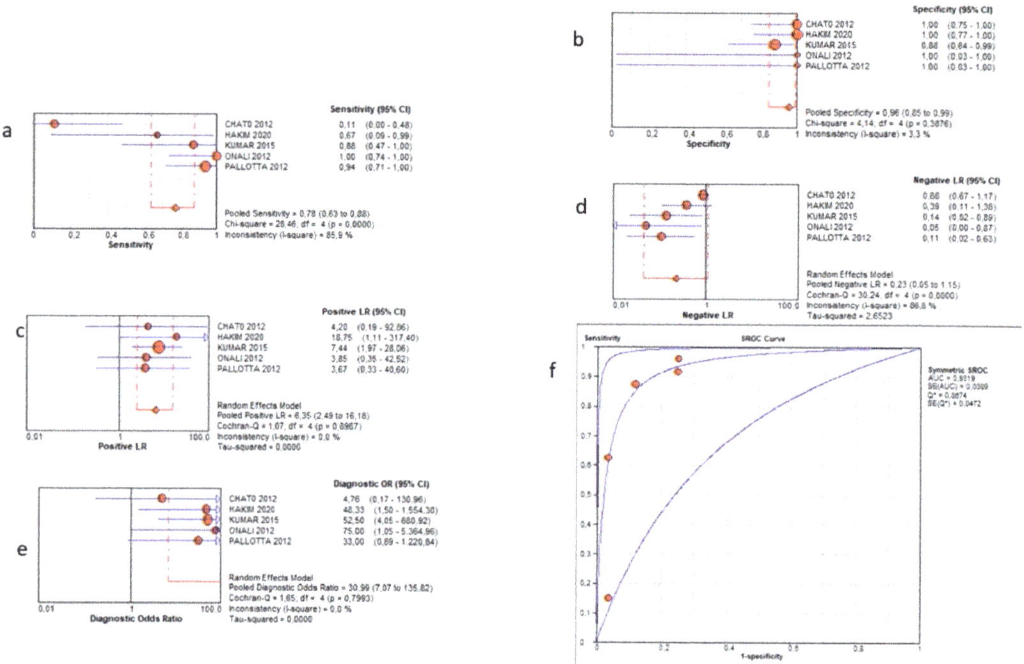

Figure 3. Sensitivity (**a**), specificity (**b**), positive likelihood ratio (**c**), negative likelihood ratio (**d**), diagnostic odd ratio (**e**), and AUC (**f**) for stenosis detection.

3.4. Abscesses

This analysis was possible for only forty patients overall in three studies [13–15]. SICUS demonstrated a pooled sensitivity of 100% (95% CI 59–100%), a specificity of 90% (95% CI 74–98%), a positive LR of 6.34 (1.94–21.17), a negative LR of 0.13 (0.02–0.84), and a DOR = 53.08 (5.07–555.11). It was not possible to calculate the AUC of SROC. Such results are reported in the plots of Figure 4. Of note, since one study provided several zero values, the corresponding diamond in the plots was not drawn in the figures.

3.5. Fistulae

This outcome was evaluated in 55 patients overall across three studies [13–15]. SICUS showed a pooled sensitivity of 77% (95% CI 46–95%), a specificity of 92% (95% CI 75–99%), a positive LR of 8.82 (2.23–34.88), a negative LR of 0.29 (0.08–1.11), and a DOR = 33.75 (3.13–363.90). It was not possible to calculate the AUC of SROC. Such results are reported in the plots of Figure 5. Of note, since one study provided several zero values, the corresponding diamond in the plots was not drawn in the figures.

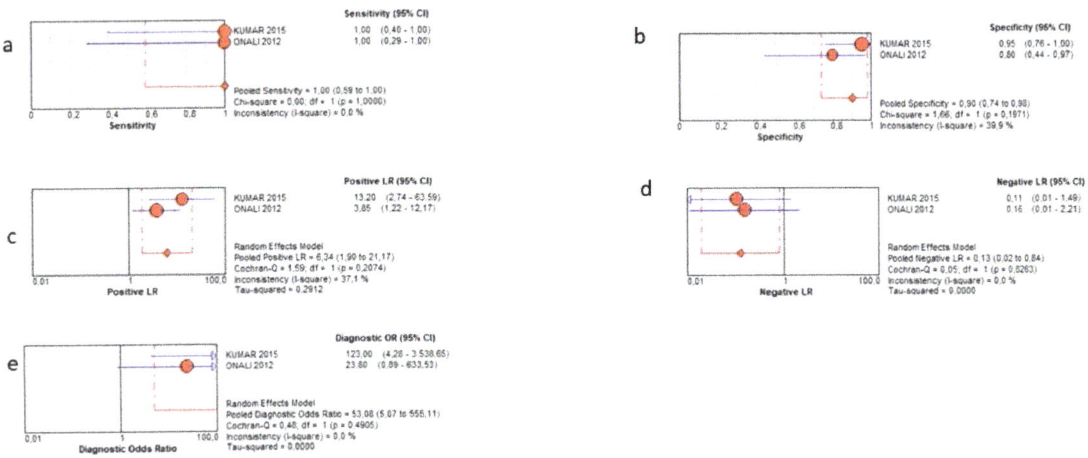

Figure 4. Sensitivity (**a**), specificity (**b**), positive likelihood ratio (**c**), negative likelihood ratio (**d**), and diagnostic odd ratio (**e**) for abscess detection.

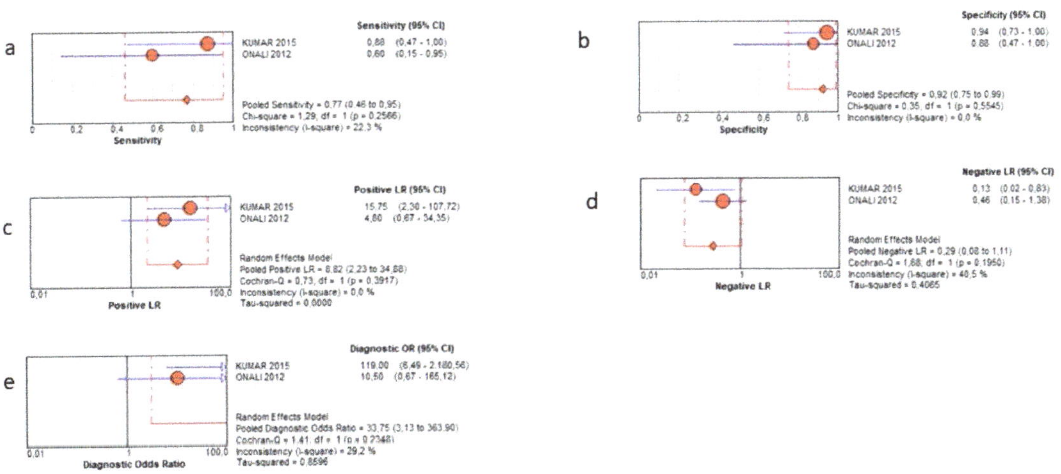

Figure 5. Sensitivity (**a**), specificity (**b**), positive likelihood ratio (**c**), negative likelihood ratio (**d**), and diagnostic odd ratio (**e**) for fistulae detection.

3.6. Dilation

Three studies [12–14] investigated the presence of pre-stenotic luminal dilation in 61 patients. We found a pooled sensitivity of 100% (95% CI 80–100%), a specificity of 80% (95% CI 65–90%), a positive LR of 3.99 (2.30–6.94), a negative LR of 0.10 (0.02–0.49) and a DOR of 41.03 (6.62–254.27). The AUC of the SROC curve was 0.91. Such results are summarized in the plots of Figure 6.

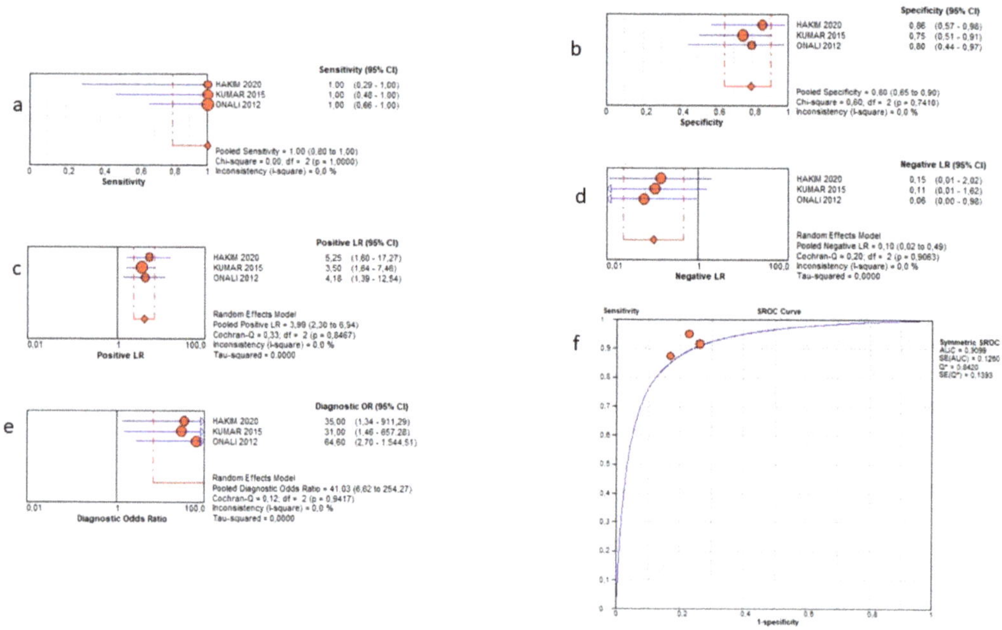

Figure 6. Sensitivity (**a**), specificity (**b**), positive likelihood ratio (**c**), negative likelihood ratio (**d**), diagnostic odd ratio (**e**), and AUC (**f**) for bowel dilation diagnosis.

4. Discussion

Since CD may affect every segment of the digestive system, with transmural involvement, endoscopy techniques are not always adequate for the investigation of the whole bowel length. Imaging procedures with panoramic spatial resolution are necessary to integrate clinical and endoscopic. MRE is considered the gold standard nowadays, but it has some drawbacks. For example, it is not available in all centers, and it is time consuming. CT enterography has emerged as an alternative as it is more widespread and more rapid, despite radiation exposure being a relevant limit. SICUS is an ultrasound-based method that explores bowel loops and is able to identify wall thickness, intestinal motility, perfusion using a Doppler scan, and possible complications such as stenosis, dilation, fistulae, and abscesses [16]. Oral ingestion of a contrast (usually PEG dissolved in a volume of water ranging from 250 to 1000 mL) may help to increase the sensitivity of ultrasound since it may enhance some characteristics such as pre-stenotic dilation; furthermore, lumen distension is useful to better evaluate the thickness of the wall and the feature of its layers. Another advantage of SICUS is its dynamic peculiarity, which allows one to focus on a detail and analyze it under several planes and direct motion. Conversely, artifacts, interposition of air and loops, and power of resolution might be intrinsic limitations of this method. Bowel ultrasound is a highly acceptable and well-tolerated tool for monitoring disease activity in IBD patients [17].

SICUS is a safe technique: side effects were described only in the articles by Onali and Pallotta, and no side effects were recorded in any patients in these two studies. Nevertheless, it could be argued that in case of clinically significant strictures, a liquid overload may elicit subocclusion symptoms; therefore, particular care should be taken into account.

The first relevant finding of our meta-analysis was a very high sensitivity (95%) for CD diagnosis, while the specificity was slightly lower (77%). This could be justified by the use of a cut-off value of 3 mm for bowel wall thickness in most studies [11,14,15]. Indeed, some Authors have proposed higher cut-offs of 4 mm [18] or 5 mm [19] to increase specificity. On the other hand, we found a sensitivity of 78% for stenosis detection. This finding is in agreement with previous studies, showing that the sensitivity of ultrasound for stenosis detection may range around 80% [20]; therefore, some stenotic areas may have been missed at SICUS. Apart from such results, most studies confirmed that SICUS has a good agreement with gold standard procedures. The perspective is different for fistulae. The ultrasound pattern evocating a possible fistula may not be univocal, and several possible signs have been proposed, often related to the experience of the examiner [21]. Indeed, some further evidence showed a sensitivity close to 70% for detecting fistulae, even when other ancillary techniques, such as water immersion, were adopted [22]. However, results are conflicting in the literature, as an additional study showed a sensitivity of 100% and a specificity of 98% [23], thus underlining that the expertise of the observer may be a main issue and a bias to be highlighted when reporting results in a systematic review. Rectum may be difficult to examine by ultrasound, and this may explain why some cases of fistulae or abscesses may be missed by SICUS [24]. A different approach in this case, i.e., trans-perineal ultrasound examination, could add sensitivity to SICUS, as shown in some evidence from literature [25], provided that the operator has a sufficient level of expertise when scanning the perineal and perirectal areas.

In pediatric populations, sensitivity and specificity were even higher, >90% [26,27]. This could be explained as CD commonly affects the small bowel in children [28]. In this regard, the pediatric population could be the ideal target for SICUS due to non-invasiveness and lack of radiation exposure. A recent expert consensus clearly underlined this point and promoted the standardization of the technique, as basic equipment requirements, patient selection, preparation and positioning, technical considerations, and limitations may cause a lack of reproducibility among operators [29]. In this regard, the Simple Pediatric Activity Ultrasound Score has been published, demonstrating a substantial agreement between ultrasound and endoscopy for all disease locations (weighted $k = 0.85$) and substantial agreement for ileocolonic disease (weighted $k = 0.96$) [30]. In children, a bowel wall thickness superior to 1.9 mm had a sensitivity of 64%, a specificity of 76%, and an area under the curve of 0.743 for detecting inflammation, compared to ileo-colonoscopy [31].

A previous meta-analysis from 2016 comparing imaging and endoscopy has already been published on the topic [32], showing a pooled sensitivity of 88.3% and specificity of 86.1%. However, such meta-analysis was enclosed as the gold standard for both imaging techniques and endoscopy; therefore, it was hampered by a relevant heterogeneity. Moreover, comparing ileopancolonoscopy and SICUS is possible only for colonic or ileal disease; therefore, the remaining segments of the small bowel cannot be taken into account. In the present analysis, we recruited only studies in which the gold standard could provide a panoramic and transmural evaluation of the whole intestine, thus providing a more homogeneous and punctual comparison. The comparison between colonoscopy and SICUS may be useful only for assessing the activity of terminal ileum or to predict disease reactivation after ileo-cecal resection; in this regard, another meta-analysis confirmed a very good sensitivity (99%) and specificity (74%) to detect post-surgical recurrence [8].

Despite the accuracy of the methodological approach, the current meta-analysis has some limitations. The most important one is that for some outcomes, the total amount of patients analyzed is low (about 50 for fistulae and abscesses). Another limitation is that we were not able to sub-analyze the localization of the disease (proximal or distal small bowel) because such data were not available in all the studies included.

In conclusion, our meta-analysis confirmed that SICUS has a very good performance compared to the gold standard as well as the evident advantage of its easy availability and feasibility. Some disadvantages might be the level of operator experience and the risk of missing some pictures. For these reasons, the present study supports SICUS's usefulness for the periodic monitoring of CD evolution; nevertheless, a panoramic MRE should be performed upon initial classification and in the event of significant progression of the disease. Some authors have suggested that the diagnostic accuracy of intestinal ultrasound could be optimized using contrast-enhanced ultrasonography [33], and this might be an additional step to reach an effectiveness comparable to current imaging gold standards.

Supplementary Materials: The following supporting information can be downloaded at https://www.mdpi.com/article/10.3390/jcm12247714/s1, Supplementary Material S1. PRISMA-DTA checklist. Supplementary Material S2. Quality Assessment of Diagnostic Accuracy Studies version 2 (QUADAS-2) instrument.

Author Contributions: Conceptualization, G.L., A.D.L. and M.P.; methodology, G.L, P.D., M.P., R.R., A.I. and M.D.B.; software, G.L.; validation, M.P, A.D.L. and E.I.; formal analysis, G.L., R.R. and M.D.B.; investigation, M.D.B., R.R. and C.M.P.; resources, P.D.; data curation, A.I. and C.M.P.; writing—original draft preparation, C.M.P. and G.L.; writing—review and editing, E.I. and M.P. All authors have read and agreed to the published version of the manuscript.

Funding: This research received no external funding.

Conflicts of Interest: The authors declare no conflict of interest.

References

1. Torres, J.; Mehandru, S.; Colombel, J.F.; Peyrin-Biroulet, L. Crohn's disease. *Lancet* **2017**, *389*, 1741–1755. [CrossRef]
2. Gomollón, F.; Dignass, A.; Annese, V.; Tilg, H.; Van Assche, G.; Lindsay, J.O.; Peyrin-Biroulet, L.; Cullen, G.J.; Daperno, M.; Kucharzik, T.; et al. 3rd European Evidence-based Consensus on the Diagnosis and Management of Crohn's Disease 2016: Part 1: Diagnosis and Medical Management. *J. Crohn's Colitis* **2017**, *11*, 3–25. [CrossRef] [PubMed]
3. Mocci, G.; Migaleddu, V.; Cabras, F.; Sirigu, D.; Scanu, D.; Virgilio, G.; Marzo, M. SICUS and CEUS imaging in Crohn's disease: An update. *J. Ultrasound* **2017**, *20*, 1–9. [CrossRef] [PubMed]
4. Roda, G.; Chien Ng, S.; Kotze, P.G.; Argollo, M.; Panaccione, R.; Spinelli, A.; Kaser, A.; Peyrin-Biroulet, L.; Danese, S. Crohn's disease. *Nat. Rev. Dis. Primers* **2020**, *6*, 22. [CrossRef] [PubMed]
5. Rispo, A.; Imperatore, N.; Testa, A.; Nardone, O.M.; Luglio, G.; Caporaso, N.; Castiglione, F. Diagnostic Accuracy of Ultrasonography in the Detection of Postsurgical Recurrence in Crohn's Disease: A Systematic Review with Meta-analysis. *Inflamm. Bowel Dis.* **2018**, *24*, 977–988. [CrossRef] [PubMed]
6. Liberati, A.; Altman, D.G.; Tetzlaff, J.; Mulrow, C.; Gøtzsche, P.C.; Ioannidis, J.P.A.; Clarke, M.; Devereaux, P.J.; Kleijnen, J.; Moher, D. The PRISMA statement for reporting systematic reviews and meta-analyses of studies that evaluate health care interventions: Explanation and elaboration. *PLoS Med.* **2009**, *6*, e1000100. [CrossRef] [PubMed]
7. McInnes, M.D.; Moher, D.; Thombs, B.D.; McGrath, T.A.; Bossuyt, P.M.; Clifford, T.; Cohen, J.F.; Deeks, J.J.; Gatsonis, C.; Hooft, L.; et al. Preferred Reporting Items for a Systematic Review and Meta-analysis of Diagnostic Test Accuracy Studies: The PRISMA-DTA Statement. *JAMA* **2018**, *319*, 388–396. [CrossRef]
8. Leandro, G. *Meta Analysis: The Handbook for Understanding and Practice of Meta Analysis in Medical Research*; The Bridge Publishing: Milan, Italy, 2018.
9. Zamora, J.; Abraira, V.; Muriel, A.; Khan, K.; Coomarasamy, A. Meta-DiSc: A software for meta-analysis of test accuracy data. *BMC Med. Res. Methodology* **2006**, *6*, 31. [CrossRef]
10. Whiting, P.F.; Rutjes, A.W.S.; Westwood, M.E.; Mallett, S.; Deeks, J.J.; Reitsma, J.B.; Leeflang, M.M.G.; Sterne, J.A.C.; Bossuyt, P.M.M.; QUADAS-2 Group. QUADAS-2: A Revised Tool for the Quality Assessment of Diagnostic Accuracy Studies. *Ann. Intern. Med.* **2011**, *155*, 529–536. [CrossRef]
11. Chatu, S.; Pilcher, J.; Saxena, S.; Fry, D.; Pollok, R. Diagnostic accuracy of small intestine ultrasonography using an oral contrast agent in Crohn's disease: Comparative study from the UK. *Clin. Radiol.* **2012**, *67*, 553–559. [CrossRef]
12. Hakim, A.; Alexakis, C.; Pilcher, J.; Tzias, D.; Mitton, S.; Paul, T.; Saxena, S.; Pollok, R.; Kumar, S. Comparison of small intestinal contrast ultrasound with magnetic resonance enterography in pediatric Crohn's disease. *JGH Open* **2019**, *4*, 126–131. [CrossRef] [PubMed]
13. Kumar, S.; Hakim, A.; Alexakis, C.; Chhaya, V.; Tzias, D.; Pilcher, J.; Vlahos, J.; Pollok, R. Small intestinal contrast ultrasonography for the detection of small bowel complications in Crohn's disease: Correlation with intraoperative findings and magnetic resonance enterography. *J. Gastroenterol. Hepatol.* **2015**, *30*, 86–91. [CrossRef] [PubMed]
14. Onali, S.; Calabrese, E.; Petruzziello, C.; Zorzi, F.; Sica, G.; Fiori, R.; Ascolani, M.; Lolli, E.; Condino, G.; Palmieri, G.; et al. Small intestine contrast ultrasonography vs computed tomography enteroclysis for assessing ileal Crohn's disease. *World J. Gastroenterol.* **2012**, *18*, 6088–6095. [CrossRef] [PubMed]
15. Pallotta, N.; Vincoli, G.; Montesani, C.; Chirletti, P.; Pronio, A.; Caronna, R.; Ciccantelli, B.; Romeo, E.; Marcheggiano, A.; Corazziari, E. Small intestine contrast ultrasonography (SICUS) for the detection of small bowel complications in crohn's disease: A prospective comparative study versus intraoperative findings. *Inflamm. Bowel Dis.* **2012**, *18*, 74–84. [CrossRef]
16. Kucharzik, T.; Maaser, C. Intestinal ultrasound and management of small bowel Crohn's disease. *Ther. Adv. Gastroenterol.* **2018**, *11*, 1756284818771367. [CrossRef]
17. Rajagopalan, A.; Sathananthan, D.; An, Y.; Van De Ven, L.; Martin, S.; Fon, J.; Costello, S.P.; Begun, J.; Bryant, R.V. Gastrointestinal ultrasound in inflammatory bowel disease care: Patient perceptions and impact on disease-related knowledge. *JGH Open* **2019**, *4*, 267–272. [CrossRef]

18. Goodsall, T.M.; Jairath, V.; Feagan, B.G.; Parker, C.E.; Nguyen, T.M.; Guizzetti, L.; Asthana, A.K.; Begun, J.; Christensen, B.; Friedman, A.B.; et al. Standardisation of intestinal ultrasound scoring in clinical trials for luminal Crohn's disease. *Aliment. Pharmacol. Ther.* **2021**, *53*, 873–886. [CrossRef]
19. Neye, H.; Voderholzer, W.; Rickes, S.; Weber, J.; Wermke, W.; Lochs, H. Evaluation of criteria for the activity of Crohn's disease by power Doppler sonography. *Dig. Dis.* **2004**, *22*, 67–72. [CrossRef]
20. Sleiman, J.; Chirra, P.; Gandhi, N.S.; Baker, M.E.; Lu, C.; Gordon, I.O.; Viswanath, S.E.; Rieder, F. Crohn's disease related strictures in cross-sectional imaging: More than meets the eye? *United Eur. Gastroenterol. J.* **2022**, *10*, 1167–1178. [CrossRef]
21. de la Portilla, F.; Sojo, V.; Vázquez-Monchul, J.M.; Pintor, J.; Dios, S.; Reyes-Díaz, M.L. Description of a new ultrasound sign to distinguish Crohn's anal fistula from cryptoglandular fistula: The rosary sign. *Colorectal Dis.* **2023**, *25*, 1446–1452. [CrossRef]
22. Wang, F.; Numata, K.; Yonezawa, H.; Sato, K.; Ishii, Y.; Yaguchi, K.; Kume, N.; Hashimoto, Y.; Nishio, M.; Nakamori, Y.; et al. Consistency of Trans-Abdominal and Water-Immersion Ultrasound Images of Diseased Intestinal Segments in Crohn's Disease. *Diagnostics* **2020**, *10*, 267. [CrossRef] [PubMed]
23. Allocca, M.; Fiorino, G.; Bonifacio, C.; Furfaro, F.; Gilardi, D.; Argollo, M.; Peyrin-Biroulet, L.; Danese, S. Comparative Accuracy of Bowel Ultrasound Versus Magnetic Resonance Enterography in Combination With Colonoscopy in Assessing Crohn's Disease and Guiding Clinical Decision-making. *J. Crohn's Colitis* **2018**, *12*, 1280–1287. [CrossRef] [PubMed]
24. Girlich, C.; Ott, C.; Strauch, U.; Schacherer, D.; Obermeier, F.; Jung, E.M.; Schölmerich, J.; Schreyer, A.G.; Klebl, F. Clinical feature and bowel ultrasound in Crohn's disease—Does additional information from magnetic resonance imaging affect therapeutic approach and when does extended diagnostic investigation make sense? *Digestion* **2011**, *83*, 18–23. [CrossRef]
25. Terracciano, F.; Scalisi, G.; Bossa, F.; Scimeca, D.; Biscaglia, G.; Mangiacotti, M.; Valvano, M.R.; Perri, F.; Simeone, A.; Andriulli, A. Transperineal ultrasonography: First level exam in IBD patients with perianal disease. *Dig. Liver Dis.* **2016**, *48*, 874–879. [CrossRef]
26. Oliva, S.; Cucchiara, S.; Civitelli, F.; Casciani, E.; Di Nardo, G.; Hassan, C.; Papoff, P.; Cohen, S.A. Colon capsule endoscopy compared with other modalities in the evaluation of pediatric Crohn's disease of the small bowel and colon. *Gastrointest. Endosc.* **2015**, *83*, 975–983. [CrossRef] [PubMed]
27. Aloi, M.; Di Nardo, G.; Romano, G.; Casciani, E.; Civitelli, F.; Oliva, S.; Viola, F.; Maccioni, F.; Gualdi, G.; Cucchiara, S. Magnetic resonance enterography, small-intestine contrast US, and capsule endoscopy to evaluate the small bowel in pediatric Crohn's disease: A prospective, blinded, comparison study. *Gastrointest. Endosc.* **2015**, *81*, 420–427. [CrossRef] [PubMed]
28. Van Limbergen, J.; Russell, R.K.; Drummond, H.E.; Aldhous, M.C.; Round, N.K.; Nimmo, E.R.; Smith, L.; Gillett, P.M.; McGrogan, P.; Weaver, L.T.; et al. Definition of Phenotypic Characteristics of Childhood-Onset Inflammatory Bowel Disease. *Gastroenterology* **2008**, *135*, 1114–1122. [CrossRef]
29. Kellar, A.M.; Dolinger, M.M.; Novak, K.L.M.; Chavannes, M.M.M.; Dubinsky, M.; Huynh, H. Intestinal Ultrasound for the Pediatric Gastroenterologist: A Guide for Inflammatory Bowel Disease Monitoring in Children: Expert Consensus on Behalf of the International Bowel Ultrasound Group (IBUS) Pediatric Committee. *J. Pediatr. Gastroenterol. Nutr.* **2022**, *76*, 142–148. [CrossRef]
30. Kellar, A.; Wilson, S.; Kaplan, G.; DeBruyn, J.; Tanyingoh, D.; Novak, K.L. The Simple Pediatric Activity Ultrasound Score (SPAUSS) for the Accurate Detection of Pediatric Inflammatory Bowel Disease. *J. Pediatr. Gastroenterol. Nutr.* **2019**, *69*, e1–e6. [CrossRef]
31. Chavannes, M.; Hart, L.; Rezvan, P.H.; Dillman, J.R.; Polk, D.B. Bedside Intestinal Ultrasound Predicts Disease Severity and the Disease Distribution of Pediatric Patients with Inflammatory Bowel Disease: A Pilot Cross-sectional Study. *Inflamm. Bowel Dis.* **2023**, izad083. [CrossRef]
32. Zhu, C.; Ma, X.; Xue, L.; Xu, J.; Li, Q.; Wang, Y.; Zhang, J. Small intestine contrast ultrasonography for the detection and assessment of Crohn disease: A meta-analysis. *Medicine* **2016**, *95*, e4235. [CrossRef] [PubMed]
33. Białecki, M.; Białecka, A.; Laskowska, K.; Liebert, A.; Kłopocka, M.; Serafin, Z. Contrast-Enhanced Ultrasonography in Crohn's Disease Diagnostics. *Hepatogastroenterology* **2015**, *62*, 927–932. [PubMed]

Journal of
Clinical Medicine

MDPI

Review

Role of Device-Assisted Enteroscopy in Crohn's Disease

Giulia Catassi [1,2,*], Clelia Marmo [1], Antonio Gasbarrini [3] and Maria Elena Riccioni [1,*]

1 Digestive Endoscopy Unit, IRCCS "Agostino Gemelli" University Hospital, Catholic University of Rome, Largo A. Gemelli 8, 00168 Rome, Italy; clelia.marmo@outlook.it
2 Pediatric Gastroenterology and Liver Unit, Umberto I Hospital, Sapienza University of Rome, Largo A. Gemelli 8, 00168 Rome, Italy
3 Internal Medicine, Gastroenterology and Liver Unit, "Agostino Gemelli" University Hospital, Catholic University of Rome, Largo A. Gemelli 8, 00168 Rome, Italy; antonio.gasbarrini@policlinicogemelli.it
* Correspondence: giulia.catassi@gmail.com (G.C.); mariaelena.riccioni@policlinicogemelli.it (M.E.R.)

Abstract: Crohn's Disease (CD) is a chronic inflammatory disorder of the gastrointestinal tract, posing diagnostic and management challenges due to its potential involvement of any segment from the mouth to the anus. Device-assisted enteroscopy (DAE) has emerged as a significant advancement in the management of CD, particularly for its ability to access the small intestine—a region difficult to evaluate with conventional endoscopic methods. This review discusses the pivotal role of DAE in the nuanced management of CD, emphasizing its enhanced diagnostic precision and therapeutic efficacy. DAE techniques, including double-balloon enteroscopy (DBE), single-balloon enteroscopy (SBE), and the now-withdrawn spiral enteroscopy, enable comprehensive mucosal assessment, targeted biopsies, and therapeutic interventions like stricture dilation, bleeding control, and foreign body removal. Despite its benefits, DAE carries risks such as perforation, bleeding, and pancreatitis, which require careful procedural planning and a skilled execution. The review highlights DAE's impact on reducing surgical interventions and improving patient outcomes through minimally invasive approaches, thereby enhancing the quality of life for patients with CD. Continuous improvement and research are essential in order to maximize DAE's utility and safety in clinical practice.

Keywords: enteroscopy; Crohn's Disease

1. Introduction

Crohn's Disease (CD) is a chronic, inflammatory condition of the gastrointestinal tract, classified under the umbrella of inflammatory bowel diseases (IBDs). The etiology of CD is complex, involving an interplay of genetic factors, environmental triggers, immune system responses, and microbiota composition [1,2]. CD is distinguished by its potential to affect any part of the gastrointestinal tract, from the mouth to the anus, and presents a discontinuous, segmental distribution, which complicates both diagnosis and management [3]. Small-bowel (SB) lesions are recognized in 30 to 60% of CD patients, and 10% to 30% of individuals have isolated SB disease [4]. Because these lesions cannot be recognized with upper and lower endoscopy alone—the conventional endoscopic methods—isolated SB CD is challenging to identify [4]. The development of device-assisted enteroscopy (DAE) techniques in the early 21st century have substantially impacted the diagnosis and treatment of Crohn's, particularly with its capacity to access and assess the small intestine, a region elusive to conventional endoscopic methods, such as push enteroscopy and capsule endoscopy [5].

The evolution of DAE techniques marks a significant milestone, shifting from limited traditional methods to enabling direct visualization and intervention across the entire small bowel. This advancement has been crucial for a more accurate and comprehensive diagnosis and treatment of small-bowel diseases, particularly CD, where direct mucosal evaluation, targeted biopsies, and therapeutic interventions like stricture dilation, bleeding control, and foreign bodies removal are now possible [6].

2. Purpose of the Review

The primary aim of this review is to discuss the substantial role DAE plays in the nuanced management of CD. It will examine the enhanced diagnostic precision DAE brings to the table, as well as its therapeutic efficacy in managing this intricate disease. The review will highlight DAE's ability to visualize the entire small intestine, which is frequently involved in CD; facilitate targeted biopsies and thorough mucosal assessments; and identify complications such as strictures, fistulas, and areas of active inflammation. Moreover, the review will emphasize the impact of DAE on therapeutic interventions, from the dilation of strictures to the control of bleeding, removal of foreign bodies, and application of local therapy to inflammatory lesions. By detailing these aspects, the review intends to demonstrate the integral role DAE plays in offering an advanced approach to CD management, potentially leading to enhanced patient outcomes and an improved quality of life.

3. Procedure Overview and Technique

DAE has significantly evolved, with various techniques offering unique benefits and limitations in the management of small-bowel diseases, including Crohn's Disease. DAE encompasses double-balloon enteroscopy (DBE), single-balloon enteroscopy (SBE), and spiral enteroscopy, each offering unique access to the small intestine [7].

3.1. Double-Balloon Enteroscopy (DBE)

The DBE technique uses two balloons, one on the endoscope and another on a flexible overtube, which alternately inflate and deflate to pleat the small intestine over the overtube and endoscope, allowing a deep traversal of the small bowel [8]. Despite its utility, DBE has limitations, particularly in terms of the extent of the bowel that can be examined in a single session [9]. A complete small-bowel enteroscopy with DBE is time-consuming and often requires full anesthesia, making it less practical for extensive examinations [10]. However, DBE is particularly advantageous for patients with prior surgeries, as it allows for the easier navigation through postoperative adhesions and altered anatomy compared to spiral enteroscopy techniques [11].

3.2. Single-Balloon Enteroscopy (SBE)

SBE uses a single balloon on an overtube to assist in guiding the endoscope through the small intestine by advancing and stabilizing the overtube sequentially [12]. While SBE offers a simpler setup compared to DBE, it may not achieve the same depth of insertion [13]. However, SBE has proven effective for both diagnostic and therapeutic purposes and is often preferred for its relative ease of use and shorter procedure times. SBE is advantageous in patients where full anesthesia might be a concern, as it can often be performed under deep sedation [14]. There is also a modality of SBE where the balloon is inserted through the scope itself, eliminating the need for an overtube. This approach involves a balloon catheter that can be passed through the working channel of the endoscope, which is then inflated to help advance and stabilize the endoscope. This method simplifies the procedure further and can reduce the time required for setup and execution [15,16].

3.3. Spiral Enteroscopy (SE)

SE employs a spiral-shaped overtube that, when rotated, pleats the small intestine onto the overtube, propelling the endoscope forward [17]. Initially, SE was "manual", meaning manually rotated by the endoscopist. It was particularly advantageous for patients with upper intestinal polyps. The spiral-shaped overtube allowed the endoscope to be withdrawn through it, facilitating the easy harvesting of polyps. This feature provided a distinct advantage over other enteroscopy techniques. Then, recent developments have introduced motorized spiral enteroscopy (MSE). which represents an evolution of the manual spiral technique, incorporating a motorized system to automate the rotation of the spiral overtube. The motorized system offers several advantages over its manual predecessor, including a more controlled and consistent rotation, a reduced physical strain on the endoscopist, and potentially shorter procedure times. MSE uses an electric motor to rotate the overtube, allowing for the precise and continuous advancement of the endoscope through the small intestine. Studies have demonstrated its effectiveness in reaching deep segments of the small bowel, making it a valuable tool in the management of Crohn's Disease (CD) [12,18]. However, SE has been withdrawn from the market in July 2023 due to severe adverse events [19].

DAE is commonly performed under deep sedation or general anesthesia to ensure patient comfort and facilitate a thorough examination. X-ray surveillance, typically fluoroscopy, is often used during DAE to guide the procedure, particularly in complex cases where navigation through the small intestine is challenging [20]. Fluoroscopy can help in accurately positioning the endoscope and overtube, especially when dealing with anatomical variations or postoperative adhesions. However, the necessity of X-ray surveillance is not absolute for all DAE procedures [21]. In many cases, experienced endoscopists can perform DAE without the need for continuous fluoroscopic guidance, relying instead on anatomical landmarks and tactile feedback to navigate the small intestine. This approach can reduce radiation exposure to both the patient and the medical team [21] The decision to use X-ray surveillance depends on various factors, including the complexity of the case, the experience of the endoscopist, and the specific clinical scenario [21].

The choice between DBE and SBE depends on clinical indications, operator expertise, and device availability [22]. The procedural approach, anterograde (oral) or retrograde (anal), is chosen based on the small-intestine segment requiring examination, as suggested by symptoms and imaging, or WCE [23]. Certain symptoms and clinical presentations can help localize the disease burden within the small intestine, thus informing the choice of approach: patients with jejunal involvement often present with symptoms such as upper abdominal pain, bloating, and early satiety; ileal involvement is commonly associated with symptoms such as lower abdominal pain, cramping, diarrhea, and sometimes blood in the stool [24,25]. In some cases, if the exact location of the disease is unclear, imaging can be performed first. For patients without suspicion or evidence of stenoses, it is possible to precede DAE with a capsule endoscopy to identify the level or area of interest. If the area of interest is within the first 75% of the small-bowel transit time, an oral approach is recommended. Conversely, if it is beyond 75%, an anal approach is indicated. This strategy is particularly useful when addressing small-intestinal ulcers and bleeding [26].

The duration of DAE is variable, depending on the complexity of the case and the extent of the small bowel that needs to be examined [27]. Following the procedure, patients typically undergo a recovery phase to offset the effects of sedation or anesthesia. The majority of patients are discharged on the same day, provided there are no complications or need for extended observation. Post-procedural care includes dietary advice and monitoring for signs of potential complications such as abdominal pain, fever, or bleeding, which require prompt medical attention [28]. For dietary advice, there are no specific guidelines; however, the same dietary recommendations as those used post-procedure are followed: immediately after the procedure, patients are advised to start with clear liquids such as water, clear broths, or tea. If clear liquids are well-tolerated, patients can gradually progress to a soft diet within the first 24 h. Soft foods include mashed potatoes, yogurt, applesauce, and well-cooked vegetables. These dietary guidelines can help minimize the risk of post-procedural complications and improve patient outcomes.

The patients eligible for DAE are as follows:

- Patients who have undergone an endoscopy with negative results but have indications of Crohn's Disease (CD) based on MRI or small-bowel capsule endoscopy findings—device-assisted enteroscopy can be utilized for endoscopic and histological confirmation of the diagnosis [2];
- When clinical symptoms suggest small-bowel involvement that remains unexplained after initial non-invasive investigations [2];

- When therapeutic maneuvers such as stricture dilation, control of bleeding, or removal of foreign bodies are needed [2].

In these scenarios, DAE serves as a strategic choice to bridge the gap between initial non-invasive imaging and the need for a more definitive diagnosis and therapeutic intervention [29].

4. Advantages of Device-Assisted Enteroscopy (DAE) over Other Methods

DAE has shown numerous advantages over other diagnostic methods in Crohn's Disease, such as magnetic resonance enterography (MRE), computed tomography enterography (CTE), and wireless capsule endoscopy (WCE) [30]. It should be considered complementary to a non-invasive examination of the small intestine, as it provides not only a direct and detailed visualization of the mucosal surface (with a sensitivity for detecting small-bowel lesions in Crohn's Disease of 65%), but also the unique opportunity for biopsy and therapeutic interventions [31]. While MRE and CTE are critical for a comprehensive structural assessment and initial suspicion of Crohn disease, they cannot offer a direct mucosal assessment and histological examination [32]. WCE allows for a broader visualization of the mucosal surface and is sensitive for detecting small-bowel lesions, but it has limitations due to the inability to take biopsies, its diagnostic-only capacity, and the risk of capsule retention [33].

MRE, in particular, is a non-invasive sectional imaging modality that is highly useful for following up on inflammatory activity. It can detect fistulas or strictures with a high sensitivity and specificity, making it an excellent tool for monitoring disease progression and complications. The sensitivity of MRE for detecting small-bowel active inflammation in Crohn's Disease is approximately 68%, with a specificity of approximately 95% [34]. These rates highlight MRE's effectiveness in non-invasively assessing disease activity and complications. Moreover, MRE also serves as a valuable prognostic tool in Crohn's Disease. The Magnetic Resonance Index of Activity (MaRIA) score is a validated scoring system used in MRE to quantify disease activity: it incorporates parameters such as bowel wall thickness, edema, ulceration, and contrast enhancement, providing an objective measure of inflammatory activity in Crohn's Disease. Studies have shown that the MaRIA score correlates well with endoscopic findings and can predict the risk of surgery, making it an effective tool for guiding treatment strategies and monitoring disease progression over time [35].

Despite these strengths, MRE and CTE lack the capability for a direct mucosal visualization and histological examination. This limitation is where DAE excels, offering not just a detailed visualization but also the ability to perform therapeutic interventions. This is especially significant in Crohn's Disease management, where the accurate assessment of the disease extent, activity, and complications can directly influence treatment decisions and patient outcomes. DAE allows for the biopsy of suspicious areas, dilation of strictures, and treatment of bleeding lesions, providing a comprehensive approach to disease management that cannot be matched by non-invasive imaging techniques alone [36].

5. Role of DAE in Diagnosing Crohn's Disease

The role of DAE in diagnosing Crohn's Disease is multifaceted, offering significant advantages over traditional diagnostic methods. First, it is unparalleled in its ability to visually access the entire small intestine, providing a favorable diagnostic yield of up to 80%, with a low complication rate which underscores its safety [37–39]. It, indeed, enables the detection of early mucosal changes that are indicative of Crohn's Disease and are often missed by other diagnostics, including minor erosions, aphthous ulcers, or early inflammatory lesions [40]. The ability to perform targeted biopsies is instrumental in confirming the diagnosis, as the histopathological examination of biopsy samples can reveal granulomas or other microscopic features characteristic of CD, thus enhancing diagnostic precision [41]. Moreover, DAE can predict the risk of surgery in Crohn's Disease patients, with the small-bowel simple endoscopic score for Crohn's Disease (SES-CD) serving as a key prognostic tool, thus influencing treatment decisions and patient management strategies. Research carried out at Samsung Medical Center discovered a significant rise in the likelihood of surgical complications in patients with a small-bowel simple endoscopic score for Crohn's Disease (SES-CD) of 7, as opposed to those with a small-bowel SES-CD of 6 [42].

While DAE provides a high diagnostic yield, there are instances where the procedure may not be able to visualize the entire small intestine. In such cases, alternative or complementary diagnostic methods (imaging or WCE) can be employed to achieve a comprehensive evaluation.

6. Therapeutic Applications of DAE in Crohn's Disease

DAE not only plays a pivotal role in the diagnosis of Crohn's Disease but also offers a range of therapeutic applications such as balloon stricture dilation, steroid injections, the treatment of bleeding ulcers, and the removal of foreign bodies. These interventions can directly address complications associated with the disease, potentially reducing the need for surgical interventions and improving patient outcomes [43].

6.1. *Stricture Dilation*

Strictures in Crohn's Disease, characterized by the narrowing of the intestinal lumen due to inflammation, fibrosis, or both, can lead to obstructive symptoms such as abdominal pain, bloating, and nausea [44]. Before considering dilation, it is important to perform magnetic resonance imaging to accurately determine the length and characteristics of the stricture. DAE can directly approach stenoses that are fibrotic, less than 5 cm, and without prestenotic dilation, allowing for endoscopic dilation [45]. This procedure involves the use of a balloon which is guided to the site of the stricture, and then expanded to widen the narrowed area [46]. Dilation can alleviate obstructive symptoms and restore bowel patency, improving the quality of life for patients with symptomatic strictures [47]. DAE has been shown to be an effective and relatively safe therapeutic option; a pooled analysis of individual data from 1463 patients revealed a technical success rate of 89.1%, clinical efficacy in 80% of patients, and a major complication rate of 2.8%, with symptomatic recurrence observed in 75% over a mean follow-up period of 24 months. A stricture length of 5 cm or less was correlated with a successful result without the need for surgery [48]. Further studies including metanalysis corroborate the efficacy and safety of endoscopic dilation for small-bowel Crohn's Disease strictures, emphasizing its role in delaying surgical interventions and improving patient outcomes in the short term; however, up to two-thirds of patients need re-dilation or surgery [48,49].

6.2. *Removal of Foreign Bodies*

In the context of Crohn's Disease, foreign bodies typically refer to undigested food particles or medication bezoars that can accumulate in areas of the intestine narrowed by strictures [50,51]. DAE allows for the direct visualization and removal of these foreign bodies, which can alleviate obstructive symptoms and prevent the progression to more severe complications, such as bowel obstruction or perforation [52]. DAE is also a feasible, relatively safe, and effective method to remove retained video capsule endoscopes. A recent systematic review demonstrated that the pooled successful retrieval rate using DBE was 86.5%, with a higher success for capsules retained in the jejunum or higher in the small bowel (100% retrieval success rate), and lower for those in the ileum (success rate of 74.1%). Successful capsule retrieval significantly reduced the need for subsequent surgeries. Only 7.2% of successful retrievals required surgery compared to 38.5% in unsuccessful cases, highlighting the benefit of effective DBE use [53].

6.3. *Treatment of Bleeding Lesions*

Bleeding in the small intestine can originate from disease-associated lesions and anastomotic ulcers, potentially causing significant blood loss and leading to anemia [54]. DAE enables the precise localization and treatment of these bleeding lesions, employing techniques such as argon plasma coagulation (APC) [55], endoscopic clipping [56], or the injection of hemostatic agents [47].

These endoscopic treatments can effectively manage and control bleeding, reducing the need for transfusions, further diagnostic testing, or surgical intervention [57]. The choice of technique is influenced by the lesion's location, severity of bleeding, presence of associated complications (e.g., strictures), and the patient's overall condition [58].

In cases where the bleeding is severe, a prior CT angiography may be relevant. CT angiography can help identify the precise bleeding site and assess the vascular anatomy, which is crucial for planning an appropriate treatment [59]. Some severe cases of bleeding can be more effectively managed with intravascular coiling, a minimally invasive procedure performed by interventional radiologists. Intravascular coiling involves the placement of coils to occlude the bleeding vessel, providing rapid hemostasis and minimizing the risk of recurrent bleeding [60].

For cases of severely bleeding ulcers, an endovascular radiological approach may also be preferable. This approach allows for the targeted delivery of embolic agents or coiling directly to the bleeding site, offering an alternative to endoscopic treatments when bleeding is not controlled or accessible via DAE [61,62]. The integration of endovascular techniques in the management of small-intestinal bleeding underscores the importance of a multidisciplinary approach, combining the expertise of gastroenterologists, interventional radiologists, and surgeons to optimize patient outcomes.

6.4. Steroid Injection

Endoscopic steroid injections have been studied as a treatment for Crohn's Disease, particularly focusing on strictures and inflammation management [63]. Singh et al. highlight the use of intramural steroid injections in conjunction with endoscopic dilation, presenting a promising approach to managing CD-related strictures, indicating high success rates and suggesting the potential for reduced fibrosis and improved clinical outcomes [64]. Alesandra Lavy and colleague affirm the beneficial outcomes of steroid injections in CD strictures, pointing towards improved stricture management [65]. Di Nardo et al. contribute to this body of evidence with a prospective, randomized, double-blind, controlled trial focusing on pediatric CD patients, which underscores a steroid injection following endoscopic balloon dilation, providing evidence that it is a successful approach for decreasing the need for both redilation and surgery [66]. In contrast, a controlled trial by East et al. raised doubts about its safety and efficacy: patients receiving steroid injections showed a higher incidence of the need for repeat procedures and a shorter time to recurrence of the stricture [67]. In conclusion, there is currently insufficient evidence to support routine use in clinical practice without a large-scale controlled trial, and it should be noted that this approach is still considered experimental to date [68].

7. Impact on Disease Management and Patient Outcomes

The incorporation of DAE into the management of Crohn's Disease has had a profound impact on disease strategy and patient outcomes. The ability to perform targeted interventions for complications that would otherwise require surgery has led to a reduction in surgical intervention rates [39]. This shift towards less invasive management options can have profound implications for patients, including reduced morbidity associated with surgery, the preservation of bowel length (crucial in preventing short bowel syndrome in a disease prone to multiple interventions over time), and decreased recovery times [69]. Furthermore, avoiding surgery can significantly impact the patient's overall health trajectory, reducing the risks of post-operative complications and the potential for subsequent surgeries. Double-balloon enteroscopy (DBE) has been shown to have a substantial impact on the management and outcomes of CD by enabling a detailed examination and intervention within the small intestine [70]. A multicenter retrospective study highlighted its findings and management implications, showing DBE's role in altering treatment strategies for many patients. The findings from DBE affected management in a high percentage of patients with documented and suspected CD (82% and 79%, respectively) [39].

8. Improvement in Symptoms and Quality of Life

DAE's role in directly treating the complications of Crohn's Disease contributes significantly to symptom relief. For instance, the dilation of strictures can immediately relieve obstructive symptoms such as abdominal pain, vomiting, and bloating, while the control of bleeding lesions can prevent anemia and associated fatigue, improving overall well-being [71]. Beyond the physical symptom relief, the minimally invasive nature of DAE, coupled with its efficacy in managing specific disease complications, contributes to an overall improvement in the quality of life. Patients may experience fewer disease flare-ups, reduced anxiety about their health, and greater engagement in social and professional activities, contributing to a more positive outlook on life despite living with a chronic condition [72].

9. Challenges and Limitations of DAE in Crohn's Disease

While DAE offers significant advantages in diagnosing and managing Crohn's Disease, it is not without its challenges and potential complications, especially perforation and bleeding. These factors must be carefully considered when opting for DAE as a diagnostic or therapeutic tool.

9.1. Risk of Perforation, Bleeding, and Pancreatitis

The major adverse events related to DAE are perforation, bleeding, and pancreatitis. One of the most serious complications in Crohn's Disease is the risk of perforation. This risk is inherent to the nature of the procedure, which involves navigating and, sometimes, dilating the small intestine, an organ that may already be compromised by disease-related damage, including the thinning or weakening of the intestinal walls due to inflammation or fibrosis [73]. A recent systematic review found that the per-procedure perforation rate for diagnostic BAE in CD was 0.15%, which is comparable to the rate for diagnostic BAE across all indications. For therapeutic BAE in CD, the perforation rate was 1.74% per procedure. The majority of these therapeutic perforations, 86%, occurred as a result of stricture dilation [74]. Similarly, a multicenter survey in Portugal reported a perforation risk of 0.28% associated with DAE, indicating a relatively low but significant risk [75]. Perforation can lead to severe outcomes, requiring emergency surgical intervention and potentially leading to further complications such as infection or sepsis. DAE also carries a risk of inducing bleeding, especially when a procedure such as stricture dilation are performed. While bleeding is often less severe than perforation and can frequently be managed endoscopically, it nonetheless represents a significant risk, particularly in patients with Crohn's Disease who may already be at an increased risk of bleeding due to their underlying condition. A retrospective study on 776 dilations performed on patients with Crohn's Disease reported a risk of major bleeding, i.e., requiring blood transfusion, of 1% [76]. The estimated risk of acute pancreatitis is 0.3–1%; the proposed explanations for the onset of acute pancreatitis from enteroscopy include the rise in intraluminal pressure within the duodenum during the procedure, which causes duodenal fluids to flow back into the pancreatic duct [77].

The complication rate was evaluated in a large retrospective multicenter US study, which aimed to assess the safety, diagnostic, and therapeutic yields of DAE over a five-year period. Over 1787 instances of DAE, only 0.9% encountered complications, including two perforations (0.1%), six cases with bleeding (0.3%), and one episode of pancreatitis (0.1%) [78]. Similar results emerged from a large cohort study that examined 3894 cases, revealing an overall complication rate of approximately 1%, with pancreatitis as the most frequent complication in diagnostic exams [79].

9.2. Sedation Risks

DAE must be performed under deep sedation or general anesthesia, which carries inherent risks, especially in patients with compromised health [80]. A large German registry indicated that 0.5% of complications during DAE were associated with sedation. While DAE can be safely performed on an outpatient basis, it is recommended that we conduct the procedure as an inpatient procedure with extended monitoring for patients with significant comorbidities [81]. Prolonged sedation can lead to respiratory depression, hypotension, and other anesthesia-related complications. Studies have shown that the length of the procedure can increase the risk of these complications. For instance, a study examining the safety of prolonged endoscopic procedures under sedation found that an extended procedure time was associated with a higher incidence of sedation-related adverse events, including hypoxia and hypotension [82].

9.3. Skill and Experience Requirements

The successful and safe performance of DAE requires a high degree of skill and expertise. This is because DAE procedures involve complex techniques for navigating the small intestine, a challenging and lengthy part of the gastrointestinal tract. The ability to effectively manage the equipment, recognize and navigate around potential complications, and perform therapeutic interventions requires extensive training and experience. The outcomes of DAE, including both its diagnostic yield and the success rate of therapeutic interventions, are closely linked to the operator's experience. Studies have shown that higher volumes of procedures are associated with improved outcomes and reduced complication rates. This necessitates a concentrated effort to train gastroenterologists in these techniques, which may not be available in all healthcare settings, potentially limiting access to DAE for some patients.

9.4. Addressing the Challenges

The challenges and limitations of DAE underscore the need for careful patient selection, thorough pre-procedural planning, and the judicious use of DAE by skilled and experienced practitioners. Strategies to mitigate these risks include the use of pre-procedural imaging to assess the feasibility and safety of DAE, ongoing training and education for endoscopists, and the development of guidelines to standardize the procedure and manage complications effectively [83,84].

In conclusion, while DAE represents a significant advancement in the management of Crohn's Disease, its technical challenges and potential complications require a careful and considered approach. Through specialized training, experience, and the adherence to best practices, the risks associated with DAE can be minimized, maximizing its benefits for patients with Crohn's Disease [85].

10. Conclusions

DAE has solidified its role as a pivotal tool in the management of Crohn's Disease by providing comprehensive insights into the small intestine and offering both diagnostic and therapeutic capabilities. As the technology and techniques of DAE continue to evolve, the potential to further improve patient care and outcomes in Crohn's Disease remains significant. Ongoing research and development are vital to maximizing the utility of DAE, ensuring patient safety, and expanding its therapeutic applications. The continuous improvement of DAE technology and techniques is essential in order to enhance its safety profile, reduce procedural risks, and expand its therapeutic capabilities.

Author Contributions: Conceptualization, G.C.; methodology, G.C.; validation, G.C. and C.M.; data curation, G.C., C.M. and M.E.R.; writing—original draft preparation, G.C.; writing—review and editing, G.C, C.M., A.G. and M.E.R. All authors have read and agreed to the published version of the manuscript.

Funding: No external funding was received to support this research.

Institutional Review Board Statement: Not applicable.

Informed Consent Statement: Not applicable.

Data Availability Statement: Not applicable.

Conflicts of Interest: AG reports personal fees received for consultancy for Eisai S.r.l., 3PSolutions, Real Time Meeting, Fondazione Istituto Danone, Sinergie S.r.l. Board MRGE, and Sanofi S.p.A; personal fees for acting as a speaker for Takeda S.p.A, AbbVie, and Sandoz S.p.A; and personal fees for acting on advisory boards for VSL3 and Eisai. The other authors have no potential competing interests to disclose.

References

1. Roda, G.; Chien Ng, S.; Kotze, P.G.; Argollo, M.; Panaccione, R.; Spinelli, A.; Kaser, A.; Peyrin-Biroulet, L.; Danese, S. Crohn's Disease. *Nat. Rev. Dis. Primers* **2020**, *6*, 1–19. [CrossRef] [PubMed]
2. Maaser, C.; Sturm, A.; Vavricka, S.R.; Kucharzik, T.; Fiorino, G.; Annese, V.; Calabrese, E.; Baumgart, D.C.; Bettenworth, D.; Borralho Nunes, P.; et al. ECCO-ESGAR Guideline for Diagnostic Assessment in IBD Part 1: Initial Diagnosis, Monitoring of Known IBD, Detection of Complications. *J. Crohn's Colitis* **2019**, *13*, 144K–164K. [CrossRef]
3. Cushing, K.; Higgins, P.D.R. Management of Crohn Disease: A Review. *JAMA* **2021**, *325*, 69–80. [CrossRef] [PubMed]
4. Voderholzer, W.A.; Beinhoelzl, J.; Rogalla, P.; Murrer, S.; Schachschal, G.; Lochs, H.; Ortner, M.A. Small Bowel Involvement in Crohn's Disease: A Prospective Comparison of Wireless Capsule Endoscopy and Computed Tomography Enteroclysis. *Gut* **2005**, *54*, 369–373. [CrossRef]
5. Lee, H.H.; Kim, J.S.; Goong, H.J.; Lee, S.H.; Oh, E.H.; Park, J.; Kim, M.C.; Nam, K.; Yang, Y.J.; Kim, T.J.; et al. Use of Device-Assisted Enteroscopy in Small Bowel Disease: An Expert Consensus Statement by the Korean Association for the Study of Intestinal Diseases. *Intest. Res.* **2023**, *21*, 3–19. [CrossRef] [PubMed]
6. Moreels, T.G. Small Bowel Enteroscopy in Crohn's Disease. *Ann. Gastroenterol.* **2012**, *25*, 14. [PubMed]
7. Tharian, B. Enteroscopy in Small Bowel Crohn's Disease: A Review. *World J. Gastrointest. Endosc.* **2013**, *5*, 476. [CrossRef] [PubMed]
8. Lee, S.P.; Jang, H.J.; Kae, S.H.; Lee, J.G.; Kwon, J.H. Indication, Location of the Lesion, Diagnostic Yield, and Therapeutic Yield of Double-Balloon Enteroscopy: Seventeen Years of Experience. *Diagnostics* **2022**, *12*, 2224. [CrossRef] [PubMed]
9. Mehdizadeh, S.; Ross, A.; Gerson, L.; Leighton, J.; Chen, A.; Schembre, D.; Chen, G.; Semrad, C.; Kamal, A.; Harrison, E.M.; et al. What Is the Learning Curve Associated with Double-Balloon Enteroscopy? Technical Details and Early Experience in 6 U.S. Tertiary Care Centers. *Gastrointest. Endosc.* **2006**, *64*, 740–750. [CrossRef]
10. Messer, I.; May, A.; Manner, H.; Ell, C. Prospective, Randomized, Single-Center Trial Comparing Double-Balloon Enteroscopy and Spiral Enteroscopy in Patients with Suspected Small-Bowel Disorders. *Gastrointest. Endosc.* **2013**, *77*, 241–249. [CrossRef]
11. Patel, M.K.; Horsley-Silva, J.L.; Gómez, V.; Stauffer, J.A.; Stark, M.E.; Lukens, F.J. Double Balloon Enteroscopy Procedure in Patients with Surgically Altered Bowel Anatomy: Analysis of a Large Prospectively Collected Database. *J. Laparoendosc. Adv. Surg. Tech. A* **2013**, *23*, 409–413. [CrossRef] [PubMed]
12. Morita, Y.; Bamba, S.; Inatomi, O.; Takahashi, K.; Imai, T.; Murata, M.; Ohno, M.; Sasaki, M.; Tsujikawa, T.; Andoh, A. Prototype Single-Balloon Enteroscopy with Passive Bending and High Force Transmission Improves Depth of Insertion in the Small Intestine. *Intest. Res.* **2020**, *18*, 229–237. [CrossRef] [PubMed]
13. Upchurch, B.R.; Sanaka, M.R.; Lopez, A.R.; Vargo, J.J. The Clinical Utility of Single-Balloon Enteroscopy: A Single-Center Experience of 172 Procedures. *Gastrointest. Endosc.* **2010**, *71*, 1218–1223. [CrossRef] [PubMed]
14. Manno, M.; Barbera, C.; Dabizzi, E.; Mussetto, A.; Conigliaro, R. Safety of Single-Balloon Enteroscopy: Our Experience of 72 Procedures. *Endoscopy* **2010**, *42*, 773. [CrossRef]
15. Manno, M.; Barbera, C.; Bertani, H.; Manta, R.; Mirante, V.G.; Dabizzi, E.; Caruso, A.; Pigo, F.; Olivetti, G.; Conigliaro, R. Single Balloon Enteroscopy: Technical Aspects and Clinical Applications. *World J. Gastrointest. Endosc.* **2012**, *4*, 28. [CrossRef] [PubMed]
16. Ali, R.; Wild, D.; Shieh, F.; Diehl, D.L.; Fischer, M.; Tamura, W.; Rubin, D.T.; Kumbhari, V.; Okolo, P.; Storm, A.; et al. Deep Enteroscopy with a Conventional Colonoscope: Initial Multicenter Study by Using a through-the-Scope Balloon Catheter System. *Gastrointest. Endosc.* **2015**, *82*, 855–860. [CrossRef] [PubMed]
17. Mans, L.; Arvanitakis, M.; Neuhaus, H.; Devière, J. Motorized Spiral Enteroscopy for Occult Bleeding. *Dig. Dis.* **2018**, *36*, 325–327. [CrossRef]
18. Pal, P.; Ramchandani, M.; Banerjee, R.; Viswakarma, P.; Singh, A.P.; Reddy, M.; Rughwani, H.; Patel, R.; Sekaran, A.; Kanaganti, S.; et al. Technical Performance and Diagnostic Yield of Motorised Spiral Enteroscopy Compared with Single-Balloon Enteroscopy in Suspected Crohn's Disease: A Randomised Controlled, Open-Label Study (the MOTOR-CD Trial). *Gut* **2023**, *72*, 1866–1874. [CrossRef]
19. Yamamoto, H.; Despott, E.J.; González-Suárez, B.; Pennazio, M.; Mönkemüller, K. The Evolving Role of Device-Assisted Enteroscopy: The State of the Art as of August 2023. *Best Pract. Res. Clin. Gastroenterol.* **2023**, *64–65*, 101858. [CrossRef]
20. Schneider, A.W.; Vogell, H.; Rost, M.; Grebe-Schultheis, G. Fluoroscopy in Double-Balloon Enteroscopy. *Gastrointest. Endosc.* **2006**, *63*, AB162. [CrossRef]

21. Manner, H.; May, A.; Pohl, J.; Färber, M.; Ell, C. Impact of Fluoroscopy on Oral Double-Balloon Enteroscopy: Results of a Randomized Trial in 156 Patients. *Endoscopy* **2010**, *42*, 820–826. [CrossRef] [PubMed]
22. Lipka, S.; Rabbanifard, R.; Kumar, A.; Brady, P. Single Versus Double Balloon Enteroscopy for Small Bowel Diagnostics: A Systematic Review and Meta-Analysis. *J. Clin. Gastroenterol.* **2015**, *49*, 177–184. [CrossRef]
23. Sanaka, M.R.; Navaneethan, U.; Kosuru, B.; Yerneni, H.; Lopez, R.; Vargo, J.J. Antegrade Is More Effective than Retrograde Enteroscopy for Evaluation and Management of Suspected Small-Bowel Disease. *Clin. Gastroenterol. Hepatol.* **2012**, *10*, 910–916. [CrossRef]
24. Kidambi, T.D.; Liang, Y.; Motarjem, P.; Mirza, R.; Han, A.; Hein, M.; Singh, D.; Lin, J.L.; Banciu-Odell, C.; Toroussian, R.; et al. Episodic, Severe Abdominal Pain Due to Isolated Jejunal Crohn's Disease. *Clin. J. Gastroenterol.* **2021**, *14*, 1084–1089. [CrossRef]
25. Zhang, D.; Chen, N.; Yang, J.; Guo, S. Crohn's Disease with Multiple Jejunum and Ileum Lesions: A Case Report. *J. Pak. Med. Assoc.* **2024**, *74*, 158–160. [CrossRef] [PubMed]
26. Nakamura, M.; Ohmiya, N.; Shirai, O.; Takenaka, H.; Morishima, K.; Miyahara, R.; Ando, T.; Watanabe, O.; Kawashima, H.; Itoh, A.; et al. Route Selection for Double-Balloon Endoscopy, Based on Capsule Transit Time, in Obscure Gastrointestinal Bleeding. *J. Gastroenterol.* **2010**, *45*, 592–599. [CrossRef] [PubMed]
27. Hale, M.F.; Davison, C.; Panter, S.; Drew, K.; Sanders, D.S.; Sidhu, R.; McAlindon, M.E. Review: Practical Aspects of Delivering a Small Bowel Endoscopy Service in the UK. *Frontline Gastroenterol.* **2015**, *6*, 132. [CrossRef]
28. Hadj, A.K.; Nikfarjam, M. Post-Procedural Considerations. *Princ. Flex. Endosc. Surg.* **2013**, 55–62. [CrossRef]
29. Aloi, M.; Di Nardo, G.; Romano, G.; Casciani, E.; Civitelli, F.; Oliva, S.; Viola, F.; Maccioni, F.; Gualdi, G.; Cucchiara, S. Magnetic Resonance Enterography, Small-Intestine Contrast US, and Capsule Endoscopy to Evaluate the Small Bowel in Pediatric Crohn's Disease: A Prospective, Blinded, Comparison Study. *Gastrointest. Endosc.* **2015**, *81*, 420–427. [CrossRef]
30. Hijaz, N.M.; Attard, T.M.; Colombo, J.M.; Mardis, N.J.; Friesen, C.A. Comparison of the Use of Wireless Capsule Endoscopy with Magnetic Resonance Enterography in Children with Inflammatory Bowel Disease. *World J. Gastroenterol.* **2019**, *25*, 3808. [CrossRef]
31. Carter, D.; Eliakim, R. Current Role of Endoscopy in Inflammatory Bowel Disease Diagnosis and Management. *Curr. Opin. Gastroenterol.* **2014**, *30*, 370–377. [CrossRef] [PubMed]
32. Zammit, S.C.; Ellul, P.; Sidhu, R. The Role of Small Bowel Endoscopy for Crohn's Disease. *Curr. Opin. Gastroenterol.* **2019**, *35*, 223–234. [CrossRef] [PubMed]
33. Sara, I.; Saverio, M.; Paolo, Q.; Beatrice, L.; Cucchiara, S. Review on Advances in Pediatric Endoscopy in the Management of Inflammatory Bowel Disease. *Curr. Pediatr. Rev.* **2024**, *20*. [CrossRef]
34. Taylor, S.A.; Mallett, S.; Bhatnagar, G.; Baldwin-Cleland, R.; Bloom, S.; Gupta, A.; Hamlin, P.J.; Hart, A.L.; Higginson, A.; Jacobs, I.; et al. Diagnostic Accuracy of Magnetic Resonance Enterography and Small Bowel Ultrasound for the Extent and Activity of Newly Diagnosed and Relapsed Crohn's Disease (METRIC): A Multicentre Trial. *Lancet Gastroenterol. Hepatol.* **2018**, *3*, 548–558. [CrossRef] [PubMed]
35. Amitai, M.M.; Ben-Horin, S.; Eliakim, R.; Kopylov, U. Magnetic Resonance Enterography in Crohn's Disease: A Guide to Common Imaging Manifestations for the IBD Physician. *J. Crohn's Colitis* **2013**, *7*, 603–615. [CrossRef] [PubMed]
36. Takenaka, K.; Ohtsuka, K.; Kitazume, Y.; Nagahori, M.; Fujii, T.; Saito, E.; Naganuma, M.; Araki, A.; Watanabe, M. Comparison of Magnetic Resonance and Balloon Enteroscopic Examination of the Small Intestine in Patients with Crohn's Disease. *Gastroenterology* **2014**, *147*, 334–342.e3. [CrossRef]
37. Lee, Y.J. Is Paradigm for the Role of Balloon-Assisted Enteroscopy Changing in Crohn's Disease? *Gut Liver* **2021**, *15*, 325–326. [CrossRef]
38. Bourreille, A.; Ignjatovic, A.; Aabakken, L.; Loftus, E., Jr.; Eliakim, R.; Pennazio, M.; Bouhnik, Y.; Seidman, E.; Keuchel, M.; Albert, J.; et al. Role of Small-Bowel Endoscopy in the Management of Patients with Inflammatory Bowel Disease: An International OMED–ECCO Consensus. *Endoscopy* **2009**, *41*, 618–637. [CrossRef]
39. Rahman, A.; Ross, A.; Leighton, J.A.; Schembre, D.; Gerson, L.; Lo, S.K.; Waxman, I.; Dye, C.; Semrad, C. Double-Balloon Enteroscopy in Crohn's Disease: Findings and Impact on Management in a Multicenter Retrospective Study. *Gastrointest. Endosc.* **2015**, *82*, 102–107. [CrossRef]
40. Jeon, S.R.; Kim, J.-O.; Byeon, J.-S.; Yang, D.-H.; Ko, B.M.; Goong, H.J.; Jang, H.J.; Park, S.J.; Kim, E.R.; Hong, S.N.; et al. Enteroscopy in Crohn's Disease: Are There Any Changes in Role or Outcomes Over Time? A KASID Multicenter Study. *Gut Liver* **2021**, *15*, 375–382. [CrossRef]
41. Goong, H.J.; Kim, T.J.; Nam, K.; Park, J.; Kim, J.O.; Kim, H.G.; Ko, B.M.; Jeon, S.R. Histological Diagnostic Yield and Clinical Significance of the First Biopsy in Device-Assisted Enteroscopy in Patients with Small Bowel Diseases: A KASID Multicenter Study. *Diagnostics* **2022**, *12*, 964. [CrossRef] [PubMed]
42. Na, J.E.; Kim, H.S.; Hong, S.N.; Song, K.D.; Kim, J.E.; Kim, E.R.; Kim, Y.H.; Chang, D.K. Comparison of an Endoscopic Scoring System and the Simplified Magnetic Resonance Index of Activity in Patients with Small Bowel Crohn's Disease. *Gut Liver* **2024**, *18*, 97–105. [CrossRef] [PubMed]
43. Di Nardo, G.; Ziparo, C.; Villa, M.P.; Parisi, P.; Esposito, G.; Micheli, F.; Baccini, F.; Corleto, V.D.; Masoni, L.; Manca, M.B. Enteroscopy in Children and Adults with Inflammatory Bowel Disease. *World J. Gastroenterol.* **2020**, *26*, 5944–5958. [CrossRef] [PubMed]

44. Alfredsson, J.; Wick, M.J. Mechanism of Fibrosis and Stricture Formation in Crohn's Disease. *Scand. J. Immunol.* **2020**, *92*, e12990. [CrossRef] [PubMed]
45. Yang, H.; Kurban, M.; Li, M.; Huang, Z.; Lin, H.; Hu, P.; Gao, X.; Shen, B.; Guo, Q. Device-Assisted Enteroscopy-Based Stricturotomy for Small Bowel Strictures Associated with Crohn's Disease (with Video). *Gastroenterol. Rep.* **2022**, *10*, goac073. [CrossRef] [PubMed]
46. Baars, J.E.; Theyventhiran, R.; Aepli, P.; Saxena, P.; Kaffes, A.J. Double-Balloon Enteroscopy-Assisted Dilatation Avoids Surgery for Small Bowel Strictures: A Systematic Review. *World J. Gastroenterol.* **2017**, *23*, 8073. [CrossRef] [PubMed]
47. Shen, B. Interventional Inflammatory Bowel Disease: Endoscopic Therapy of Complications of Crohn's Disease. *Gastroenterol. Rep.* **2022**, *10*, goac045. [CrossRef] [PubMed]
48. Bettenworth, D.; Gustavsson, A.; Atreja, A.; Lopez, R.; Tysk, C.; Van Assche, G.; Rieder, F. A Pooled Analysis of Efficacy, Safety, and Long-Term Outcome of Endoscopic Balloon Dilation Therapy for Patients with Stricturing Crohn's Disease. *Inflamm. Bowel Dis.* **2017**, *23*, 133–142. [CrossRef] [PubMed]
49. Halloran, B.P.; Melmed, G.Y.; Jamil, L.H.; Lo, S.K.; Vasiliauskas, E.a.; Mann, N.K. Sa1649 Double Balloon Enteroscopy-Assisted Stricture Dilation Delays Surgery in Patients with Small Bowel Crohn's Disease. *Gastrointest. Endosc.* **2013**, *77*, AB280. [CrossRef]
50. Serpa, E.; Luciano, E.; Pacheco, F.; Solh, W. Phytobezoar Causing Small Bowel Obstruction in a Patient with Crohn's Disease: A Case Report. *Int. J. Surg. Case Rep.* **2022**, *99*, 107615. [CrossRef]
51. Sleiman, J.; Chirra, P.; Gandhi, N.S.; Baker, M.E.; Lu, C.; Gordon, I.O.; Viswanath, S.E.; Rieder, F. Crohn's Disease Related Strictures in Cross-sectional Imaging: More than Meets the Eye? *United Eur. Gastroenterol. J.* **2022**, *10*, 1167. [CrossRef] [PubMed]
52. Kim, J.; Lee, B.J.; Ham, N.S.; Oh, E.H.; Choi, K.D.; Ye, B.D.; Byeon, J.S.; Eun, C.S.; Kim, J.S.; Yang, D.H. Balloon-Assisted Enteroscopy for Retrieval of Small Intestinal Foreign Bodies: A KASID Multicenter Study. *Gastroenterol. Res. Pract.* **2020**, *2020*, 3814267. [CrossRef] [PubMed]
53. Gao, Y.; Xin, L.; Wang, Y.X.; Dong, Y.H.; Liao, Z.; Li, Z.S.; Du, Y.Q. Double-Balloon Enteroscopy for Retrieving Retained Small-Bowel Video Capsule Endoscopes: A Systematic Review. *Scand. J. Gastroenterol.* **2020**, *55*, 105–113. [CrossRef] [PubMed]
54. Podugu, A.; Tandon, K.; Castro, F.J. Crohn's Disease Presenting as Acute Gastrointestinal Hemorrhage. *World J. Gastroenterol.* **2016**, *22*, 4073. [CrossRef] [PubMed]
55. Olmos, J.; Marcolongo, M.; Pogorelsky, V.; Herrera, L.; Tobal, F.; Davolos, J.R. Push Enteroscopy and Argon Plasma Coagulation in the Prevention of Recurrent Bleeding from Small Bowel Angiodysplasia. *Gastrointest. Endosc.* **2005**, *61*, AB177. [CrossRef]
56. Nitta, K.; Matsui, A.; Araki, A.; Kikuchi, D.; Hoteya, S. Clipping with Double-Balloon Endoscopy for Small Intestinal Venous Malformations in a Patient with Blue Rubber Bleb Nevus Syndrome. *Clin. J. Gastroenterol.* **2022**, *15*, 901–906. [CrossRef] [PubMed]
57. Liu, J.J.; Saltzman, J.R. Endoscopic Hemostasis Treatment: How Should You Perform It? *Can. J. Gastroenterol.* **2009**, *23*, 484. [CrossRef]
58. Pasha, S.F.; Leighton, J.A. Enteroscopy in the Diagnosis and Management of Crohn Disease. *Gastrointest. Endosc. Clin. N. Am.* **2009**, *19*, 427–444. [CrossRef]
59. Anthony, S.; Uberoi, R. CT Imaging of Acute Gastrointestinal Haemorrhage. *Imaging* **2009**, *21*, 32–37. [CrossRef]
60. Wells, M.L.; Hansel, S.L.; Bruining, D.H.; Fletcher, J.G.; Froemming, A.T.; Barlow, J.M.; Fidler, J.L. CT for Evaluation of Acute Gastrointestinal Bleeding. *Radiographics* **2018**, *38*, 1089–1107. [CrossRef]
61. Ali, H.; Sana, M.; Pamarthy, R.; Rahat, E.; Sarfraz, S. Use of Endovascular Coiling to Stop Gastric Ulcer Bleeding in a Patient with Extensive Risk Factors. *Cureus* **2021**, *13*, e16164. [CrossRef] [PubMed]
62. Loffroy, R.; Favelier, S.; Pottecher, P.; Estivalet, L.; Genson, P.Y.; Gehin, S.; Cercueil, J.P.; Krausé, D. Transcatheter Arterial Embolization for Acute Nonvariceal Upper Gastrointestinal Bleeding: Indications, Techniques and Outcomes. *Diagn. Interv. Imaging* **2015**, *96*, 731–744. [CrossRef] [PubMed]
63. Van Assche, G. Intramural Steroid Injection and Endoscopic Dilation for Crohn's Disease. *Clin. Gastroenterol. Hepatol.* **2007**, *5*, 1027–1028. [CrossRef] [PubMed]
64. Singh, V.V.; Draganov, P.; Valentine, J. Efficacy and Safety of Endoscopic Balloon Dilation of Symptomatic Upper and Lower Gastrointestinal Crohn's Disease Strictures. *J. Clin. Gastroenterol.* **2005**, *39*, 284–290. [CrossRef] [PubMed]
65. Lavy, A. Steroid Injection Improves Outcome in Crohn's Disease Strictures. *Endoscopy* **1994**, *26*, 366. [CrossRef] [PubMed]
66. Di Nardo, G.; Oliva, S.; Passariello, M.; Pallotta, N.; Civitelli, F.; Frediani, S.; Gualdi, G.; Gandullia, P.; Mallardo, S.; Cucchiara, S. Intralesional Steroid Injection after Endoscopic Balloon Dilation in Pediatric Crohn's Disease with Stricture: A Prospective, Randomized, Double-Blind, Controlled Trial. *Gastrointest. Endosc.* **2010**, *72*, 1201–1208. [CrossRef] [PubMed]
67. East, J.E.; Brooker, J.C.; Rutter, M.D.; Saunders, B.P. A Pilot Study of Intrastricture Steroid versus Placebo Injection after Balloon Dilatation of Crohn's Strictures. *Clin. Gastroenterol. Hepatol.* **2007**, *5*, 1065–1069. [CrossRef] [PubMed]
68. Bevan, R.; Rees, C.J.; Rutter, M.D.; Macafee, D.A.L. Review: Review of the Use of Intralesional Steroid Injections in the Management of Ileocolonic Crohn's Strictures. *Frontline Gastroenterol.* **2013**, *4*, 238. [CrossRef] [PubMed]
69. Navaneethan, U.; Vargo, J.J.; Menon, K.V.N.; Sanaka, M.R.; Tsai, C.-J. Impact of Balloon-Assisted Enteroscopy on the Diagnosis and Management of Suspected and Established Small-Bowel Crohn's Disease. *Endosc. Int. Open* **2014**, *2*, E201–E206. [CrossRef]
70. Holleran, G.; Valerii, G.; Tortora, A.; Scaldaferri, F.; Conti, S.; Amato, A.; Gasbarrini, A.; Costamagna, G.; Riccioni, M.E. The Use of Single Balloon Enteroscopy in Crohn's Disease and Its Impact on Clinical Outcome. *Scand. J. Gastroenterol.* **2018**, *53*, 925–929. [CrossRef]

71. Esaki, M.; Sakata, Y. Clinical Impact of Endoscopic Evaluation of the Small Bowel in Crohn's Disease. *Digestion* **2023**, *104*, 51–57. [CrossRef] [PubMed]
72. Bellone, F.; Morace, C.; Impalà, G.; Viola, A.; Gullo, A.L.; Cinquegrani, M.; Fries, W.; Sardella, A.; Scolaro, M.; Basile, G.; et al. Quality of Life (QoL) in Patients with Chronic Inflammatory Bowel Diseases: How Much Better with Biological Drugs? *J. Pers. Med.* **2023**, *13*, 947. [CrossRef] [PubMed]
73. Despott, E.J.; Gupta, A.; Burling, D.; Tripoli, E.; Konieczko, K.; Hart, A.; Fraser, C. Effective Dilation of Small-Bowel Strictures by Double-Balloon Enteroscopy in Patients with Symptomatic Crohn's Disease (with Video). *Gastrointest. Endosc.* **2009**, *70*, 1030–1036. [CrossRef] [PubMed]
74. Arulanandan, A.; Dulai, P.S.; Singh, S.; Sandborn, W.J.; Kalmaz, D. Systematic Review: Safety of Balloon Assisted Enteroscopy in Crohn's Disease. *World J. Gastroenterol.* **2016**, *22*, 8999–9011. [CrossRef] [PubMed]
75. Pinho, R.; Mascarenhas-Saraiva, M.; Mão-De-Ferro, S.; Ferreira, S.; Almeida, N.; Figueiredo, P.; Rodrigues, A.; Cardoso, H.; Marques, M.; Rosa, B.; et al. Multicenter Survey on the Use of Device-Assisted Enteroscopy in Portugal. *UEG J.* **2016**, *4*, 264–274. [CrossRef] [PubMed]
76. Gustavsson, A.; Magnuson, A.; Blomberg, B.; Andersson, M.; Halfvarson, J.; Tysk, C. Endoscopic Dilation Is an Efficacious and Safe Treatment of Intestinal Strictures in Crohn's Disease. *Aliment. Pharmacol. Ther.* **2012**, *36*, 151–158. [CrossRef] [PubMed]
77. Chavalitdhamrong, D.; Adler, D.G.; Draganov, P.V. Complications of Enteroscopy: How to Avoid Them and Manage Them When They Arise. *Gastrointest. Endosc. Clin. N. Am.* **2015**, *25*, 83–95. [CrossRef] [PubMed]
78. Noujaim, M.G.; Parish, A.; Raines, D.; Gross, S.A.; Cave, D.; Vance, I.; Beyer, D.; Liu, D.; Hoffman, B.; Lawrence, Z.; et al. Use, Yield, and Risk of Device-Assisted Enteroscopy in the United States: Results from a Large Retrospective Multicenter Cohort. *J. Clin. Gastroenterol.* **2021**, *55*, 792–797. [CrossRef]
79. Möschler, O.; May, A.; Müller, M.K.; Ell, C. Complications in and Performance of Double-Balloon Enteroscopy (DBE): Results from a Large Prospective DBE Database in Germany. *Endoscopy* **2011**, *43*, 484–489. [CrossRef]
80. Sidhu, R.; Turnbull, D.; Haboubi, H.; Leeds, J.S.; Healey, C.; Hebbar, S.; Collins, P.; Jones, W.; Peerally, M.F.; Brogden, S.; et al. British Society of Gastroenterology Guidelines on Sedation in Gastrointestinal Endoscopy. *Gut* **2024**, *73*, 219. [CrossRef]
81. Mason, K.P.; Roback, M.G.; Chrisp, D.; Sturzenbaum, N.; Freeman, L.; Gozal, D.; Vellani, F.; Cavanaugh, D.; Green, S.M. Results from the Adverse Event Sedation Reporting Tool: A Global Anthology of 7952 Records Derived from >160,000 Procedural Sedation Encounters. *J. Clin. Med.* **2019**, *8*, 2087. [CrossRef] [PubMed]
82. Sidhu, R.; Turnbull, D.; Newton, M.; Thomas-Gibson, S.; Sanders, D.S.; Hebbar, S.; Haidry, R.J.; Smith, G.; Webster, G. Review: Deep Sedation and Anaesthesia in Complex Gastrointestinal Endoscopy: A Joint Position Statement Endorsed by the British Society of Gastroenterology (BSG), Joint Advisory Group (JAG) and Royal College of Anaesthetists (RCoA). *Frontline Gastroenterol.* **2019**, *10*, 141. [CrossRef] [PubMed]
83. Mensink, P.B.F.; Haringsma, J.; Kucharzik, T.; Cellier, C.; Pérez-Cuadrado, E.; Mönkemüller, K.; Gasbarrini, A.; Kaffes, A.J.; Nakamura, K.; Yen, H.H.; et al. Complications of Double Balloon Enteroscopy: A Multicenter Survey. *Endoscopy* **2007**, *39*, 613–615. [CrossRef] [PubMed]
84. Kappelman, M.D.; Palmer, L.; Boyle, B.M.; Rubin, D.T. Quality of Care in Inflammatory Bowel Disease: A Review and Discussion. *Inflamm. Bowel Dis.* **2010**, *16*, 125–133. [CrossRef]
85. Yamamoto, H.; Ogata, H.; Matsumoto, T.; Ohmiya, N.; Ohtsuka, K.; Watanabe, K.; Yano, T.; Matsui, T.; Higuchi, K.; Nakamura, T.; et al. Clinical Practice Guideline for Enteroscopy. *Dig. Endosc.* **2017**, *29*, 519–546. [CrossRef]

Journal of
Clinical Medicine

MDPI

Review

Eosinophils, Eosinophilic Gastrointestinal Diseases, and Inflammatory Bowel Disease: A Critical Review

Giulia Migliorisi [1,2,†], Elisabetta Mastrorocco [1,2,†], Arianna Dal Buono [1], Roberto Gabbiadini [1], Gaia Pellegatta [2,3], Paola Spaggiari [4], Francesca Racca [2,5], Enrico Heffler [2,5], Edoardo Vincenzo Savarino [6], Cristina Bezzio [1,2], Alessandro Repici [2,3] and Alessandro Armuzzi [1,2,*]

1 IBD Center, IRCCS Humanitas Research Hospital, Via Manzoni 56, 20089 Rozzano, Italy; giulia.migliorisi@humanitas.it (G.M.); elisabetta.mastrorocco@humanitas.it (E.M.); arianna.dalbuono@humanitas.it (A.D.B.); roberto.gabbiadini@humanitas.it (R.G.); cristina.bezzio@hunimed.eu (C.B.)
2 Department of Biomedical Sciences, Humanitas University, Via Rita Levi Montalcini 4, 20072 Pieve Emanuele, Italy; gaia.pellegatta@humanitas.it (G.P.); francesca.racca@humanitas.it (F.R.); enrico.heffler@hunimed.eu (E.H.); alessandro.repici@hunimed.eu (A.R.)
3 Endoscopic Unit, Department of Gastroenterology, IRCCS Humanitas Research Hospital, 20089 Rozzano, Italy
4 Department of Pathology, Humanitas Research Hospital, 20089 Rozzano, Italy; paola.spaggiari@humanitas.it
5 Personalized Medicine, Asthma and Allergy, IRCCS—Humanitas Research Hospital, 20089 Rozzano, Italy
6 Department of Surgery, Oncology and Gastroenterology, Department of Medical and Surgical Specialties, University of Padua, 35122 Padova, Italy; edoardosavarino@gmail.com
* Correspondence: alessandro.armuzzi@hunimed.eu; Tel.: +39-(0)282245555; Fax: +39-(0)282242591
† These authors contributed equally to this work.

Abstract: Background/Objectives: Inflammatory bowel disease (IBD) and eosinophilic gastrointestinal diseases (EGIDs) are complex, multifactorial chronic inflammatory disorders affecting the gastrointestinal tract. Their epidemiology, particularly for eosinophilic esophagitis (EoE), is increasing worldwide, with a rise in the co-diagnosis of IBD and EGIDs. Both disorders share common risk factors, such as early exposure to antibiotics or specific dietary habits. Moreover, from a molecular perspective, eosinophilic infiltration is crucial in the diagnosis of eosinophilic disorders, and it also plays a pivotal role in IBD histological diagnosis. Indeed, recent evidence highlights the significant role of eosinophils in the health of the intestinal mucosal barrier and as mediators between innate and acquired immunity, even indicating a potential role in IBD pathogenesis. This narrative review aims to summarize the current evidence regarding the common clinical and molecular aspects of EGIDs and IBD and the current state of knowledge regarding overlap conditions and their pathogenesis. Methods: Pubmed was searched until May 2023 to assess relevant studies describing the epidemiology, pathophysiology, and therapy of EGIDs in IBD. Results: The immune pathways and mechanisms underlying both EGIDs and IBD remain partially known. An improved understanding of the role of eosinophils in overlapping conditions could lead to enhanced diagnostic precision, the development of more effective future therapeutic strategies, and a more accurate prediction of patient response. Consequently, the identification of red flags indicative of an eosinophilic disorder in IBD patients is of paramount importance and must be evaluated on a case-by-case basis.

Keywords: inflammatory bowel disease; eosinophilic gastrointestinal disease; eosinophilic esophagitis; eosinophils

1. Introduction

Inflammatory bowel diseases (IBDs) and eosinophilic gastrointestinal diseases (EGIDs) are multifactorial chronic inflammatory disorders of the gastrointestinal (GI) tract. Their epidemiology is increasing worldwide, particularly in newly industrialized countries, placing a great burden on the healthcare system [1,2]. IBDs, encompassing Crohn's disease (CD) and ulcerative colitis (UC), are mainly characterized by abdominal pain, fatigue, diarrhea, and rectal bleeding. These disorders are typically managed with immune-modulating drugs, although in severe cases and complications, surgery may be required [3–5]. EGIDs are further distinguished into eosinophilic esophagitis (EoE), the most prevalent disease of this group, and non-EoE-EGIDs. Non-EoE-EGIDs are less common and include eosinophilic gastritis (EoG), eosinophilic enteritis (EoN) and eosinophilic colitis (EoC) [6]. EoE is a type 2 associated inflammatory disorder characterized by eosinophilic infiltration of the esophageal wall, which may lead to fibrosis and dysfunction of esophageal function in some patients [7]. This results in adult patients with dysphagia, food bolus impaction, chest pain and heartburn. Management includes elimination diets, conventional medications such as proton pump inhibitors and swallowed topical corticosteroids (STCs) or biologic drugs targeting interleukin 4 (IL-4) (e.g., Dupilumab), and endoscopic dilation in cases of fibrotic stenosis [8]. EGIDs and IBD share certain similarities in terms of potential etiologies and risk factors, and they may coexist simultaneously in the same patient [9]. The pathogenesis of both conditions remains unclear, although it is widely acknowledged that they result from the interaction between genetic predisposition, environmental factors, and alterations in the gut microbiota, which can lead to an aberrant immune response and chronic inflammation of the GI system [10]. It has been demonstrated that early-life exposure to antibiotics during gestation, particularly during the first years of life, is associated with an increased risk of developing both EGIDs and IBD, with a particular association with Crohn's disease in adulthood [11–13]. Furthermore, a recent meta-analysis has demonstrated that exclusive breastfeeding confers protection against the development of both IBD and EoE [14,15]. Moreover, dietary habits are considered relevant environmental risk factors for both disorders and, most importantly, specific diet restrictions are paramount in treating EGIDs. Indeed, high-fat diets and ultra-processed foods are associated with an increased risk of developing CD [16,17]. Furthermore, as previously stated, food elimination diets that avoid specific food allergens (e.g., milk, gluten, soy, fish, tree nuts/peanuts, eggs) represent a primary therapeutic approach for EoE, particularly in the pediatric population [18]. Additionally, dysbiosis and the reduction of microbiota species diversity have been reported to impact on the origin and maintenance of both inflammatory disorders [19–21]. The role of dysbiosis in the pathogenesis of these diseases may explain the higher risk of developing IBD, especially CD associated with previous PPI use [22,23], which is not observed with other anti-secretory drugs [24]. The interaction between PPIs and EGIDs is controversial, as PPIs are considered a first-line pharmaceutical therapy together with STCs; however, the resulting interference in peptic digestion may increase esophageal exposure to food allergens [25]. Furthermore, from a molecular point of view, the upregulation of shared inflammatory molecules, such as specific subtypes of Toll-like receptors (TLRs), has been observed in both non-treated EoE and in active IBD [26,27]. Similarly, pro-inflammatory cytokines (e.g., interleukin-5, IL-5), which are involved in the activation and recruitment of eosinophils, are overexpressed in the intestinal mucosa of patients with UC and active CD [28,29].

The aim of this narrative review is to provide a critical summary of the common clinical and molecular aspects of EGIDs and IBD and the role of eosinophils in their pathogenesis and to present the current state of knowledge regarding the overlapping of these conditions.

2. Eosinophils in the Gut: Their Role in EGIDs and IBD

Eosinophils are a subtype of polymorphonuclear leukocytes derived from bone marrow pluripotential hematopoietic stem cells under the influence of several cytokines, including interleukin 3 (IL-3), 13 (IL-13), IL-5 and granulocyte macrophage colony-stimulating factor (GM-CSF) [30]. Their presence is not limited to the blood and the hematopoietic organs; indeed, tissue eosinophils can be found under physiologic conditions in the mammary glands, uterus, the non-esophageal part of the gastrointestinal tract, and in adipose tissue [31]. Their physiological distribution is uneven in the GI tract [32], with a greater prevalence in the lamina propria of the small bowel, ileum, and colon and almost absent in the esophagus [32,33]. Historically, their known functions were limited to the protection against parasitic infections and food allergy phenomena [34,35]. Nevertheless, the current evidence, although limited to animal models, indicates that eosinophils play a significant role in the immune homeostasis of the entire digestive system [36]. This is particularly evident in the maintenance of the integrity of the intestinal mucosal barrier, in the interaction with gut microbiota, and in the mediation between type I and II immunity. In this context, Jung et al. [37] and Ignacio et al. [38] observed that eosinophil-deficient mice exhibited a significant decrease in the integrity of the mucosal barrier, major villous architecture abnormalities, and intestinal permeability in response to microbial colonization. Eosinophils play a pivotal role in the survival of plasma cells, as evidenced by the release of proliferation-inducing ligand (APRIL) and interleukin-6 (IL-6) in the bone marrow and inducible nitric oxide synthase (iNOS), lymphotoxin, and interleukin-1β (IL-1β) in the GI system. The aforementioned factors are responsible for the T-cell independent IgA switching class and the development of gut-associated lymphoid tissue (GALT) in Peyer patches [37,39]. Furthermore, eosinophils act as intermediaries between the innate and adaptive immune responses, increasing the number of Th2 cells [40,41] and T-regulatory cells such as Th17 [42]. Moreover, in balanced conditions, eosinophils, in conjunction with mast cells, have bidirectional communication with the enteric nervous system (ENS) [41]. This communication influences contractility and secretory bowel function through the release of vasoactive intestinal peptide (VIP) and substance P [43]. It also stimulates nervous growth and participates in the recruitment of immune cells when activated [41,44].

The recruitment of eosinophils in the intestinal mucosa is mediated by several cytokines (e.g., IL-5, IL-13 and interleukin 33 (IL-33) and chemokines (particularly eotaxines) released by white, endothelial, and epithelial cells of the GI tract. Eotaxines (principally eotaxin 1, followed by eotaxines 2 and 3) are chemokines that bind to eosinophils' surface receptor CCR3, resulting in eosinophil migration and homing in the lamina propria of the bowel mucosa [45,46]. Eosinophilic infiltration is a prominent histological feature in both IBD [47] and in EGID patients [48]. It has been demonstrated that an upregulation of eotaxines, regardless of disease activity, occurs due to overexpression of CCR3 in UC patients [49]. Furthermore, IL-1 and IL-33 have been identified in both animal and human models of colitis [50,51]. The relationship between eosinophils and UC is well supported by the well-defined assumption that UC is characterized by a disorder of the Th2 immune response rather than the enhanced Th1 profile observed in CD patients [52]. However, eosinophils in surgical specimens of resected ileum of CD patients have been linked to an increased risk of early recurrence [29], while peripheral blood eosinophilia has been shown to predict clinically active disease in pediatric CD patients [53] and has been associated with increased disease severity in both CD and UC [54,55].

Eosinophils are directly responsible for intestinal tissue damage through the degranulation of eosinophil-derived neurotoxin (EDN), eosinophil cationic protein (ECP), major basic proteins (MBP-1 and MBP-2), and eosinophil peroxidase (EPO). ECP is a ribonucleasis protein that provides apoptosis signals [56], while MBPs alter cell membrane functions, leading to increased intestinal permeability in the inflamed intestine [57]. MBP, in conjunction with EDN, may also affect the cholinergic pathways of the ENS, resulting in motility dysfunction [56]. Furthermore, elevated levels of MBP and EDN in the feces have been associated with disease activity in both CD and UC and may serve as additional biomarkers, particularly for detecting early responses to biological and steroid therapies [58,59]. Smyth et al. [60] observed that eosinophils were selectively localized near the ENS nerves in the mucosa, extending to the muscle layer in patients with CD. This resulted in enhanced substance P release and choline acetyltransferase nerve function. Moreover, eosinophils can contribute to the perpetuation of inflammation by synthesizing chemokine CXCL8, which has been observed to be responsible for neutrophil infiltration in the intestinal lamina propria, which is directly related to the severity of disease in UC patients [61]. Finally, recent evidence has shown the potential role of eosinophils in the development of fibrosis. Although eosinophil infiltration has been associated with fibrosis in other districts [57] and an abnormal distribution of eosinophils and overexpression of IL-33 has been observed in

CD ileum stricture in a pediatric population [62], more recent studies have demonstrated that eosinophil depletion can protect against chronic inflammation but does not influence collagen deposition and fibrosis development [63].

EGIDs and specifically EoE are type 2-associated inflammatory disorders that result from the interaction of genetic predisposition, food sensitization and the abnormal infiltration of eosinophil cells in the mucosa layers. Genetic variants and polymorphisms of genes involved in eosinophil homing (e.g., CCL26, eotaxin 3) and eosinophil activation and differentiation in Th2 cells (TSLP, WDR36) have been associated with an increased risk of developing EoE [64]. Chemokines involved in eosinophil migration, particularly eotaxin-3, are overexpressed in the epithelium of EoE patients as well as in IBD patients and may represent a potential therapeutic target [65]. Eosinophil degranulation products directly damage the mucosa layer and mucosal barrier function. Furthermore, in IBD, ECP and MBP can alter membrane permeability and mucosal barrier function, while EDN is involved in the activation and recruitment of dendritic cells, which in turn promotes the production of Th2 profile immune cytokines, such as IL-33, IL-5, IL-13, which sustain the inflammatory process [7,66]. Recent evidence suggests a potential role of eosinophils in esophageal motility disorders observed in EoE. For instance, MBP interferes with the cholinergic nervous pathway, while the release of IL-13 and IL-6 causes relaxation of the esophageal sphincter. Cytotoxic eosinophilic granules can cause neural apoptosis with irreversible alterations to nervous function [67]. In this regard, a recent retrospective study observed esophageal dysmotility and achalasia in almost 15% of EoE patients [68], and a recent systematic review by Visaggi et al. highlighted the resolution of motility disorders in EoE patients on treatment, supporting the hypothesis of an interaction between eosinophils and pathological functions of the ENS [69]. Nevertheless, eosinophils produce transforming growth factor-β (TGF-β), which induces the expression of collagen and fibronectin, resulting in fibrotic tissue remodeling [70]. Another potentially important factor in the pathogenesis of eosinophilic disorders is the microbiota of the gastrointestinal tract. A recent systematic review examined current knowledge regarding the role of the microbiota in EoE pathogenesis. It highlighted similarities between the oral and esophageal microbiota and microbial products, as well as a higher microbiota load in EoE patients compared to controls [71]. Furthermore, Massimino et al. [20] reported a potential correlation between microbe species and alimentary allergens triggering the inflammatory process. Finally, Facchin et al. showed that members of the Actinobacillus, Bergeyella, Porphyromonas and Alloprevotella genera were positively associated with biological samples with eos/HPF > 15 [72]. Figure 1 elucidates the molecular mechanisms possibly shared by IBD and EGIDs.

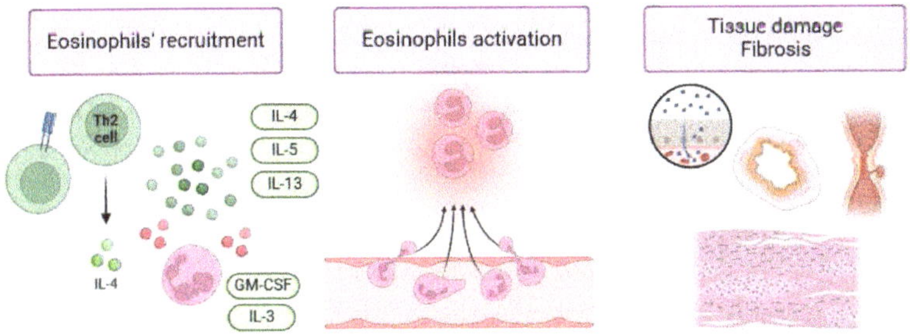

Figure 1. Molecular pathways shared by IBD and EGIDs. Different chemokines and cytokines are involved in eosinophils activation. While IL-3 and GM-CSF are responsible for activation and promoting eosinophils maturation in bone marrow, many other molecules are mainly involved in eosinophils' recruitment, such as IL-5, IL-4, IL13 and IL-33. The activation and eosinophils' degranulation can directly cause tissue damage, altering membrane permeability and barrier function.

Moreover, the products of eosinophils' degranulation can alter nervous pathways and cause neural apoptosis with irreversible altered nervous functions of the enteric nervous system. Additionally, eosinophils can induce the deposition of collagen with fibrotic tissue remodeling by the release of tumor-growing factor-β (TGF- β).

3. Diagnosis and Endoscopy: Differences and Similarities

The accurate assessment of disease severity and prognosis in both EGIDs and IBD is contingent upon a comprehensive description and quantification of endoscopic alterations, complemented by the collection of bioptic samples for diagnostic purposes. In detail, endoscopic scores of activities currently recommended for EoE and EoG (EREFS and EG-REFS, respectively) include description/evaluation of both inflammatory and fibrotic aspects [73]. EoE is endoscopically characterized by the presence of edema, rings, exudates, furrows, and strictures. However, according to the literature, in a variable proportion of patients (5–32%), these typical endoscopic features are not visible in EoE, and the esophageal mucosa may appear normal [74,75]. In contrast, the EG-REFS is based on the presence of erosions/ulcers, raised lesions, fold thickening, and pyloric stenosis or friability, erythema, and granularity of the gastric mucosa [76–79]. EoC and EoN are typically characterized by a normal mucosa appearance, with non-specific edema, erythematous areas, or aphthous lesions [80].

In UC, endoscopy mostly reveals a homogenous and continuous inflammation that originates in the rectum and extends proximally. The presence of erythema, friability and bleeding of the mucosa, erosions, and ulcers are evaluated and included as core items in the Mayo endoscopic score (MES) and the Ulcerative Colitis Endoscopic Index of Severity (UCEIS). Conversely, CD is characterized by a patchy and transmural inflammatory behavior, often with normal mucosa. Typical endoscopic features of CD include aphthous ulcers and deep serpiginous ulcers, strictures, pseudopolyps, and fistulas. In the evaluation of disease activity and severity, as recommended by the European Crohn's and Colitis Organization (ECCO), either the Simple Endoscopic Score for Crohn's Disease (SES-CD) or the Crohn's Disease Endoscopic Index of Severity (CDEIS) can be adopted [81–84].

Documenting eosinophilic infiltration is a diagnostic and necessary parameter for EGIDs and is based on an adequate and extensive bioptic sampling (i.e., at least two biopsies from the distal, mid, and upper esophagus in case of suspected EoE) [85]. The diagnosis of EGIDs requires the presence of eosinophilic infiltration above specific thresholds depending on the disease location. The diagnostic threshold for EoE is a peak of at least 15 eosinophils per high-power field (HPF) [85–87]. There is no consensus regarding the definition of eosinophil thresholds for non-EoE EGIDs. However, it is widely acknowledged that non-EoE EGIDs have higher eosinophilic infiltration cut-offs. For EoG and EoN, the proposed threshold is greater than or equal to 30 eosinophils per HPF for the stomach, greater than or equal to 50 eosinophils in the duodenum, and greater than 56 eosinophils per HPF in the ileum [88]. Eosinophils are typically absent from the left colon and rectum and are rarely observed in the right colon. In adults, normal values range from 1 to 3 cells per HPF, while in children, they range from 50 to 100 cells per HPF [89]. The pathological threshold for EoC in adults is defined as greater than 40 cells per HPF in at least two colonic segments [90]. Eosinophils in EoC are mainly located in the submucosa and within the crypt epithelium. Such instances are rare and do not result in the formation of crypt abscesses or extensive degranulation, as observed in patients with IBD [91]. If IBD is suspected, it is recommended that at least two biopsies be taken from the terminal ileum and each segment of the colon (cecum, ascending colon, transverse colon, descending colon, sigmoid colon, and rectum) [92]. This is regardless of whether the mucosa appears endoscopically normal [93,94]. In case of suspected involvement of the upper digestive tract, esophageal, gastric, and duodenal biopsies are indicated in patients with known IBD [93]. However, it is important to underline that abnormalities in the upper digestive tract have been described in almost 80% of CD patients of pediatric age [95]. The number of eosinophils present in UC colon samples is variable, but their coexistence with basal plasmacytosis (more than three cells at the base and lateral part of the crypts) increases the likelihood of a correct diagnosis [96]. Furthermore, eosinophilia (more than 60 cells HPF), especially in the left colon at diagnosis, may be predictive of non-response to medical treatment [97,98]. In contrast to UC samples, eosinophils are less characteristic in CD samples. For instance, eosinophils can be observed in conjunction with neutrophils on the surface of the intestinal epithelium in the early CD ileum [99,100]. Conversely, their presence alongside T lymphocytes within the submucosal or intramuscular plexus (ganglionitis) in surgical specimens is a distinctive histological feature of transmural inflammation and a prognostic factor for disease recurrence when present in the resection margins [101]. Esophageal involvement in CD is exceedingly rare and is typically characterized by erosions and ulcerations. Conversely, endoscopic pathognomonic features in EoE are furrows, rings, and exudates [102]. Eosinophilic infiltration is uncommon in CD esophagitis. A 14 years study conducted by the Mayo Clinic found that no esophageal biopsies in CD esophagitis showed eosinophilic infiltration [103]. Involvement of the stomach and duodenum in CD occurs in 0.5–4% of patients with CD and is usually associated with a concomitant ileal or ileo-colonic disease. The histological examination of such cases reveals non-caseating granulomas as the most common finding [104].

4. Overlapping Syndrome: EGIDs and IBD

Non-esophageal EGIDs are still considered rare diseases, and there is currently a lack of data from large retrospective and prospective studies about the potential for overlapping syndrome with IBD. The available data come from anecdotal case reports, which suggests a potential correlation with anti-TNF medications. For example, a 10-year-old patient with Crohn's disease who was exposed to infliximab developed worsening abdominal pain and diarrhea, along with peripheral eosinophilia and eosinophilic infiltration in the duodenum and stomach. These symptoms improved when the patient was taken off the infliximab [105]. In a more recent case report published by Konstantinos et al. [106], a 67-year-old female patient was diagnosed with both EoC and CD in the absence of other potential precipitating factors such as infections or medications. Symptoms of EGIDs mainly involving small and/or large bowel include chronic diarrhea, while endoscopy shows diffuse erythema of the colonic mucosa with sparing of the ileal mucosa and the presence of a mixed CD/EoC pattern on histological examination. In Figure 2, we report the clinical case of a young female patient affected by ileo-colonic CD who was referred to the emergency department for anemia and emesis with blood streaks.

Regarding the overlap between IBD and EoE, Limketkai et al. [107] in a 7-year prospective study found a risk ratio of 5.4 and 3.3, respectively, for CD and UC patients developing EoE. A pre-existing diagnosis of EoE increased the risk of a new and later IBD diagnosis with similar risk ratios. Male and younger IBD patients were more likely to develop EoE, whereas among EoE patients, male gender was only associated with a higher risk of developing UC [107]. In addition, in a recent Swedish national study, Uchida et al. [9] reported a 4-fold increased risk of developing IBD in EoE patients, while IBD patients had up to 15 times increased odds of a subsequent diagnosis of EoE. Interestingly, EoE was more commonly associated with CD, although it shares type 2 inflammatory pathways with UC [9]. Similar results were found in a retrospective pediatric study, which also reported a difference in the timing of EoE diagnosis between UC and CD; while EoE was frequently diagnosed during CD follow-up, the onset of EoE was concomitant in 64.7% of UC patients [108]. Furthermore, 83% of the co-diagnoses of EoE-CD were made during CD remission or mild activity, and 10 CD patients developed EoE during clinical remission after anti-TNF therapy, supporting the hypothesis of a correlation between anti-TNF therapy and GI eosinophilia. A possible explanation may be that CD is driven by Th1 immunity, and the resulting suppression may lead to uncontrolled upregulation of the Th2 immune pathway [108,109]. In addition, the severity and extent of disease in overlapping syndromes differ from those in isolated forms. For example, histological remission of EoE with PPI treatment is estimated to be around 50.5% [110,111] and could reach up to 57.8–64.9% with STCs in two recent systematic reviews [112,113]. However, Urquhart et al. [114] found that in overlapping syndromes, eosinophilic disease had a more severe and fibro-stenotic pattern, with more than half of the patients presenting rings and strictures at the diagnosis. In more detail, the rate of histological remission after undergoing PPI and STCs was, respectively, 8.7% and 16.7% in the UC cohort and 38.7% and 31.8% in the CD cohort. Over half of the UC patients exhibited pancolitis, while 46.8% of the CD patients displayed ileo-colonic involvement. Although data are limited, no great differences in symptoms characteristics and severity and endoscopic features have been reported between patients with co-diagnosis of IBD and EoE and patients affected by EoE alone [115]. Nevertheless, some authors reported a major prevalence of dysphagia in patients with overlap syndrome and an early diagnosis of IBD [116]. The evidence basis for the clinical outcomes of co-diagnosis of IBD and EoE is limited, and the available data are not entirely consistent. In this context, Limketkai et al. [107] evaluated an elevated risk of IBD complications in co-diagnosis of IBD and EoE, with an increased likelihood of requiring systemic steroids and biological treatment. The study found a reduced risk of bowel resection in both CD and UC. Similarly, Malik et al. [117] reported in a recent retrospective cohort study that there was an increased composite risk of IBD-related complications for both CD and UC [(CD: adjusted HR (aHR) 1.14, $p < 0.005$; UC: aHR 1.17, $p < 0.01$)], as well as a need for biologic treatment for IBD. However, there were no significant differences in surgical resection and the need for systemic steroids [117]. EoE in the context of concurrent IBD was found to be significantly associated with a lower risk of food bolus impaction and a greater need for biological therapies, in comparison to non-IBD-EoE counterparts [117]. This may be attributed to the enhanced endoscopic surveillance and the concurrent administration of biological therapy in IBD treatment.

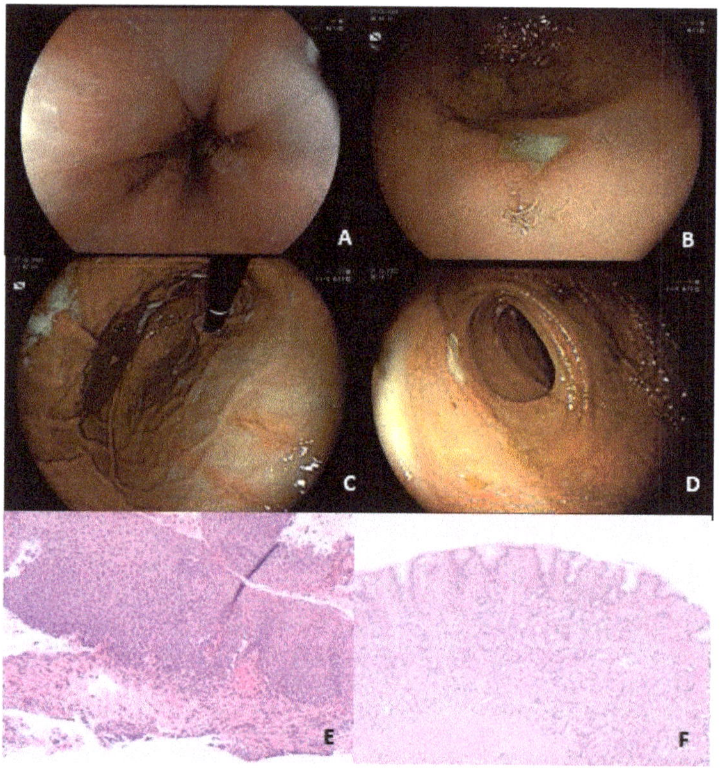

Figure 2. Concomitant Crohn's disease and EGID: during colonoscopy (**D**), peri-anastomotic mild activity of IBD was documented (Rutgeerts score i2), while the esophagogastroduodenoscopy (EGD)

revealed in the esophagus oedema, exudates and longitudinal furrows and erythema and linear erosions in the stomach (**A**,**C**) with multiple gastric clear-based ulcers (III, sec Forrest Classification) (**B**). Histological examination of the esophagus revealed diffuse eosinophilic infiltrate involving the squamous mucosa (200/HPF), basal zone hyperplasia, focal surface desquamation, and lamina propria fibrosis (**E**). Diffuse eosinophilic infiltrate involving the mucosa and the submucosa with intra-epithelial eosinophils, mucin depletion, reactive epithelial changes, and mild architectural distortion was observed in the gastric specimens (**F**).

In conclusion, patients with IBD and EoE have a higher risk of developing immune-mediated comorbidities than those with only one of the two disorders. This risk is particularly high for Th1-mediated disorders, such as coeliac disease and rheumatological IBD-related conditions, and for Th2-mediated disorders such as eczema and asthma.

5. Treatment of IBD and Overlapping EoE

To date, there is a paucity of data regarding the treatment of IBD with concomitant EoE. The optimal treatment strategies in the setting of co-occurrence remain unknown. The majority of data on treatment outcomes, escalation, and safety derive from pediatric studies. Overall, lower clinical and histologic response rates have been observed in cases of EoE and coexisting IBD, suggesting that this phenotype might be more difficult to treat [114]. Conversely, further studies have reported that patients with IBD alone have significantly higher rates of treatment escalation and hospitalization compared to those with EoE-IBD or EoE alone [118]. Biologic therapies, such as anti-TNF agents, are commonly used to treat IBD. However, they have not proven effective in treating EoE [119], despite TNF-α being upregulated and highly expressed by esophageal epithelial cells in patients with EoE [120]. Their role is controversial; as previously stated, TNF-alpha inhibitors have been associated with a higher risk of developing eosinophilic disorders in IBD patients [105,106]. However, isolated cases of steroid-dependent EoE have been reported and successfully treated with other anti-TNFα such as adalimumab, mainly in the pediatric population [121,122]. Indeed, a retrospective case–control study including pediatric patients demonstrated that the use of anti-TNFα in managing pre-existing IBD provided protection against EoE development (RR 0.314, 95% CI 0.159–0.619) [123].

Moreover, another biological drug that may be employed in the treatment of overlapping conditions is represented by vedolizumab, an anti-$\alpha 4\beta 7$ integrin agent that inhibits leukocyte trafficking in CD and CU. This drug has recently been reported for the treatment of refractory EoE [124]. In detail, clinical response, along with endoscopic and histological improvement, was observed in patients with lower gastrointestinal tract eosinophilic involvement and with eosinophilic duodenitis [125,126]. In support of the hypothesis that the two diseases operate through mechanisms of shared leukocyte trafficking, a number of studies have shown that the presence of mucosal eosinophilia is an independent predictor of a higher rate of efficacy of vedolizumab in IBD [127,128].

As previously mentioned, EoE is typically characterised by a Th2 inflammatory response, whereas IBD, especially CD, involves a Th1/Th17 response with the participation of interleukin 10 (IL-10). Nevertheless, both disease states exhibit shared cytokine and T-helper cell-mediated mechanisms. In CD, there is an elevation in mucosal IL-5 expression, while UC exhibits increased eotaxin expression, which acts as a chemoattractant for eosinophils. IL-5 has been linked to eosinophil activation in tissues and may contribute to early mucosal damage in CD [107,129]. This suggests that EoE and IBD may share similar biological pathways and therapeutic targets but may lack a definitive common inflammatory pathway that prevents a full response in patients with the two overlapping conditions. Dupilumab, a monoclonal antibody that blocks interleukin-4 (IL-4) and IL-13 and the only biologic approved for the treatment of EoE, has not been studied in patients with IBD and concomitant EoE. Nevertheless, dupilumab has been demonstrated to be safe and efficacious in the treatment of atopic dermatitis among patients with IBD, including primary atopic dermatitis and dermatitis triggered or exacerbated by anti-TNF therapy [130,131]. A Phase 2 clinical trial is currently enrolling participants to assess the efficacy and safety of dupilumab therapy in patients with UC with an eosinophilic phenotype [132]. Finally, combination treatment with monoclonal antibodies targeting hyper-eosinophilic syndrome in overlapping EoE and IBD syndrome has been reported without safety concerns [133].

6. Discussion

IBD, EoE, and non-EoE EGIDs are examples of gastrointestinal diseases characterized by underlying immune dysregulation. Current research is making a significant effort to understand their shared pathogenic pathways. Preclinical and clinical data indicate and support that these disorders hold common genetic and early environmental factors. The association of IBD and EGIDs appears to be bidirectional. Indeed, recent nationwide cohort studies have reported a nearly 4-fold increased risk of later IBD diagnosis in patients with established EoE and 15-fold increased odds of later EoE diagnosis in patients with established IBD [9]. The diagnosis of an overlapping IBD and EGID poses several challenges for physicians; recognizing possible 'red flags' (disease-specific signs and symptoms) of an adjunctive inflammatory disorder in the context of an established disease with a known GI involvement may be tricky and delay further diagnostic work-up and referral. Secondly, medications used for the underlying chronic disease may confound the onset of the later IBD/EGIDs, and finally, some patients might have an initial misclassification of the first IBD/EGID. Regarding IBD, after many years of collaborative research across multiple societies, so-called 'red flags' have been identified and standardized for the appropriate referral of patients to specialists. This process has not yet been initiated for associations with concurrent, even rarer, conditions such as EGIDs. In Figure 3, we propose an algorithm for suspecting and ruling out EGIDs in case of known IBD. The occurrence of extra-intestinal symptoms (i.e., dysphagia, weight loss, rapid dose escalation or swapping of therapies) requires further investigation in IBD patients. The preliminary characterization of coexistent IBD and EGIDs, particularly EoE, has shown that these patients may present accelerated organ remodeling (i.e., esophageal rings and strictures), displaying a modified phenotype and natural history [114]. Coexistent IBD and EGIDs may configurate a sub-set of yet unidentified difficult-to-treat patients. Preclinical data have shown clinical efficacy and achievement of therapeutic goals in both conditions selectively blocking the IL-4, IL-5 and IL-13 pathways. Still, a precise characterization of these molecular pathways, especially that of Th-2 inflammation (which is involved in the creation of organ damage) is necessary to identify and develop new therapeutic targets. In our view, to fully comprehend the complex relationship between IBD and EGIDs, larger studies incorporating genetic and environmental data are needed. Awareness of and education on coexisting IBD and EGIDs must be promoted by healthcare professionals and require multidisciplinary management.

Demographic features	Symptoms	Disease course
male gender younger age (pediatric, < 15 years old) family history of EGIDs personal history of asthma	dysphagia weight loss atypical chest pain	rapid dose escalation rapid swapping of therapies pediatric onset of IBD

Figure 3. Red flags for suspecting and ruling out EGIDs in cases of known IBD.

Author Contributions: Guarantor of the article: A.A., G.M., E.M. and A.D.B. equally wrote the manuscript. A.A., R.G., P.S., C.B., A.R., E.H., F.R., E.V.S. and G.P. critically reviewed the content of the paper. A.A. conceived the subject of the paper, contributed to the critical interpretation, and supervised the project. All authors have read and agreed to the published version of the manuscript.

Funding: This research received no external funding.

Institutional Review Board Statement: Not applicable.

Informed Consent Statement: Endoscopic images from the clinical case have been collected and published after written informed consent was given by the patients, following Italian privacy legislation.

Data Availability Statement: Data sharing is not applicable. No new data were created or analyzed in this study.

Conflicts of Interest: A. Armuzzi has received consulting fees from AbbVie, Allergan, Amgen, Arena, Biogen, Boehringer Ingelheim, Bristol-Myers Squibb, Celgene, Celltrion, Eli-Lilly, Ferring, Galapagos, Gilead, Janssen, MSD, Mylan, Pfizer, Protagonist Therapeutics, Roche, Samsung Bioepis, Sandoz and Takeda; speaker's fees from AbbVie, Amgen, Arena, Biogen, Bristol-Myers Squibb, Eli-Lilly, Ferring, Galapagos, Gilead, Janssen, MSD, Novartis, Pfizer, Roche, Samsung Bioepis, Sandoz, Takeda, and Tigenix; and research support from Biogen, MSD, Takeda, and Pfizer. C. Bezzio received lecture fees and served as a consultant for Takeda, MSD, Ferring, Abbvie, Galapagos and Janssen. R. Gabbiadini has received speaker's fees from Pfizer, MSD and Celltrion. A. Dal Buono has received speaker's fees from AbbVie, Galapagos and Celltrion. E.V. Savarino has served as speaker for Abbvie, Abivax, Agave, AGPharma, Alfasigma, CaDiGroup, Celltrion, Dr Falk, EG Stada Group, Fenix Pharma, Galapagos, Johnson&Johnson, JB Pharmaceuticals, Innovamedica/Adacyte, Eli Lilly, Malesci, Mayoly Biohealth, Omega Pharma, Pfizer, Reckitt Benckiser, Sandoz, SILA, Sofar, Takeda, Tillots, Unifarco; has served as consultant for Abbvie, Agave, Alfasigma, Biogen, Bristol-Myers Squibb, Celltrion, Dr. Falk, Eli Lilly, Fenix Pharma, Johnson&Johnson, JB Pharmaceuticals, Merck & Co, Nestlè, Pfizer, Reckitt Benckiser, Regeneron, Sanofi, SILA, Sofar, Takeda, Unifarco; he received research support from Bonollo, Difass, Pfizer, Reckitt Benckiser, SILA, Sofar, Unifarco, Zeta Farmaceutici; G. Pellegatta has received speaker's fees from Sanofi, DrFalk Pharma, Malesci. F. Racca has received consulting fees from Sanofi and DrFalk. E. Heffler, A. Repici, G. Migliorisi, E. Mastrorocco and P. Spaggiari declare no conflicts of interest.

References

1. Low, E.E.; Dellon, E.S. Review Article: Emerging Insights into the Epidemiology, Pathophysiology, Diagnostic and Therapeutic Aspects of Eosinophilic Oesophagitis and Other Eosinophilic Gastrointestinal Diseases. *Aliment. Pharmacol. Ther.* **2024**, *59*, 322–340. [CrossRef] [PubMed]
2. Ng, S.C.; Shi, H.Y.; Hamidi, N.; Underwood, F.E.; Tang, W.; Benchimol, E.I.; Panaccione, R.; Ghosh, S.; Wu, J.C.Y.; Chan, F.K.L.; et al. Worldwide Incidence and Prevalence of Inflammatory Bowel Disease in the 21st Century: A Systematic Review of Population-Based Studies. *Lancet* **2017**, *390*, 2769–2778. [CrossRef] [PubMed]
3. Le Berre, C.; Honap, S.; Peyrin-Biroulet, L. Ulcerative Colitis. *Lancet* **2023**, *402*, 571–584. [CrossRef] [PubMed]
4. Dolinger, M.; Torres, J.; Vermeire, S. Crohn's Disease. *Lancet* **2024**, *403*, 1177–1191. [CrossRef]
5. Solina, G.; Mandalà, S.; La Barbera, C.; Mandalà, V. Current Management of Intestinal Bowel Disease: The Role of Surgery. *Updates Surg.* **2016**, *68*, 13–23. [CrossRef] [PubMed]
6. Dellon, E.S.; Gonsalves, N.; Abonia, J.P.; Alexander, J.A.; Arva, N.C.; Atkins, D.; Attwood, S.E.; Auth, M.K.H.; Bailey, D.D.; Biederman, L.; et al. International Consensus Recommendations for Eosinophilic Gastrointestinal Disease Nomenclature. *Clin. Gastroenterol. Hepatol.* **2022**, *20*, 2474–2484.e3. [CrossRef] [PubMed]
7. O'Shea, K.M.; Aceves, S.S.; Dellon, E.S.; Gupta, S.K.; Spergel, J.M.; Furuta, G.T.; Rothenberg, M.E. Pathophysiology of Eosinophilic Esophagitis. *Gastroenterology* **2018**, *154*, 333–345. [CrossRef] [PubMed]
8. Dellon, E.S.; Collins, M.H.; Katzka, D.A.; Hudgens, S.; Lan, L.; Williams, J.; Vera-Llonch, M.; Hirano, I. Improvements in Dysphagia and Pain with Swallowing in Patients with Eosinophilic Esophagitis Receiving Budesonide Oral Suspension. *Clin. Gastroenterol. Hepatol.* **2021**, *19*, 699–706.e4. [CrossRef] [PubMed]
9. Uchida, A.M.; Garber, J.J.; Pyne, A.; Peterson, K.; Roelstraete, B.; Olén, O.; Halfvarson, J.; Ludvigsson, J.F. Eosinophilic Esophagitis Is Associated with Increased Risk of Later Inflammatory Bowel Disease in a Nationwide Swedish Population Cohort. *Eur. Gastroenterol. J.* **2024**, *12*, 34–43. [CrossRef] [PubMed]
10. Vuyyuru, S.K.; Kedia, S.; Sahu, P.; Ahuja, V. Immune-Mediated Inflammatory Diseases of the Gastrointestinal Tract: Beyond Crohn's Disease and Ulcerative Colitis. *JGH Open* **2022**, *6*, 100–111. [CrossRef]
11. Canova, C.; Ludvigsson, J.F.; Di Domenicantonio, R.; Zanier, L.; Amidei, C.B.; Zingone, F. Perinatal and Antibiotic Exposures and the Risk of Developing Childhood-Onset Inflammatory Bowel Disease: A Nested Case-Control Study Based on a Population-Based Birth Cohort. *Int. J. Environ. Res. Public Health* **2020**, *17*, 2409. [CrossRef]
12. Örtqvist, A.K.; Lundholm, C.; Halfvarson, J.; Ludvigsson, J.F.; Almqvist, C. Fetal and Early Life Antibiotics Exposure and Very Early Onset Inflammatory Bowel Disease: A Population-Based Study. *Gut* **2019**, *68*, 218–225. [CrossRef] [PubMed]

13. Jensen, E.T.; Dai, X.; Kodroff, E.; Strobel, M.J.; Zicarelli, A.; Gray, S.; Cordell, A.; Anderson, C.; Hiremath, G.; Dellon, E.S. Early Life Exposures as Risk Factors for Non-Esophageal Eosinophilic Gastrointestinal Diseases. *Clin. Res. Hepatol. Gastroenterol.* **2023**, *47*, 102170. [CrossRef] [PubMed]
14. Agrawal, M.; Sabino, J.; Frias-Gomes, C.; Hillenbrand, C.M.; Soudant, C.; Axelrad, J.E.; Shah, S.C.; Ribeiro-Mourão, F.; Lambin, T.; Peter, I.; et al. Early Life Exposures and the Risk of Inflammatory Bowel Disease: Systematic Review and Meta-Analyses. *EClinicalMedicine* **2021**, *36*, 100884. [CrossRef] [PubMed]
15. Jensen, E.T.; Kappelman, M.D.; Kim, H.P.; Ringel-Kulka, T.; Dellon, E.S. Early Life Exposures as Risk Factors for Pediatric Eosinophilic Esophagitis. *J. Pediatr. Gastroenterol. Nutr.* **2013**, *57*, 67–71. [CrossRef]
16. Lo, C.H.; Lochhead, P.; Khalili, H.; Song, M.; Tabung, F.K.; Burke, K.E.; Richter, J.M.; Giovannucci, E.L.; Chan, A.T.; Ananthakrishnan, A.N. Dietary Inflammatory Potential and Risk of Crohn's Disease and Ulcerative Colitis. *Gastroenterology* **2020**, *159*, 873–883.e1. [CrossRef] [PubMed]
17. Lo, C.H.; Khandpur, N.; Rossato, S.L.; Lochhead, P.; Lopes, E.W.; Burke, K.E.; Richter, J.M.; Song, M.; Ardisson Korat, A.V.; Sun, Q.; et al. Ultra-Processed Foods and Risk of Crohn's Disease and Ulcerative Colitis: A Prospective Cohort Study. *Clin. Gastroenterol. Hepatol.* **2022**, *20*, e1323–e1337. [CrossRef]
18. Racca, F.; Pellegatta, G.; Cataldo, G.; Vespa, E.; Carlani, E.; Pelaia, C.; Paoletti, G.; Messina, M.R.; Nappi, E.; Canonica, G.W.; et al. Type 2 Inflammation in Eosinophilic Esophagitis: From Pathophysiology to Therapeutic Targets. *Front. Physiol.* **2022**, *12*, 815842. [CrossRef]
19. Brusilovsky, M.; Bao, R.; Rochman, M.; Kemter, A.M.; Nagler, C.R.; Rothenberg, M.E. Host–Microbiota Interactions in the Esophagus During Homeostasis and Allergic Inflammation. *Gastroenterology* **2022**, *162*, 521–534.e8. [CrossRef]
20. Massimino, L.; Barchi, A.; Mandarino, F.V.; Spanò, S.; Lamparelli, L.A.; Vespa, E.; Passaretti, S.; Peyrin-Biroulet, L.; Savarino, E.V.; Jairath, V.; et al. A Multi-Omic Analysis Reveals the Esophageal Dysbiosis as the Predominant Trait of Eosinophilic Esophagitis. *J. Transl. Med.* **2023**, *21*, 46. [CrossRef]
21. Nishida, A.; Inoue, R.; Inatomi, O.; Bamba, S.; Naito, Y.; Andoh, A. Gut Microbiota in the Pathogenesis of Inflammatory Bowel Disease. *Clin. J. Gastroenterol.* **2018**, *11*, 1–10. [CrossRef] [PubMed]
22. Shastri, S.A.; Kantamneni, R.; Rashid, M.; Chandran, V.P.; Suhita, R.; Begum, I.; Nair, S.; Thunga, G. Proton Pump Inhibitors Use and Risk of Inflammatory Bowel Diseases: A Meta-Analysis of Observational Studies. *Med. Pharm. Rep.* **2022**, *95*, 357–369. [CrossRef] [PubMed]
23. Singh, N.; Nugent, Z.; Singh, H.; Shaffer, S.R.; Bernstein, C.N. Proton Pump Inhibitor Use Before and After a Diagnosis of Inflammatory Bowel Disease. *Inflamm. Bowel Dis.* **2023**, *29*, 1871–1878. [CrossRef] [PubMed]
24. Xia, B.; Yang, M.; Nguyen, L.H.; He, Q.; Zhen, J.; Yu, Y.; Di, M.; Qin, X.; Lu, K.; Kuo, Z.C.; et al. Regular Use of Proton Pump Inhibitor and the Risk of Inflammatory Bowel Disease: Pooled Analysis of 3 Prospective Cohorts. *Gastroenterology* **2021**, *161*, 1842–1852.e10. [CrossRef] [PubMed]
25. Merwat, S.N.; Spechler, S.J. Might the Use of Acid-Suppressive Medications Predispose to the Development of Eosinophilic Esophagitis? *Am. J. Gastroenterol.* **2009**, *104*, 1897–1902. [CrossRef] [PubMed]
26. Arias, Á.; Vicario, M.; Bernardo, D.; Olalla, J.M.; Fortea, M.; Montalban-Arques, A.; Martínez-Fernández, P.; González-Castro, A.M.; Mota-Huertas, T.; Arias-González, L.; et al. Toll-like Receptors-Mediated Pathways Activate Inflammatory Responses in the Esophageal Mucosa of Adult Eosinophilic Esophagitis. *Clin. Transl. Gastroenterol.* **2018**, *9*, e147. [CrossRef] [PubMed]
27. Lu, Y.; Li, X.; Liu, S.; Zhang, Y.; Zhang, D. Toll-like Receptors and Inflammatory Bowel Disease. *Front. Immunol.* **2018**, *9*, 72. [CrossRef] [PubMed]
28. Strober, W.; Fuss, I.J. Proinflammatory Cytokines in the Pathogenesis of Inflammatory Bowel Diseases. *Gastroenterology* **2011**, *140*, 1756–1767.e1. [CrossRef] [PubMed]
29. Dubucquoi, S.; Janin, A.; Desreumaux, P.; Quandalle, P.; Cortot, A.; Capron, M.F.; Colombel, P.J. Activated Eosinophils and Interleukin 5 Expression in Early Recurrence of Crohn's Disease. *Gut* **1995**, *37*, 242–246. [CrossRef]
30. Hassani, M.; Leijte, G.; Bruse, N.; Kox, M.; Pickkers, P.; Vrisekoop, N.; Koenderman, L. Differentiation and Activation of Eosinophils in the Human Bone Marrow during Experimental Human Endotoxemia. *J. Leukoc. Biol.* **2020**, *108*, 1665–1671. [CrossRef]
31. Gigon, L.; Fettrelet, T.; Yousefi, S.; Simon, D.; Simon, H. Eosinophils from A to Z. *Allergy* **2023**, *78*, 1810–1846. [CrossRef] [PubMed]
32. Koutri, E.; Patereli, A.; Noni, M.; Gutiérrez-Junquera, C.; González-Lois, C.; Oliva, S.; Giordano, C.; Stefanaki, K.; Papadopoulou, A. Distribution of Eosinophils in the Gastrointestinal Tract of Children with No Organic Disease. *Ann. Gastroenterol.* **2020**, *33*, 508–515. [CrossRef] [PubMed]
33. Kato, M.; Kephart, G.M.; Talley, N.J.; Wagner, J.M.; Sarr, M.G.; Bonno, M.; Mcgovern, T.W.; Gleich, G.J. Eosinophil Infiltration and Degranulation in Normal Human Tissue. *Anat. Rec.* **1998**, *252*, 418–425. [CrossRef]
34. Shin, M.H.; Lee, Y.A.; Min, D.Y. Eosinophil-Mediated Tissue Inflammatory Responses in Helminth Infection. *Korean J. Parasitol.* **2009**, *47*, S125–S131. [CrossRef]
35. Tedner, S.G.; Asarnoj, A.; Thulin, H.; Westman, M.; Konradsen, J.R.; Nilsson, C. Food Allergy and Hypersensitivity Reactions in Children and Adults—A Review. *J. Intern. Med.* **2022**, *291*, 283–302. [CrossRef] [PubMed]
36. Marichal, T.; Mesnil, C.; Bureau, F. Homeostatic Eosinophils: Characteristics and Functions. *Front. Med.* **2017**, *4*, 101. [CrossRef]
37. Jung, Y.; Wen, T.; Mingler, M.K.; Caldwell, J.M.; Wang, Y.H.; Chaplin, D.D.; Lee, E.H.; Jang, M.H.; Woo, S.Y.; Seoh, J.Y.; et al. IL-1β in Eosinophil-Mediated Small Intestinal Homeostasis and IgA Production. *Mucosal Immunol.* **2015**, *8*, 930–942. [CrossRef]

38. Ignacio, A.; Shah, K.; Bernier-Latmani, J.; Köller, Y.; Coakley, G.; Moyat, M.; Hamelin, R.; Armand, F.; Wong, N.C.; Ramay, H.; et al. Small Intestinal Resident Eosinophils Maintain Gut Homeostasis Following Microbial Colonization. *Immunity* **2022**, *55*, 1250–1267.e12. [CrossRef]
39. Chu, V.T.; Beller, A.; Rausch, S.; Strandmark, J.; Zänker, M.; Arbach, O.; Kruglov, A.; Berek, C. Eosinophils Promote Generation and Maintenance of Immunoglobulin-A-Expressing Plasma Cells and Contribute to Gut Immune Homeostasis. *Immunity* **2014**, *40*, 582–593. [CrossRef]
40. Nussbaum, J.C.; Van Dyken, S.J.; Von Moltke, J.; Cheng, L.E.; Mohapatra, A.; Molofsky, A.B.; Thornton, E.E.; Krummel, M.F.; Chawla, A.; Liang, H.E.; et al. Type 2 Innate Lymphoid Cells Control Eosinophil Homeostasis. *Nature* **2013**, *502*, 245–248. [CrossRef]
41. Loktionov, A. Eosinophils in the Gastrointestinal Tract and Their Role in the Pathogenesis of Major Colorectal Disorders. *World J. Gastroenterol.* **2019**, *25*, 3503–3526. [CrossRef] [PubMed]
42. Sugawara, R.; Lee, E.J.; Jang, M.S.; Jeun, E.J.; Hong, C.P.; Kim, J.H.; Park, A.; Yun, C.H.; Hong, S.W.; Kim, Y.M.; et al. Small Intestinal Eosinophils Regulate Th17 Cells by Producing IL-1 Receptor Antagonist. *J. Exp. Med.* **2016**, *213*, 555–567. [CrossRef] [PubMed]
43. Coakley, G.; Wang, H.; Harris, N.L. Intestinal Eosinophils: Multifaceted Roles in Tissue Homeostasis and Disease. *Semin. Immunopathol.* **2021**, *43*, 307–317. [CrossRef] [PubMed]
44. Salvo-Romero, E.; Rodiño-Janeiro, B.K.; Albert-Bayo, M.; Lobo, B.; Santos, J.; Farré, R.; Martinez, C.; Vicario, M. Eosinophils in the Gastrointestinal Tract: Key Contributors to Neuro-Immune Crosstalk and Potential Implications in Disorders of Brain-Gut Interaction. *Cells* **2022**, *11*, 1644. [CrossRef] [PubMed]
45. Weller, P.F.; Spencer, L.A. Functions of Tissue-Resident Eosinophils. *J. Exp. Med.* **2023**, *220*, e20221435. [CrossRef] [PubMed]
46. Gurtner, A.; Borrelli, C.; Gonzalez-Perez, I.; Bach, K.; Acar, I.E.; Nùnez, N.G.; Crepaz, D.; Handler, K.; Vu, V.P.; Lafzi, A.; et al. Active eosinophils regulate host defence and immune responses in colitis. *Nature* **2023**, *615*, 151–157. [CrossRef] [PubMed]
47. Villanacci, V.; Reggiani-Bonetti, L.; Salviato, T.; Leoncini, G.; Cadei, M.; Albarello, L.; Caputo, A.; Aquilano, M.C.; Battista, S.; Parente, P. Histopathology of IBD Colitis. A Practical Approach from the Pathologists of the Italian Group for the Study of the Gastrointestinal Tract (GIPAD). *Pathologica* **2021**, *113*, 39–53. [CrossRef] [PubMed]
48. Barchi, A.; Vespa, E.; Passaretti, S.; Dell'Anna, G.; Fasulo, E.; Yacoub, M.-R.; Albarello, L.; Sinagra, E.; Massimino, L.; Ungaro, F.; et al. The Dual Lens of Endoscopy and Histology in the Diagnosis and Management of Eosinophilic Gastrointestinal Disorders—A Comprehensive Review. *Diagnostics* **2024**, *14*, 858. [CrossRef]
49. Manousou, P.; Kolios, G.; Valatas, V.; Drygiannakis, I.; Bourikas, L.; Pyrovolaki, K.; Koutroubakis, I.; Papadaki, H.A.; Kouroumalis, E. Increased Expression of Chemokine Receptor CCR3 and Its Ligands in Ulcerative Colitis: The Role of Colonic Epithelial Cells in in Vitro Studies. *Clin. Exp. Immunol.* **2010**, *162*, 337–347. [CrossRef]
50. Schmitz, J.; Owyang, A.; Oldham, E.; Song, Y.; Murphy, E.; McClanahan, T.K.; Zurawski, G.; Moshrefi, M.; Qin, J.; Li, X.; et al. IL-33, an Interleukin-1-like Cytokine That Signals via the IL-1 Receptor-Related Protein ST2 and Induces T Helper Type 2-Associated Cytokines. *Immunity* **2005**, *23*, 479–490. [CrossRef]
51. Shakerian, L.; Kolahdooz, H.; Garousi, M.; Keyvani, V.; Kamal Kheder, R.; Abdulsattar Faraj, T.; Yazdanpanah, E.; Esmaeili, S.-A. IL-33/ST2 Axis in Autoimmune Disease. *Cytokine* **2022**, *158*, 156015. [CrossRef] [PubMed]
52. Li, J.; Ueno, A.; Gasia, M.F.; Luider, J.; Wang, T.; Hirota, C.; Jijon, H.B.; Deane, M.; Tom, M.; Chan, R.; et al. Profiles of Lamina Propria T Helper Cell Subsets Discriminate between Ulcerative Colitis and Crohn's Disease. *Inflamm. Bowel Dis.* **2016**, *22*, 1779–1792. [CrossRef]
53. Zabrowski, D.; Abraham, D.; Rosenthal, G.; Kader, H. Development of Peripheral Eosinophilia in Inflammatory Bowel Disease Patients on Infliximab Treated at a Tertiary Pediatric Inflammatory Bowel Disease Center Is Associated with Clinically Active Disease but Does Not Result in Loss of Efficacy or Adverse Outcomes. *JGH Open* **2020**, *4*, 636–641. [CrossRef]
54. Click, B.; Anderson, A.M.; Koutroubakis, I.E.; Ramos Rivers, C.; Babichenko, D.; Machicado, J.D.; Hartman, D.J.; Hashash, J.G.; Dunn, M.A.; Schwartz, M.; et al. Peripheral Eosinophilia in Patients With Inflammatory Bowel Disease Defines an Aggressive Disease Phenotype. *Am. J. Gastroenterol.* **2017**, *112*, 1849–1858. [CrossRef]
55. Barrie, A.; El Mourabet, M.; Weyant, K.; Clarke, K.; Gajendran, M.; Rivers, C.; Park, S.Y.; Hartman, D.; Saul, M.; Regueiro, M.; et al. Recurrent Blood Eosinophilia in Ulcerative Colitis Is Associated with Severe Disease and Primary Sclerosing Cholangitis. *Dig. Dis. Sci.* **2013**, *58*, 222–228. [CrossRef]
56. Filippone, R.T.; Sahakian, L.; Apostolopoulos, V.; Nurgali, K. Eosinophils in Inflammatory Bowel Disease. *Inflamm. Bowel Dis.* **2019**, *25*, 1140–1151. [CrossRef] [PubMed]
57. Jacobs, I.; Ceulemans, M.; Wauters, L.; Breynaert, C.; Vermeire, S.; Verstockt, B.; Vanuytsel, T. Role of Eosinophils in Intestinal Inflammation and Fibrosis in Inflammatory Bowel Disease: An Overlooked Villain? *Front. Immunol.* **2021**, *12*, 754413. [CrossRef]
58. Nada, A.; Teresa, S.; Sandra, K.; Jessica, R.; Stefani, R.; Christian, T.; Konrad, S.; Gernot, S. Fecal Eosinophil Cationic Protein Is a Diagnostic and Predictive Biomarker in Young Adults with Inflammatory Bowel Disease. *J. Clin. Med.* **2019**, *8*, 2025. [CrossRef] [PubMed]
59. Ling Lundström, M.; Peterson, C.; Lampinen, M.; Hedin, C.R.H.; Keita, Å.V.; Kruse, R.; Magnusson, M.K.; Lindqvist, C.M.; Repsilber, D.; D'Amato, M.; et al. Fecal Biomarkers of Neutrophil and Eosinophil Origin Reflect the Response to Biological Therapy and Corticosteroids in Patients with Inflammatory Bowel Disease. *Clin. Transl. Gastroenterol.* **2023**, *14*, e00605. [CrossRef]

60. Smyth, C.M.; Akasheh, N.; Woods, S.; Kay, E.; Morgan, R.K.; Thornton, M.A.; O'Grady, A.; Cummins, R.; Sheils, O.; Smyth, P.; et al. Activated Eosinophils in Association with Enteric Nerves in Inflammatory Bowel Disease. *PLoS ONE* **2013**, *8*, e64216. [CrossRef]
61. Wéra, O.; Lancellotti, P.; Oury, C. The Dual Role of Neutrophils in Inflammatory Bowel Diseases. *J. Clin. Med.* **2016**, *5*, 118. [CrossRef] [PubMed]
62. Masterson, J.C.; Capocelli, K.E.; Hosford, L.; Biette, K.; McNamee, E.N.; De Zoeten, E.F.; Harris, R.; Fernando, S.D.; Jedlicka, P.; Protheroe, C.; et al. Eosinophils and IL-33 Perpetuate Chronic Inflammation and Fibrosis in a Pediatric Population with Stricturing Crohn's Ileitis. *Inflamm. Bowel Dis.* **2015**, *21*, 2429–2440. [CrossRef] [PubMed]
63. Jacobs, I.; Deleu, S.; Cremer, J.; De Hertogh, G.; Vermeire, S.; Breynaert, C.; Vanuytsel, T.; Verstockt, B. DOP09 Eosinophils Exert a Pro-Inflammatory Role in a Chronic DSS Colitis Model without an Impact on Fibrosis. *J. Crohns Colitis* **2023**, *17*, i67–i69. [CrossRef]
64. Ryu, S.; Lee, K.H.; Tizaoui, K.; Terrazzino, S.; Cargnin, S.; Effenberger, M.; Shin, J., II; Kronbichler, A. Pathogenesis of Eosinophilic Esophagitis: A Comprehensive Review of the Genetic and Molecular Aspects. *Int. J. Mol. Sci.* **2020**, *21*, 7253. [CrossRef]
65. Cheng, E.; Zhang, X.; Wilson, K.S.; Wang, D.H.; Park, J.Y.; Huo, X.; Yu, C.; Zhang, Q.; Spechler, S.J.; Souza, R.F. JAK-STAT6 Pathway Inhibitors Block Eotaxin-3 Secretion by Epithelial Cells and Fibroblasts from Esophageal Eosinophilia Patients: Promising Agents to Improve Inflammation and Prevent Fibrosis in EoE. *PLoS ONE* **2016**, *11*, e0157376. [CrossRef] [PubMed]
66. Massironi, S.; Mulinacci, G.; Gallo, C.; Elvevi, A.; Danese, S.; Invernizzi, P.; Vespa, E. Mechanistic Insights into Eosinophilic Esophagitis: Therapies Targeting Pathophysiological Mechanisms. *Cells* **2023**, *12*, 2473. [CrossRef] [PubMed]
67. Spechler, S.J. Eosinophilic Esophagitis: Novel Concepts Regarding Pathogenesis and Clinical Manifestations. *J. Gastroenterol.* **2019**, *54*, 837–844. [CrossRef]
68. Ghisa, M.; Laserra, G.; Marabotto, E.; Ziola, S.; Tolone, S.; de Bortoli, N.; Frazzoni, M.; Mauro, A.; Penagini, R.; Savarino, V.; et al. Achalasia and Obstructive Motor Disorders Are Not Uncommon in Patients with Eosinophilic Esophagitis. *Clin. Gastroenterol. Hepatol.* **2021**, *19*, 1554–1563. [CrossRef]
69. Visaggi, P.; Ghisa, M.; Barberio, B.; Marabotto, E.; de Bortoli, N.; Savarino, E. Systematic Review: Esophageal Motility Patterns in Patients with Eosinophilic Esophagitis. *Dig. Liver Dis.* **2022**, *54*, 1143–1152. [CrossRef]
70. Muir, A.B.; Wang, J.X.; Nakagawa, H. Epithelial-Stromal Crosstalk and Fibrosis in Eosinophilic Esophagitis. *J. Gastroenterol.* **2019**, *54*, 10–18. [CrossRef]
71. Angerami Almeida, K.; de Queiroz Andrade, E.; Burns, G.; Hoedt, E.C.; Mattes, J.; Keely, S.; Collison, A. The Microbiota in Eosinophilic Esophagitis: A Systematic Review. *J. Gastroenterol. Hepatol.* **2022**, *37*, 1673–1684. [CrossRef] [PubMed]
72. Facchin, S.; Calgaro, M.; Pandolfo, M.; Caldart, F.; Ghisa, M.; Greco, E.; Sattin, E.; Valle, G.; Dellon, E.S.; Vitulo, N.; et al. Salivary Microbiota Composition May Discriminate between Patients with Eosinophilic Oesophagitis (EoE) and non-EoE Subjects. *Aliment. Pharmacol. Ther.* **2022**, *56*, 450–462. [CrossRef] [PubMed]
73. Greuter, T.; Katzka, D. Endoscopic Features of Eosinophilic Gastrointestinal Diseases. *Immunol. Allergy Clin.* **2024**, *44*, 357–368. [CrossRef] [PubMed]
74. Kim, H.P.; Vance, R.B.; Shaheen, N.J.; Dellon, E.S. The Prevalence and Diagnostic Utility of Endoscopic Features of Eosinophilic Esophagitis: A Meta-Analysis. *Clin. Gastroenterol. Hepatol.* **2012**, *10*, 988–996.e5. [CrossRef] [PubMed]
75. Liacouras, C.A.; Spergel, J.M.; Ruchelli, E.; Verma, R.; Mascarenhas, M.; Semeao, E.; Flick, J.; Kelly, J.; Brown–Whitehorn, T.; Mamula, P.; et al. Eosinophilic Esophagitis: A 10-Year Experience in 381 Children. *Clin. Gastroenterol. Hepatol.* **2005**, *3*, 1198–1206. [CrossRef] [PubMed]
76. Khalaf, R.T.; Rosenwald, K.; Zhou, W.; Pan, Z.; Kramer, R.E.; Menard-Katcher, C. Quality Improvement Initiative to Improve Endoscopic Reassessment of Eosinophilic Esophagitis. *JPGN Rep.* **2021**, *2*, e104. [CrossRef] [PubMed]
77. Carlson, D.A.; Hirano, I.; Gonsalves, N.; Kahrilas, P.J.; Araujo, I.K.; Yang, M.; Tetreault, M.-P.; Pandolfino, J.E. A PhysioMechanical Model of Esophageal Function in Eosinophilic Esophagitis. *Gastroenterology* **2023**, *165*, 552–563.e4. [CrossRef]
78. Cotton, C.C.; Woosley, J.T.; Moist, S.E.; McGee, S.J.; Iuga, A.; Shaheen, N.J.; Dellon, E.S. Determination of a Treatment Response Threshold for the Eosinophilic Esophagitis Endoscopic Reference Score. *Endoscopy* **2022**, *54*, 635–643. [CrossRef] [PubMed]
79. Ma, C.; Bredenoord, A.J.; Dellon, E.S.; Alexander, J.A.; Biedermann, L.; Hogan, M.; Guizzetti, L.; Zou, G.; Katzka, D.A.; Chehade, M.; et al. Reliability and Responsiveness of Endoscopic Disease Activity Assessment in Eosinophilic Esophagitis. *Gastrointest. Endosc.* **2022**, *95*, 1126–1137.e2. [CrossRef]
80. Impellizzeri, G.; Marasco, G.; Eusebi, L.H.; Salfi, N.; Bazzoli, F.; Zagari, R.M. Eosinophilic Colitis: A Clinical Review. *Dig. Liver Dis.* **2019**, *51*, 769–773. [CrossRef]
81. Srinivasan, A.R. Treat to Target in Crohn's Disease: A Practical Guide for Clinicians. *World J. Gastroenterol.* **2024**, *30*, 50–69. [CrossRef] [PubMed]
82. Maaser, C.; Sturm, A.; Vavricka, S.R.; Kucharzik, T.; Fiorino, G.; Annese, V.; Calabrese, E.; Baumgart, D.C.; Bettenworth, D.; Borralho Nunes, P.; et al. ECCO-ESGAR Guideline for Diagnostic Assessment in IBD Part 1: Initial Diagnosis, Monitoring of Known IBD, Detection of Complications. *J. Crohns Colitis* **2019**, *13*, 144–164. [CrossRef] [PubMed]
83. Negreanu, L.; Voiosu, T.; State, M.; Voiosu, A.; Bengus, A.; Mateescu, B.R. Endoscopy in Inflammatory Bowel Disease: From Guidelines to Real Life. *Therap. Adv. Gastroenterol.* **2019**, *12*, 175628481986515. [CrossRef]
84. Neurath, M.F.; Vieth, M. Different Levels of Healing in Inflammatory Bowel Diseases: Mucosal, Histological, Transmural, Barrier and Complete Healing. *Gut* **2023**, *72*, 2164–2183. [CrossRef] [PubMed]

85. Dhar, A.; Haboubi, H.N.; Attwood, S.E.; Auth, M.K.H.; Dunn, J.M.; Sweis, R.; Morris, D.; Epstein, J.; Novelli, M.R.; Hunter, H.; et al. British Society of Gastroenterology (BSG) and British Society of Paediatric Gastroenterology, Hepatology and Nutrition (BSPGHAN) Joint Consensus Guidelines on the Diagnosis and Management of Eosinophilic Oesophagitis in Children and Adults. *Gut* **2022**, *71*, 1459–1487. [CrossRef] [PubMed]
86. Dellon, E.S.; Liacouras, C.A.; Molina-Infante, J.; Furuta, G.T.; Spergel, J.M.; Zevit, N.; Spechler, S.J.; Attwood, S.E.; Straumann, A.; Aceves, S.S.; et al. Updated International Consensus Diagnostic Criteria for Eosinophilic Esophagitis: Proceedings of the AGREE Conference. *Gastroenterology* **2018**, *155*, 1022–1033.e10. [CrossRef] [PubMed]
87. Lucendo, A.J.; Molina-Infante, J.; Arias, Á.; von Arnim, U.; Bredenoord, A.J.; Bussmann, C.; Amil Dias, J.; Bove, M.; González-Cervera, J.; Larsson, H.; et al. Guidelines on Eosinophilic Esophagitis: Evidence-based Statements and Recommendations for Diagnosis and Management in Children and Adults. *Eur. Gastroenterol. J.* **2017**, *5*, 335–358. [CrossRef] [PubMed]
88. Collins, M.H. Histopathologic Features of Eosinophilic Esophagitis and Eosinophilic Gastrointestinal Diseases. *Gastroenterol. Clin.* **2014**, *43*, 257–268. [CrossRef] [PubMed]
89. Conner, J.R.; Kirsch, R. The Pathology and Causes of Tissue Eosinophilia in the Gastrointestinal Tract. *Histopathology* **2017**, *71*, 177–199. [CrossRef] [PubMed]
90. Díaz Del Arco, C.; Taxonera, C.; Muñoz, L.E.; Olivares, D.; Fernández Aceñero, M.J. Eosinophilic Colitis: Experience in a Large Tertiary Hospital. *Rom. J. Morphol. Embryol.* **2017**, *58*, 783–789.
91. Reggiani Bonetti, L.; Leoncini, G.; Daperno, M.; Principi, M.B.; Baronchelli, C.; Manenti, S.; Caprioli, F.; Armuzzi, A.; Caputo, A.; Parente, P.; et al. Histopathology of Non-IBD Colitis Practical Recommendations from Pathologists of IG-IBD Group. *Dig. Liver Dis.* **2021**, *53*, 950–957. [CrossRef]
92. Kaltenbach, T.R.; Soetikno, R.M.; DeVivo, R.; Laine, L.A.; Barkun, A.; McQuaid, K.R.; Cheifetz, A.; Chiorean, M.; East, J.E.; Farraye, F.A.; et al. Optimizing the Quality of Endoscopy in Inflammatory Bowel Disease: Focus on Surveillance and Management of Colorectal Dysplasia Using Interactive Image- and Video-Based Teaching. *Gastrointest. Endosc.* **2017**, *86*, 1107–1117.e1. [CrossRef] [PubMed]
93. Magro, F.; Langner, C.; Driessen, A.; Ensari, A.; Geboes, K.; Mantzaris, G.J.; Villanacci, V.; Becheanu, G.; Nunes, P.B.; Cathomas, G.; et al. European Consensus on the Histopathology of Inflammatory Bowel Disease. *J. Crohns Colitis* **2013**, *7*, 827–851. [CrossRef] [PubMed]
94. Kim, E.S.; Kwon, Y.; Choe, Y.H.; Kim, M.J. Upper gastrointestinal tract involvement is more prevalent in Korean patients with pediatric Crohn's disease than in European patients. *Sci. Rep.* **2020**, *10*, 19032. [CrossRef]
95. Magro, F.; Doherty, G.; Peyrin-Biroulet, L.; Svrcek, M.; Borralho, P.; Walsh, A.; Carneiro, F.; Rosini, F.; de Hertogh, G.; Biedermann, L.; et al. ECCO Position Paper: Harmonization of the Approach to Ulcerative Colitis Histopathology. *J. Crohns Colitis* **2020**, *14*, 1503–1511. [CrossRef]
96. Canavese, G.; Villanacci, V.; Antonelli, E.; Cadei, M.; Sapino, A.; Rocca, R.; Daperno, M.; Suriani, R.; Di Santo, M.G.; Cassoni, P.; et al. Eosinophilia–Associated Basal Plasmacytosis: An Early and Sensitive Histologic Feature of Inflammatory Bowel Disease. *APMIS* **2017**, *125*, 179–183. [CrossRef]
97. Zezos, P.; Patsiaoura, K.; Nakos, A.; Mpoumponaris, A.; Vassiliadis, T.; Giouleme, O.; Pitiakoudis, M.; Kouklakis, G.; Evgenidis, N. Severe Eosinophilic Infiltration in Colonic Biopsies Predicts Patients with Ulcerative Colitis Not Responding to Medical Therapy. *Color. Dis.* **2014**, *16*, O420–O430. [CrossRef]
98. Leoncini, G.; Villanacci, V.; Marin, M.G.; Crisafulli, V.; Cadei, M.; Antonelli, E.; Leoci, C.; Bassotti, G. Colonic Hypereosinophilia in Ulcerative Colitis May Help to Predict the Failure of Steroid Therapy. *Tech. Coloproctol.* **2018**, *22*, 941–946. [CrossRef]
99. Sankey, E.A.; Dhillon, A.P.; Anthony, A.; Wakefield, A.J.; Sim, R.; More, L.; Hudson, M.; Sawyerr, A.M.; Pounder, R.E. Early Mucosal Changes in Crohn's Disease. *Gut* **1993**, *34*, 375–381. [CrossRef] [PubMed]
100. Villanacci, V.; Bassotti, G. Histopathological Findings of Extra-Ileal Manifestations at Initial Diagnosis of Crohn's Disease-Related Ileitis. *Virchows Arch.* **2017**, *470*, 595–596. [CrossRef]
101. Decousus, S.; Boucher, A.-L.; Joubert, J.; Pereira, B.; Dubois, A.; Goutorbe, F.; Déchelotte, P.J.; Bommelaer, G.; Buisson, A. Myenteric Plexitis Is a Risk Factor for Endoscopic and Clinical Postoperative Recurrence after Ileocolonic Resection in Crohn's Disease. *Dig. Liver Dis.* **2016**, *48*, 753–758. [CrossRef] [PubMed]
102. Annunziata, M.L.; Caviglia, R.; Papparella, L.G.; Cicala, M. Upper Gastrointestinal Involvement of Crohn's Disease: A Prospective Study on the Role of Upper Endoscopy in the Diagnostic Work-Up. *Dig. Dis. Sci.* **2012**, *57*, 1618–1623. [CrossRef] [PubMed]
103. De Felice, K.M.; Katzka, D.A.; Raffals, L.E. Crohn's Disease of the Esophagus. *Inflamm. Bowel Dis.* **2015**, *21*, 2106–2113. [CrossRef] [PubMed]
104. Schwartzberg, D.M.; Brandstetter, S.; Grucela, A.L. Crohn's Disease of the Esophagus, Duodenum, and Stomach. *Clin. Colon Rectal Surg.* **2019**, *32*, 231–242. [CrossRef] [PubMed]
105. Muir, A.; Surrey, L.; Kriegermeier, A.; Shaikhkalil, A.; Piccoli, D.A. Severe Eosinophilic Gastroenteritis in a Crohn's Disease Patient Treated with Infliximab and Adalimumab. *Am. J. Gastroenterol.* **2016**, *111*, 437–438. [CrossRef] [PubMed]
106. Katsanos, K.H.; Zinovieva, E.; Lambri, E.; Tsianos, E.V. Eosinophilic-Crohn Overlap Colitis and Review of the Literature. *J. Crohns Colitis* **2011**, *5*, 256–261. [CrossRef] [PubMed]
107. Limketkai, B.N.; Shah, S.C.; Hirano, I.; Bellaguarda, E.; Colombel, J.-F. Epidemiology and Implications of Concurrent Diagnosis of Eosinophilic Oesophagitis and IBD Based on a Prospective Population-Based Analysis. *Gut* **2019**, *68*, 2152–2160. [CrossRef] [PubMed]

108. Splawski, J.; Aktay, A.N.; Perry, S.; Baez-Socorro, V.; DeLozier, S.; Sferra, T.J.; Moses, J. Differences in Clinical Presentation of Eosinophilic Esophagitis in Pediatric Patients with Ulcerative Colitis and Crohn Disease. *J. Pediatr. Gastroenterol. Nutr.* **2022**, *75*, 76–80. [CrossRef] [PubMed]
109. Romagnani, S. Th1/Th2 Cells. *Inflamm. Bowel Dis.* **1999**, *5*, 285–294. [CrossRef]
110. Lucendo, A.J.; Arias, Á.; Molina-Infante, J. Efficacy of Proton Pump Inhibitor Drugs for Inducing Clinical and Histologic Remission in Patients with Symptomatic Esophageal Eosinophilia: A Systematic Review and Meta-Analysis. *Clin. Gastroenterol. Hepatol.* **2016**, *14*, 13–22.e1. [CrossRef]
111. Tomizawa, Y.; Melek, J.; Komaki, Y.; Kavitt, R.T.; Sakuraba, A. Efficacy of Pharmacologic Therapy for Eosinophilic Esophagitis. *J. Clin. Gastroenterol.* **2018**, *52*, 596–606. [CrossRef] [PubMed]
112. Murali, A.R.; Gupta, A.; Attar, B.M.; Ravi, V.; Koduru, P. Topical Steroids in Eosinophilic Esophagitis: Systematic Review and Meta-analysis of Placebo-controlled Randomized Clinical Trials. *J. Gastroenterol. Hepatol.* **2016**, *31*, 1111–1119. [CrossRef]
113. Rank, M.A.; Sharaf, R.N.; Furuta, G.T.; Aceves, S.S.; Greenhawt, M.; Spergel, J.M.; Falck-Ytter, Y.T.; Dellon, E.S.; Chachu, K.A.; Day, L.; et al. Technical Review on the Management of Eosinophilic Esophagitis: A Report from the AGA Institute and the Joint Task Force on Allergy-Immunology Practice Parameters. *Gastroenterology* **2020**, *158*, 1789–1810.e15. [CrossRef]
114. Urquhart, S.A.; Quinn, K.P.; Ravi, K.; Loftus, E. V The Clinical Characteristics and Treatment Outcomes of Concomitant Eosinophilic Esophagitis and Inflammatory Bowel Disease. *Crohns Colitis 360* **2021**, *3*, otab018. [CrossRef] [PubMed]
115. Fan, Y.C.; Steele, D.; Kochar, B.; Arsene, D.; Long, M.D.; Dellon, E.S. Increased Prevalence of Esophageal Eosinophilia in Patients with Inflammatory Bowel Disease. *Inflamm. Intest. Dis.* **2018**, *3*, 180–186. [CrossRef] [PubMed]
116. Mintz, M.J.; Ananthakrishnan, A.N. Phenotype and Natural History of Inflammatory Bowel Disease in Patients with Concomitant Eosinophilic Esophagitis. *Inflamm. Bowel Dis.* **2021**, *27*, 469–475. [CrossRef]
117. Malik, A.; Liu, B.D.; Zhu, L.; Kaelber, D.; Song, G. A Comprehensive Global Population-Based Analysis on the Coexistence of Eosinophilic Esophagitis and Inflammatory Bowel Disease. *Dig. Dis. Sci.* **2024**, *69*, 892–900. [CrossRef]
118. Aloi, M.; D'Arcangelo, G.; Rossetti, D.; Bucherini, S.; Felici, E.; Romano, C.; Martinelli, M.; Dipasquale, V.; Lionetti, P.; Oliva, S. Occurrence and Clinical Impact of Eosinophilic Esophagitis in a Large Cohort of Children with Inflammatory Bowel Disease. *Inflamm. Bowel Dis.* **2023**, *29*, 1057–1064. [CrossRef]
119. Straumann, A.; Bussmann, C.; Conus, S.; Beglinger, C.; Simon, H.-U. Anti–TNF-α (Infliximab) Therapy for Severe Adult Eosinophilic Esophagitis. *J. Allergy Clin. Immunol.* **2008**, *122*, 425–427. [CrossRef]
120. Goyal, A. Recent Discoveries and Emerging Therapeutics in Eosinophilic Esophagitis. *World J. Gastrointest. Pharmacol. Ther.* **2016**, *7*, 21. [CrossRef]
121. Fu, Y.; Choi, D.; Ronen, N.; Dalal, S. Successful Treatment of Eosinophilic Enterocolitis in an Adult Patient with Adalimumab. *ACG Case Rep. J.* **2024**, *11*, e01285. [CrossRef] [PubMed]
122. Turner, D.; Wolters, V.M.; Russell, R.K.; Shakhnovich, V.; Muise, A.M.; Ledder, O.; Ngan, B.; Friesen, C. Anti-TNF, Infliximab, and Adalimumab Can Be Effective in Eosinophilic Bowel Disease. *J. Pediatr. Gastroenterol. Nutr.* **2013**, *56*, 492–497. [CrossRef] [PubMed]
123. Moore, H.; Wechsler, J.; Frost, C.; Whiteside, E.; Baldassano, R.; Markowitz, J.; Muir, A.B. Comorbid Diagnosis of Eosinophilic Esophagitis and Inflammatory Bowel Disease in the Pediatric Population. *J. Pediatr. Gastroenterol. Nutr.* **2021**, *72*, 398–403. [CrossRef] [PubMed]
124. Mulder, D.J.; Noble, A.J.; Justinich, C.J.; Duffin, J.M. A Tale of Two Diseases: The History of Inflammatory Bowel Disease. *J. Crohns Colitis* **2014**, *8*, 341–348. [CrossRef] [PubMed]
125. Grandinetti, T.; Biedermann, L.; Bussmann, C.; Straumann, A.; Hruz, P. Eosinophilic Gastroenteritis: Clinical Manifestation, Natural Course, and Evaluation of Treatment with Corticosteroids and Vedolizumab. *Dig. Dis. Sci.* **2019**, *64*, 2231–2241. [CrossRef] [PubMed]
126. Kim, H.P.; Reed, C.C.; Herfarth, H.H.; Dellon, E.S. Vedolizumab Treatment May Reduce Steroid Burden and Improve Histology in Patients with Eosinophilic Gastroenteritis. *Clin. Gastroenterol. Hepatol.* **2018**, *16*, 1992–1994. [CrossRef] [PubMed]
127. Gabriëls, R.Y.; Bourgonje, A.R.; von Martels, J.Z.H.; Blokzijl, T.; Weersma, R.K.; Galinsky, K.; Juarez, J.; Faber, K.N.; Kats-Ugurlu, G.; Dijkstra, G. Mucosal Eosinophil Abundance in Non-Inflamed Colonic Tissue Is Associated with Response to Vedolizumab Induction Therapy in Inflammatory Bowel Disease. *J. Clin. Med.* **2022**, *11*, 4141. [CrossRef] [PubMed]
128. Kim, E.M.; Randall, C.; Betancourt, R.; Keene, S.; Lilly, A.; Fowler, M.; Dellon, E.S.; Herfarth, H.H. Mucosal Eosinophilia Is an Independent Predictor of Vedolizumab Efficacy in Inflammatory Bowel Diseases. *Inflamm. Bowel Dis.* **2020**, *26*, 1232–1238. [CrossRef]
129. Molina-Infante, J.; Schoepfer, A.M.; Lucendo, A.J.; Dellon, E.S. Eosinophilic Esophagitis: What Can We Learn from Crohn's Disease? *Eur. Gastroenterol. J.* **2017**, *5*, 762–772. [CrossRef]
130. Spencer, E.A.; Dolinger, M.T.; Dubinsky, M.C. A Single-Center Experience with Dupilumab for Atopic or Psoriasiform Dermatitis in Patients with Inflammatory Bowel Disease. *Dig. Dis. Sci.* **2023**, *68*, 1121–1124. [CrossRef]
131. Hren, M.G.; Guenin, S.; Khattri, S. Use of Dual Biologic Therapy Targeting the Th2 and Th17 Axes Simultaneously to Treat Patients with Atopic Dermatitis and Concomitant Psoriasis, Psoriatic Arthritis, or Inflammatory Bowel Disease. *J. Am. Acad. Dermatol.* **2024**, *91*, 138–140. [CrossRef] [PubMed]

132. A Study to Investigate the Efficacy and Safety of Dupilumab Therapy Compared with Placebo in Participants Aged ≥ 18 Years with Moderately to Severely Active Ulcerative Colitis with an Eosinophilic Phenotype (LIBERTY-UC SUCCEED (Study in UC for Clinical Efficacy Evaluation of Dupilumab)). Available online: https://clinicaltrials.gov/study/NCT05731128 (accessed on 11 July 2024).
133. Alegre-Bailo, A.; Sánchez-Gilo, A.; Gonzalo González, I.; Vicente Martín, F.J. Combination Treatment with Monoclonal Antibodies: Dupilumab and Ustekinumab for the Treatment of Severe Atopic Dermatitis and Crohn Disease. *Australas. J. Dermatol.* **2024**, *65*, 63–66. [CrossRef] [PubMed]

Journal of
Clinical Medicine

MDPI

Review

Crohn's Disease: Radiological Answers to Clinical Questions and Review of the Literature

Laura Maria Minordi [1,*], Francesca Bice D'Angelo [1], Giuseppe Privitera [2], Alfredo Papa [3], Luigi Larosa [1], Lucrezia Laterza [4,5], Franco Scaldaferri [4], Brunella Barbaro [1], Luigi Carbone [6] and Daniela Pugliese [4,5,7]

1 UOC di Radiologia Addomino-Pelvica, Dipartimento di Diagnostica per Immagini, Radioterapia Oncologica ed Ematologia, Fondazione Policlinico Universitario "A. Gemelli" Istituto di Ricovero e Cura a Carattere Scientifico (IRCCS), Largo Francesco Vito, 1, 00168 Roma, Italy; francescabice.dangelo01@icatt.it (F.B.D.); brunella.barbaro@policlinicogemelli.it (B.B.)
2 Dipartimento di Scienze della Salute, Università degli Studi di Milano, 20122 Milan, Italy; gpp.privitera@icloud.com
3 Unità Operativa Semplice Dipartimentale Day Hospital (UOSD DH) Medicina Interna e Malattie dell'Apparato Digerente, Fondazione Policlinico Universitario "A. Gemelli" Istituto di Ricovero e Cura a Carattere Scientifico (IRCCS), Università Cattolica del Sacro Cuore, 00168 Roma, Italy; alfredo.papa@unicatt.it
4 CEMAD Digestive Disease Center, Fondazione Policlinico Universitario "A. Gemelli" Istituto di Ricovero e Cura a Carattere Scientifico (IRCCS), Catholic University of Rome, 00168 Rome, Italy; lucrezia.laterza@policlinicogemelli.it (L.L.); franco.scaldaferri@policlinicogemelli.it (F.S.); daniela.pugliese@policlinicogemelli.it (D.P.)
5 Dipartimento di Medicina e Chirurgia Traslazionale, Università Cattolica del Sacro Cuore, L. Go A. Gemelli 8, 00168 Rome, Italy
6 UOC Pronto Soccorso, Medicina d'Urgenza e Medicina Interna, Ospedale Isola Tiberina Gemelli Isola, 00186 Rome, Italy; luigi.carbone@policlinicogemelli.it
7 UOS Gastroenterologia, Ospedale Isola Tiberina Gemelli Isola, 00186 Rome, Italy
* Correspondence: lauramaria.minordi@policlinicogemelli.it

Abstract: Background: Crohn's disease (CD) is a chronic, progressive inflammatory condition, involving primarily the bowel, characterized by a typical remitting–relapsing pattern. Despite endoscopy representing the reference standard for the diagnosis and assessment of disease activity, radiological imaging has a key role, providing information about mural and extra-visceral involvement. **Methods:** Computed Tomography and Magnetic Resonance Imaging are the most frequently used radiological techniques in clinical practice for both the diagnosis and staging of CD involving the small bowel in non-urgent settings. The contribution of imaging in the management of CD is reported on by answering the following practical questions: (1) What is the best technique for the assessment of small bowel CD? (2) Is imaging a good option to assess colonic disease? (3) Which disease pattern is present: inflammatory, fibrotic or fistulizing? (4) Is it possible to identify the presence of strictures and to discriminate inflammatory from fibrotic ones? (5) How does imaging help in defining disease extension and localization? (6) Can imaging assess disease activity? (7) Is it possible to evaluate post-operative recurrence? **Results:** Imaging is suitable for assessing disease activity, extension and characterizing disease patterns. CT and MRI can both answer the abovementioned questions, but MRI has a greater sensitivity and specificity for assessing disease activity and does not use ionizing radiation. **Conclusions:** Radiologists are essential healthcare professionals to be involved in multidisciplinary teams for the management of CD patients to obtain the necessary answers for clinically relevant questions.

Keywords: inflammatory bowel disease; Crohn's disease; Computed Tomography; Magnetic Resonance Imaging

1. Introduction

Inflammatory bowel diseases (IBDs) are chronic, progressive inflammatory diseases, involving primarily the bowel, characterized by a typical remitting-relapsing pattern. The aetiology is unknown, but the most accredited hypothesis is that environmental factors induce in genetically predisposed hosts an alteration of intestinal microbiota, gut epithelial barrier leaks and a subsequent dysregulation of the gut immune response, thus being responsible for bowel damage [1].

The incidence of IBD is quite stable in western countries, but the prevalence is progressively growing due to the low rate of disease-related mortality (stage of compounding prevalence) [2]. IBD is commonly diagnosed at a young age, with a peak of incidence between 18 and 35 years, even though it is not rare a diagnosis among paediatric and elderly populations.

Two main forms are recognized: Crohn's disease (CD), potentially affecting all gastrointestinal tracts and characterized by a transmural inflammation, and ulcerative colitis (UC), involving only the colon at the mucosa layer. If bloody diarrhoea represents the typical symptom of UC, the spectrum of clinical manifestations for CD can be quite variable. The evolution of chronic inflammation can progressively lead to the development of complications in both conditions, such as stenosis or fistulas for CD, and luminal narrowing or colorectal cancer for UC [3,4]. Endoscopy is the reference standard for the diagnosis and assessment of disease activity in both diseases, but imaging has a key role as well, providing information about parietal and extra-visceral involvement. In particular, imaging is useful for the diagnosing and staging of small bowel CD, while its role in UC is limited to the presence of complications or in cases of acute severe presentation [5].

In this setting, a strict collaboration between radiologists and gastroenterologists/surgeons is required to improve imaging performance, and radiologists are asked to answer specific clinical questions. The aim of this paper was to describe the contribution of imaging in the management of CD by answering to seven practical clinical and/or surgical questions.

2. Methods

2.1. Questions

We established 7 practical and clinically relevant questions which we tried to provide answers to, in detail:

(1) What is the best technique for the assessment of small bowel CD? (2) Is imaging a good option to assess colonic disease? (3) Which disease pattern is present; inflammatory, fibrotic or fistulizing? (4) Is it possible to identify the presence of strictures and to discriminate inflammatory from fibrotic ones? (5) How does imaging help defining disease extension and localization? (6) Can imaging assess disease activity? (7) Is it possible to evaluate post-operative recurrence?

2.2. Search on Medline Electronic Database

Accordingly, we conducted a comprehensive electronic search on the Medline electronic database through January 2024 with no language restrictions using the following search terms: ("IBD") OR ("Crohn's Disease (CD)") AND ("imaging") or ("radiology") or ("Computed Tomography") or ("Magnetic Resonance"). Two independent reviewers (LMM and LL) independently evaluated the title and abstract of studies identified in the primary search and then the full text of selected articles. Papers were selected based on their capability to provide evidence relevant to our pre-specified questions.

3. What Is the Best Technique for the Assessment of Small Bowel CD?

Computed Tomography (CT) and Magnetic Resonance Imaging (MRI) are the most frequently used radiological techniques in clinical practice for both the diagnosis and the staging of CD involving the small bowel in non-urgent settings. However, for patients presenting to the emergency room for acute abdominal pain, potentially related to an intestinal obstruction or sepsis, an abdominal CT scan with iv contrast medium and without distension of the intestinal loops is recommended [6,7]. The CT and the MRI must be performed with a rigorous technique: in particular, it is essential to have optimal distention of the intestinal loops. Accordingly, they are both performed with the administration of a contrast medium by mouth (MR-enterography, MR-E; CT-enterography, CT-E) or by naso-jejunal tube (MR-enteroclysis, MR-e; CT-enteroclysis, CT-e). The administration of the contrast medium through a naso-jejunal tube allows to obtain a better distension of the jejunum, which is often collapsed during image acquisition when the medium is administered orally [8–11] (Figure 1).

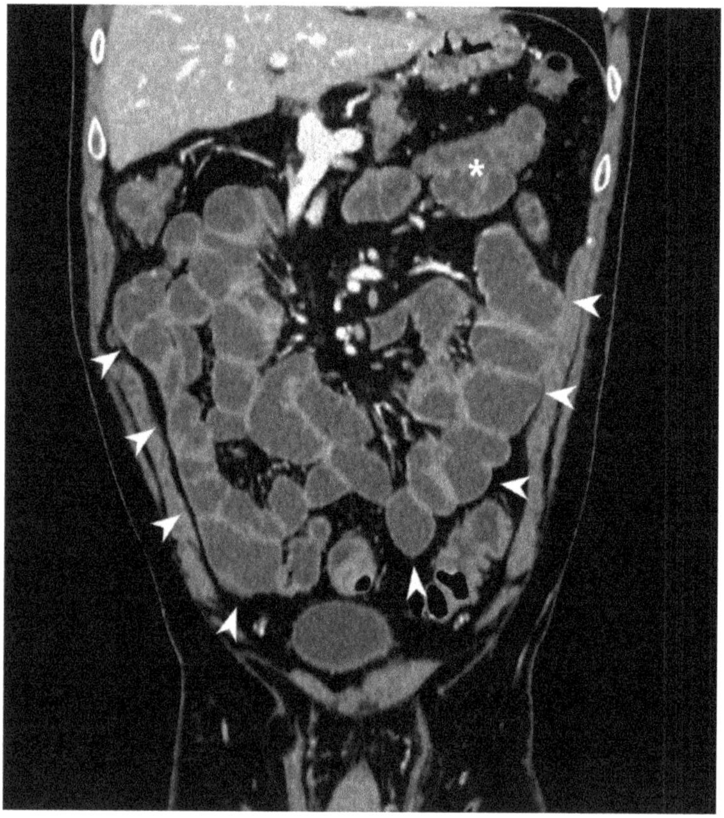

Figure 1. Coronal CT-E image after iodinated contrast medium injection: example of optimal distention of the ileal loops obtained by oral administration contrast medium (arrowheads); jejunal loops are on the top left (white asterisk). Original figures by LMM and LL.

Despite these differences in the distention of the intestinal loops, both methods of contrast administration have shown similar diagnostic accuracy for the diagnosis of CD and its complications, but patients' discomfort can be considerably higher using CT/MR-e. The values of diagnostic imaging's accuracy range from 95% to 100% for MR-e and from 72% to 98% for MR-E [12–16].

Accordingly, CT/MR-E are the most frequently used radiological techniques in clinical practice [12]. Many contrast agents are used to distend the intestine in both CT-E and MR-E, such as polyethylene glycol solution (PEG), oil emulsions, water, air, Mucofalk®, dilute barium sulphate, mannitol, sorbitol, and locust bean gum (Table 1); PEG is one of most commonly administered, due to its low cost and few side effects.

The loops can be considered adequately distended when good distension of the lumen and clear visualization of the small bowel wall are obtained; the distension can be classified into five degrees: 1, collapse; 2, distension less than 50% of the adequately distended segment; 3, distension > 50% but <80%; 4, distension in the 80–100% range; and 5, optimal distension. Use of antimotility drugs helps to reduce bowel movements that can mimic a wall thickening. These contrast agents make the lumen hypodense in CT and allow a better visualization of the small bowel internal wall and the degree of enhancement after intravenous injection of the iodinated contrast medium (Figure 2).

Table 1. Types of oral contrast agents and their advantages and disadvantages.

Oral Contrast Agents	Advantages	Disadvantage
Water	Well tolerated, biphasic properties in MRI	Rapid absorption
PEG	Better distension than water and MC	The least tolerated of all agents due to diarrhoea
MC	Better tolerated than PEG	Lower distension than PEG and dilute barium sulphate
dilute barium sulphate	Good distension	Mild side effects (gas and diarrhoea)
Oil emulsions	Grater viscosity than water	Little tolerated

PEG, polyethylene glycol solution; MC, methylcellulose.

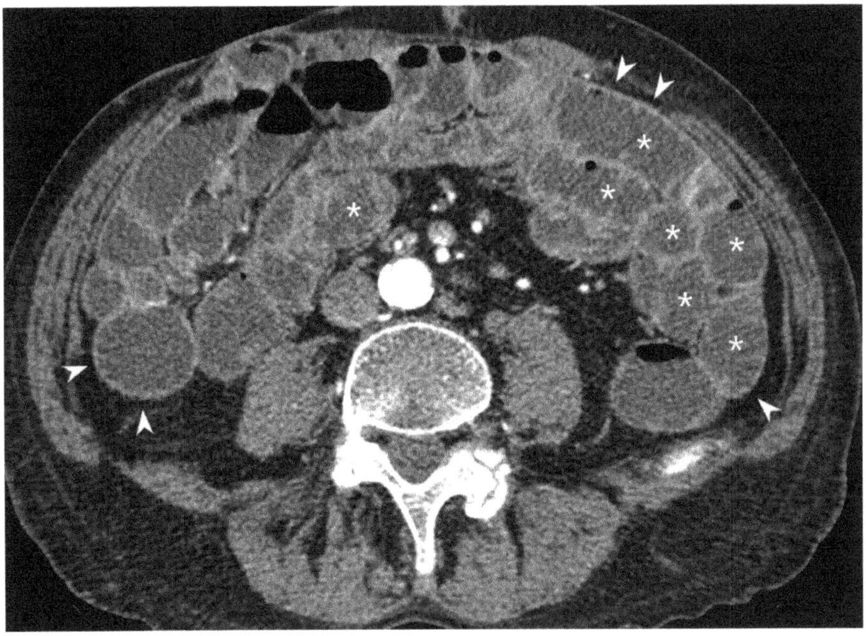

Figure 2. Axial CT-E image after iodinated contrast medium injection: example of intestinal loops' distension by a hypodense contrast medium (polyethylene glycol solution), showing the hypodensity of the jejunal lumen (asterisks) and the hyperdensity of the intestinal wall (arrowheads). Original figures by LMM and LL.

Conversely, in MRI, the appearance depends on the specific sequences of acquisition: on T2-weighted images, the intestinal lumen is hyperintense, while T1-weighted sequences after injection of gadolinium contrast medium allow to visualize the degree of enhancement of the bowel wall, thanks to the contrast between the dark bowel lumen and the hyperintense intestinal walls (Figure 3).

In CT, even if the hyperdense contrast medium (1–2% barium sulphate suspension or a 2–3% water-soluble iodinated solution) hides the normal intestinal wall and the characteristics of its enhancement, it can be used in patients with suspected intestinal perforation or fistulizing disease, as it allows better visualization of contrast medium extravasation and the fistulas (Figure 4) [17–19].

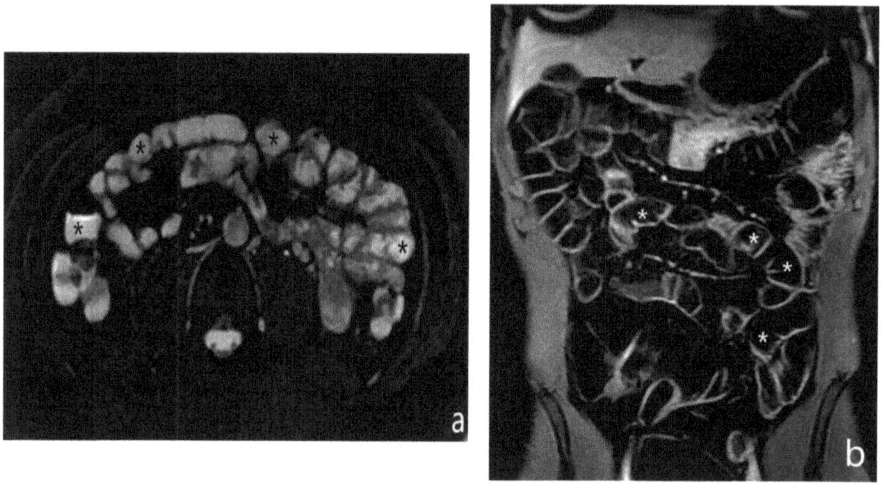

Figure 3. MR-E: example of intestinal loops' distention by biphasic contrast medium (polyethylene glycol solution). Intestinal lumen (asterisks) is hyperintense in T2-weighted axial image (**a**) and hypointense in T1-weighted coronal image after gadolinium injection (**b**). Original figures by LMM and LL.

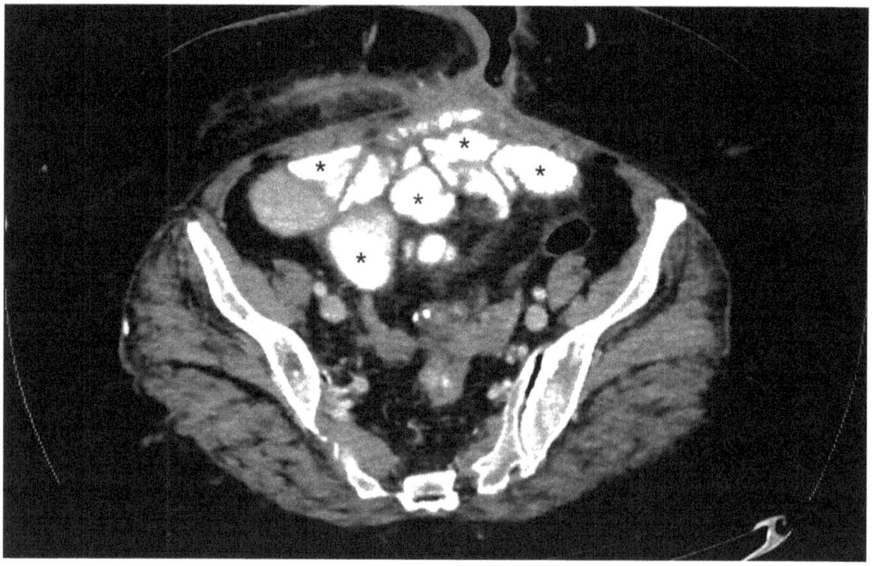

Figure 4. CT-E axial image: example of intestinal distension by oral administration of hydrosoluble iodine contrast medium in patient who has undergone intestinal resection with suspected post-surgical fistula. The image shows the hyperdense appearance of the ileal lumen (asterisks). Original figures by LMM and LL.

CT-E is still the most widely used technique; however, whenever possible, MR-E should be preferred due to the absence of ionizing radiation and the greater contrast resolution, which allows for a better visualization of the intestinal wall and its fibrotic and/or inflammatory alterations [20,21]. In fact, during their lifetime, almost 10% of patients affected by CD are exposed to a potentially harmful quantity of radiation, established as ≥50 milli-sieverts (mSv) (corresponding to five CT abdomen examinations) [22]. However, radiation exposure may significantly differ from one model of CT to another; for example, a multidetector-CT allows a reduction of radiation exposure up to 10–60%, thanks to effective detector conformation, image postprocessing algorithms, better filters, and automatic exposure controls [23]. Moreover, several techniques have been developed to reduce the radiation dose, such as moderation of exposure time, voltage, amperage, the use of noise-reduction filters and/or of concentrated oral contrast (Telebrix 9% instead of the commonly used 3% concentration) and of high noise index (MBCT—modified small bowel CT), and the absence of the administration of intravenous (iv) contrast [24]. These low-dose techniques can provide precise and useful diagnostic information, despite resulting in lower quality images [25].

4. Is Imaging a Good Option to Assess Colonic Disease?

CT-E and MR-E are usually performed for the evaluation of the small intestine, while endoscopy is preferred when it comes to colonic disease. Even though colonic distention is not routinely recommended, in specific clinical situations—such as the presence of colonic strictures—it could be helpful [26]. Bowel distension can be performed at the end of CT/MR-enterography, using air (colonography-CT) (Figure 5) or water (CT/MR-enterography with water enema or Hydro-CT/MRI) (Figure 6).

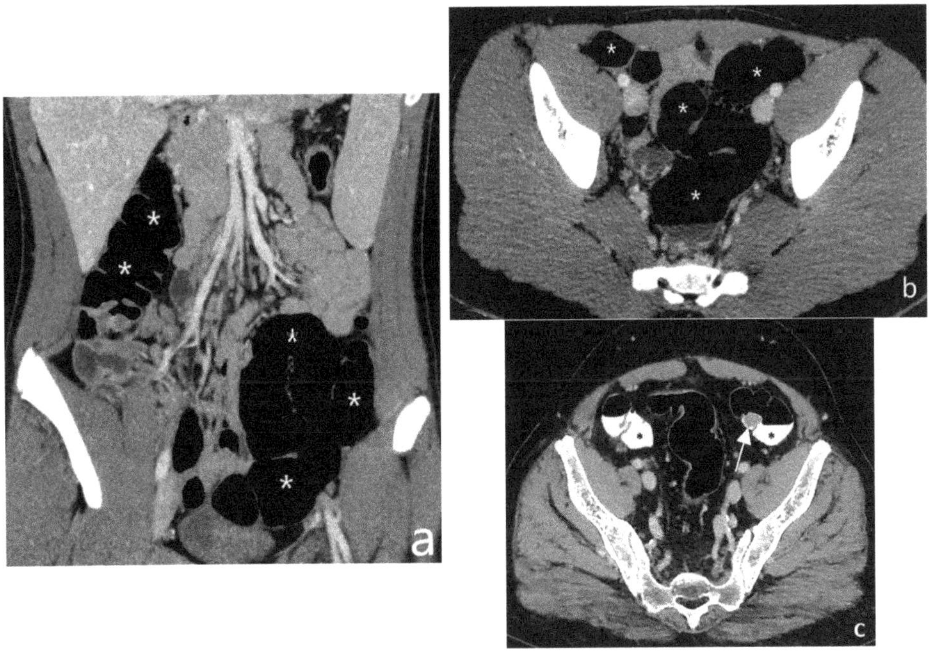

Figure 5. CT after iodinated contrast injection: example of colon distension using air by endorectal insufflation in the coronal (**a**) and axial (**b**) planes (asterisks). (**c**) Another example of colonic distension using air by endorectal insufflation in the axial plane shows a polypoid thickening of the sigmoid colon (arrow); hyperdense contrast agent for faecal tagging is also evident in the lumen (black asterisks). Original figures by LMM, LL and BB.

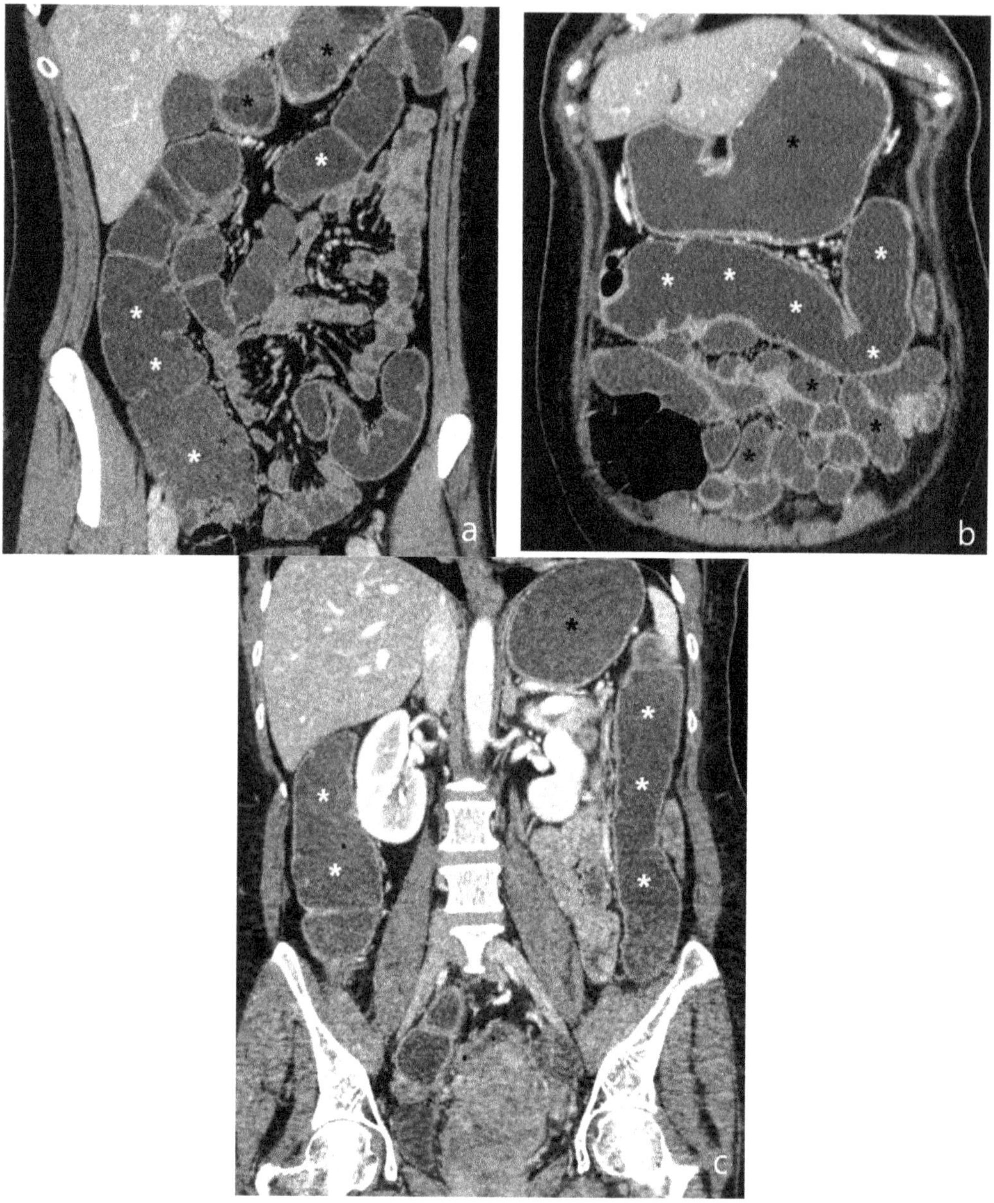

Figure 6. Hydro-CT. Coronal (**a**–**c**) images show good distension of the colon obtained by both endorectal (white asterisks) and oral (black asterisks) administration of water and hypodense contrast medium (polyethylene glycol solution). Original figures by LMM and LL.

Some studies have shown that the distention of the colon through the rectum improves the visualization of the ileo-caecal region in CT-E, thereby increasing the diagnostic accuracy of the exam, although the patient's discomfort can be considerably higher. Diagnostic accuracy values with and without colonic distension were, respectively, 92% and 81% [27]. Similar findings also emerged for MR-E, since an additional rectal enema seems to increase the confidence of radiologists in the diagnosis of bowel disease, either located in the colon or in the ileocecal region [28].

Finally, a study performed in CD patients and healthy volunteers showed that performing a synchronous colonography and MR-E guaranteed a good distension of the jejunum in around 80% and of the terminal ileum in >94% of patients in both groups [29].

5. Which Disease Pattern Is Present: Inflammatory, Fibrotic or Fistulizing?

From a radiological point of view, CD patterns can be classified into three categories: active with predominant inflammatory signs, fibro-stenotic and fistulizing/penetrating [30]. This distinction is crucial because it can influence the therapeutic approach, specifically in the choice between medical and surgical treatment.

5.1. Active Subtype

In the active subtype, the typical MR/CT-E findings are the presence of bowel thickening, oedema, mucosal ulcers, segmental parietal hyperenhancement and/or stratified contrast enhancement (CE) after the administration of iv contrast [31,32].

Thickening of the intestinal wall, measured after the distension of the loop by oral contrast medium, is considered one of the most important signs of active disease and it is found in 82% of patients with CD. The normal intestinal wall appears on CT/MR-E as a hyperdense/hyperintense line with a thickness of less than 3 mm. In the case of wall thickening, it needs to be measured at the point of greatest thickness [33]. The thickening is considered minimal if between 3 and 5 mm, moderate between 6 and 9 mm, and marked if equal to or greater than 10 mm. Some studies have shown that the degree of wall thickening correlates with disease activity: thresholds of 6 mm and 10 mm have been proposed to discriminate between mild and moderate activity, and between moderate and severe activity, respectively [28,29].

In MR-E, intestinal wall oedema is detected on T2-weighted sequences and appears as a mural hyperintense signal (compared to the signal of the skeletal muscle), more evident in fat-saturation sequences [34,35]; conversely, in CT-E, wall oedema appears as a hypodense layer of the intestinal wall, after the administration of iodinated contrast medium. Stratified CE is present when mural thickening shows a marked enhancement of the inner and outer layers (i.e., the mucosa, and the muscle layer and serosa), as a consequence of hyperaemia, while the intermediate layer (i.e., the submucosa) appears hypointense/hypodense, respectively, in CT/MR-E, due to oedema. Mucosal ulcers are usually seen in the presence of more severe inflammation, and they appear as mucosal irregularities on T2 sequences in MR-E. Finally, another frequent sign of activity is the engorgement of vasa recta, related to the hyperaemia of the near mesentery, manifesting as mesenteric arterial dilation, tortuosity, prominence and wide spacing [31]. Examples of active CD are shown in Figures 7–9.

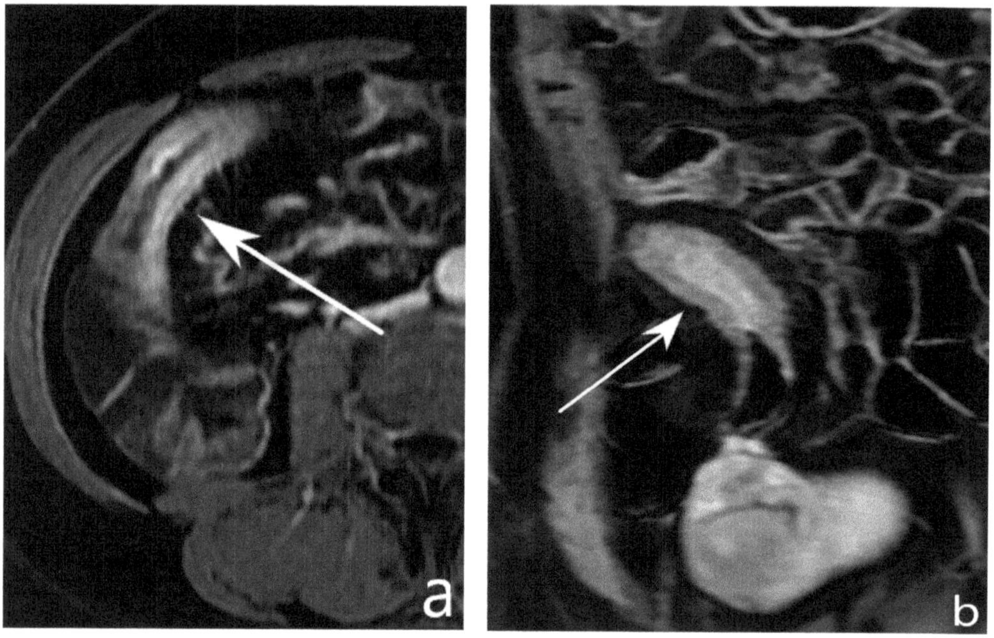

Figure 7. Assessment of disease activity. MR-E after gadolinium injection and administration of polyethylene glycol solution: axial (**a**) and coronal (**b**) images show pathological thickening of the distal ileum (arrow) with hyperintensity of the inner layer (mucosa) referred to hyperaemia, hypointensity of the intermediate layer (submucosa) referred to oedema, and hyperintensity of outer layer (serosa) referred to hyperaemia. Original figures by LMM and LL.

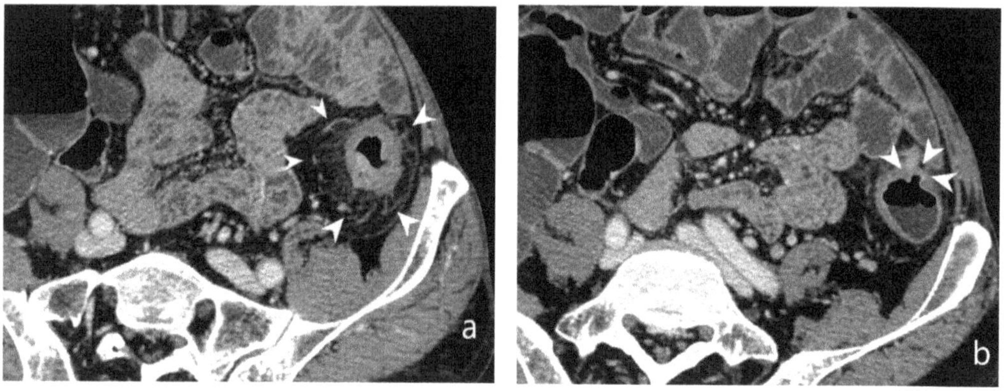

Figure 8. Assessment of disease activity. Axial CT-E after iodinated contrast injection and administration of polyethylene glycol solution (**a**,**b**) shows thickening of the descending colon with perivisceral fat stranding surrounding the pathological segment (white arrowheads in (**a**)). A bowel wall ulcer is also evident in another plane (white arrowheads in (**b**)). Original figures by LMM and LL.

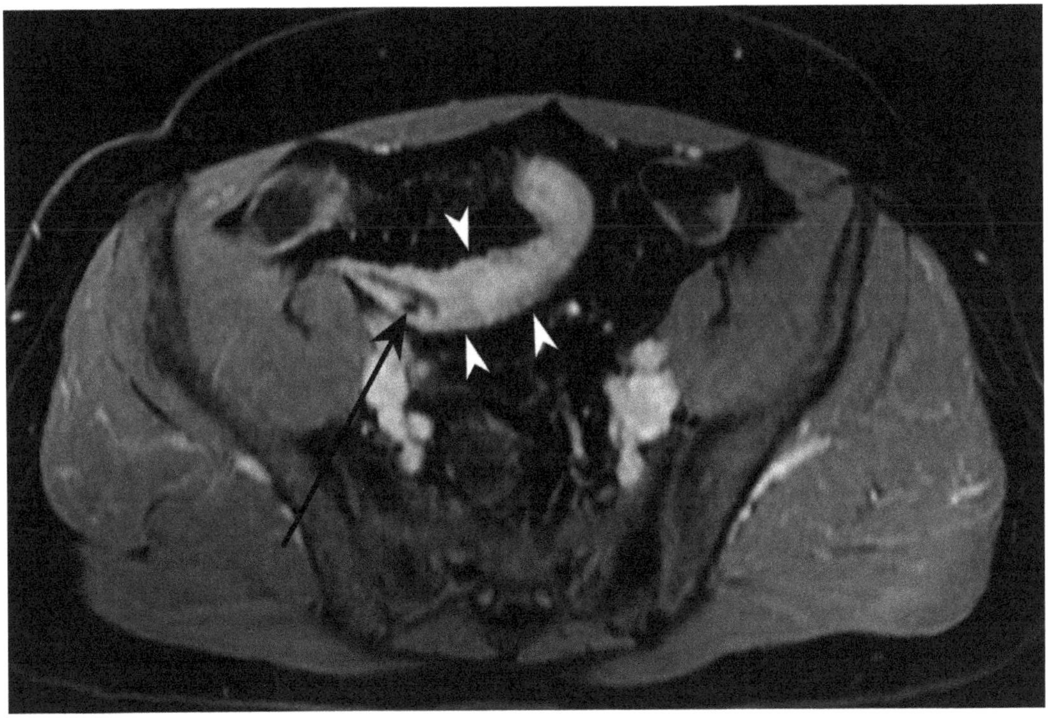

Figure 9. Assessment of disease activity. Axial MR-E after gadolinium injection image and administration of polyethylene glycol solution shows ileal thickening with stratified contrast enhancement (white arrows); a «minus» spot is present in the intestinal wall, indicative of deep parietal ulcer (black arrow). Original figures by LMM and LL.

5.2. Fibro-Stenotic Subtype

In this subtype, mural thickening is usually minimal (3–5 mm), without oedema of the bowel wall, with a homogenous, non-stratified CE after iv contrast medium administration. On MR-E, the intestinal wall shows a hypointense signal on T2-weighted sequences. In the case of stenosis, a pre-stenotic dilatation can be associated, ranging from minimal (3–4 cm) to severe (>4 cm) [33,36].

An example of fibro-stenotic disease is shown in Figure 10.

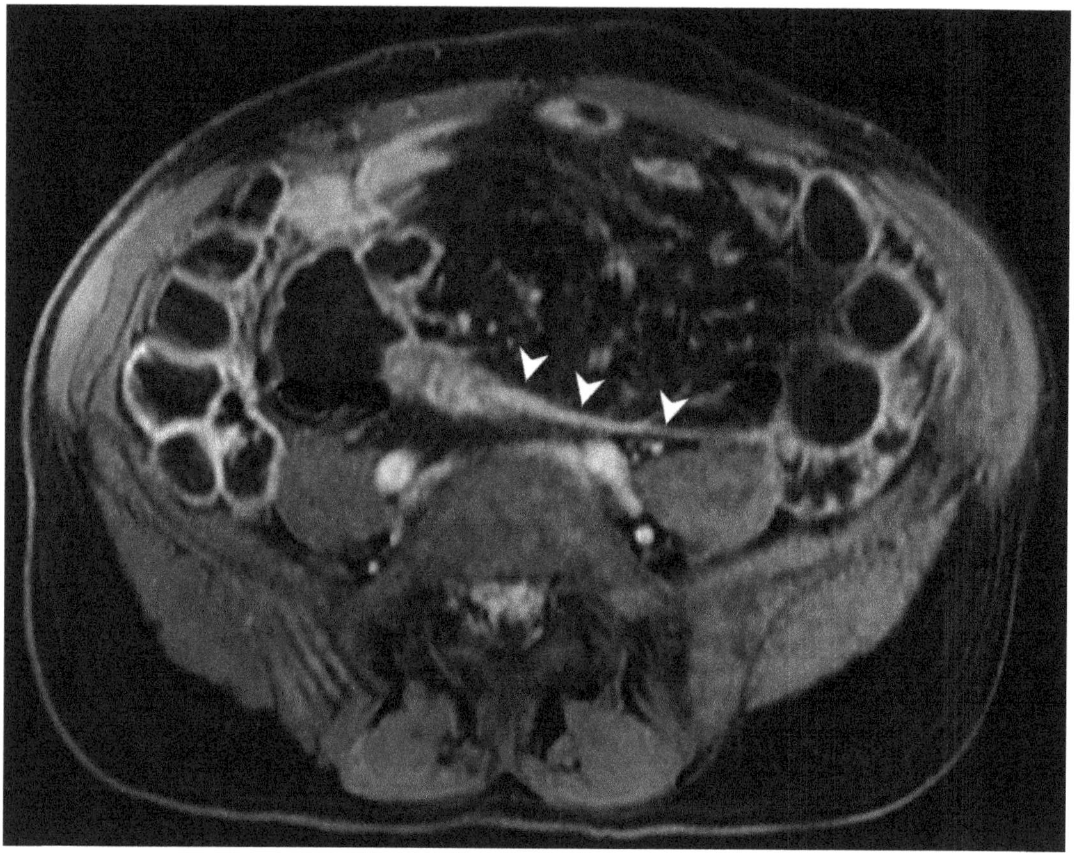

Figure 10. Fibro-stenotic subtype. MR-E after gadolinium injection and administration of polyethylene glycol solution, axial image shows fibrotic ileal loop with a stretched appearance (white arrowheads). Original figures by LMM and LL.

5.3. Fistulising/Perforating Subtype

This subtype is characterized by the presence of sinus tracts, fistulas and/or inflammatory masses. Sinus tracts are blind-ending tracts that develop when inflammation extends across the serosa layer. When a communication with another structure is established, the sinus tract generates a fistula. In radiological reports, a fistula is reported by describing the bowel loop of origin and the structure to which is connected (e.g., entero-enteric, entero-colic, entero-cutaneous or entero-vesical fistulas) (Figures 11–13).

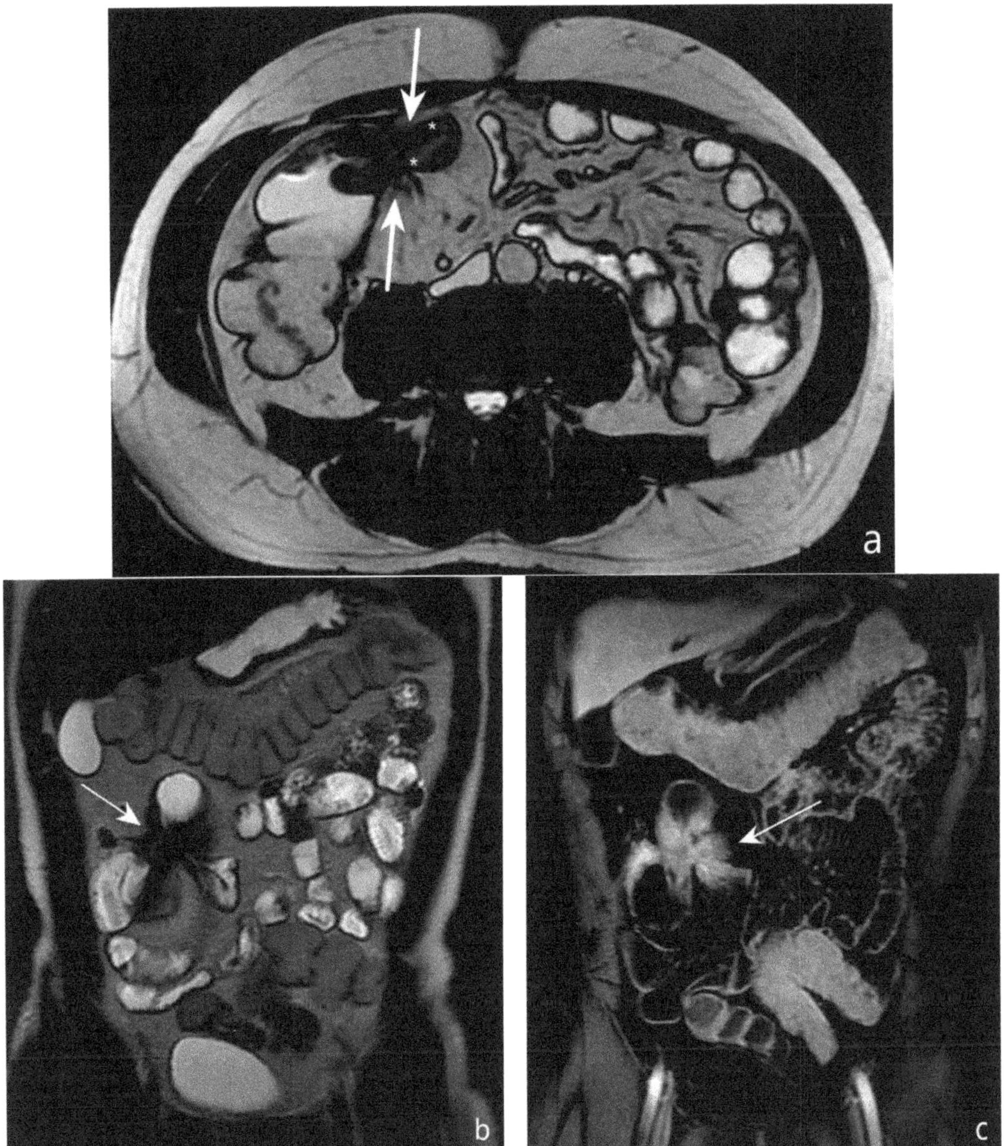

Figure 11. Fistulizing disease. MR-E after administration of polyethylene glycol solution; the T2-weighted axial image (**a**), T2-weighted coronal image (**b**) and contrast-enhanced fat-sat T1-weighted coronal image (**c**) show an ileo-ileal fistula in the distal ileum (arrows); focal fatty depositions in the submucosal layer are evident in a (asterisks). Original figures by LMM and LL.

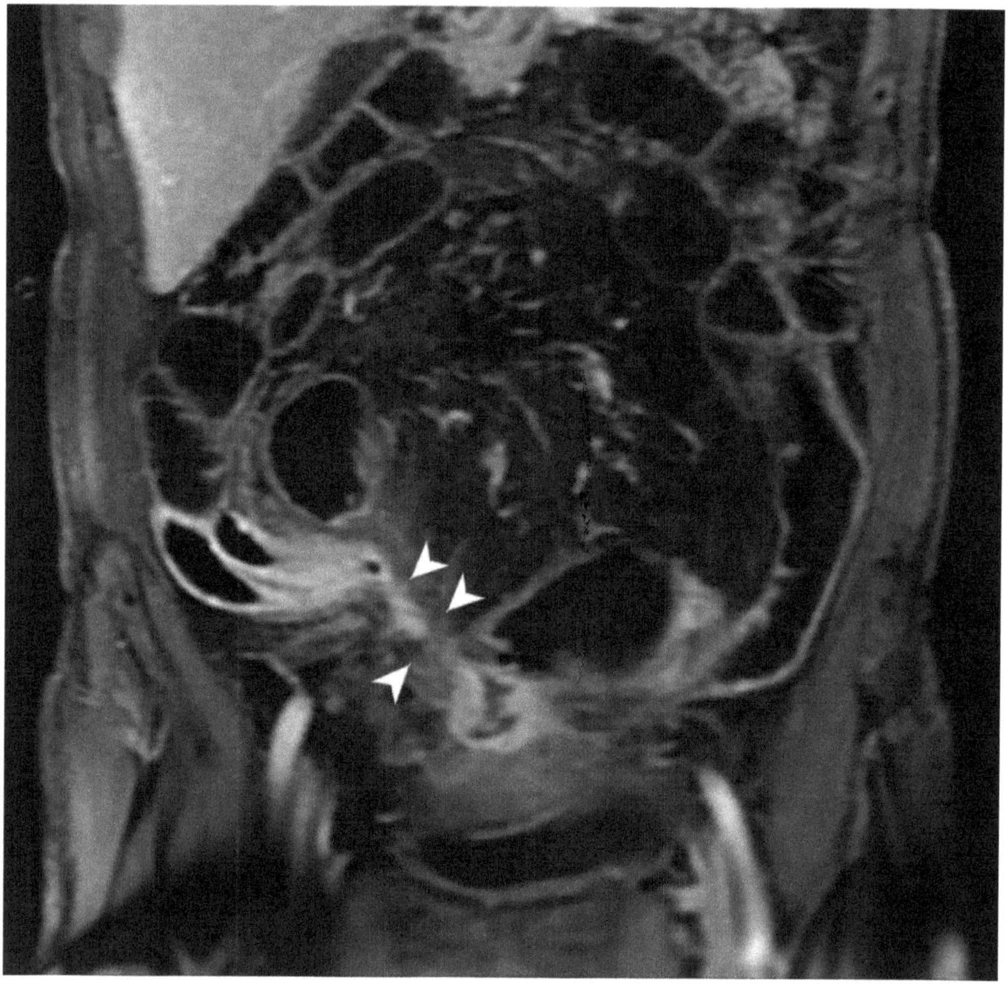

Figure 12. Fistulizing disease. MR-E after gadolinium injection and administration of polyethylene glycol solution, coronal image shows pathological intestinal loops in hypogastrium-right iliac fossa, with entero-enteric fistulas (white arrowheads). Original figures by LMM and LL.

Furthermore, a consequence of fistulising disease can be the formation of an abscess, appearing as a fluid collection delimitated by an enhanced wall and, in some cases, containing air (Figures 14–16). The accuracy of CT and MR for the detection of fistulas is similar [36].

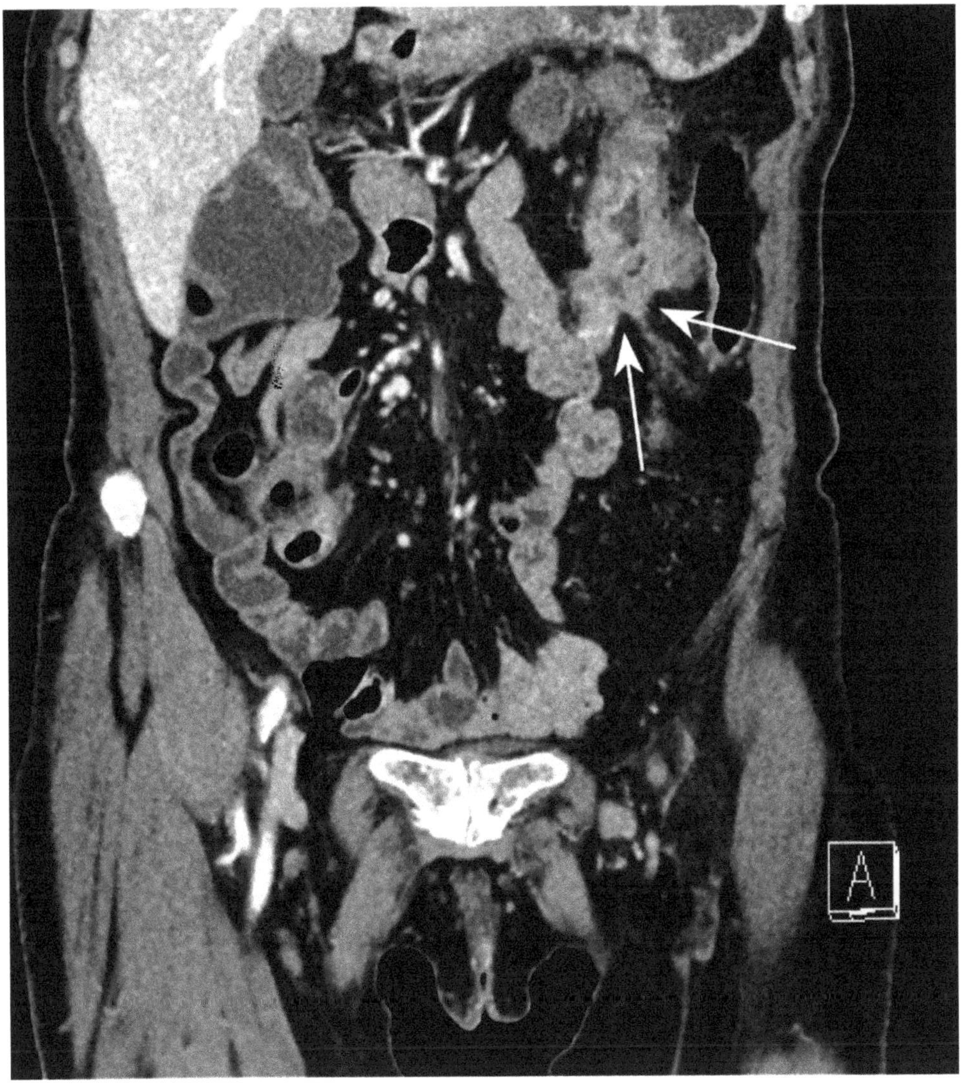

Figure 13. Entero-enteric fistula: CT-E coronal image after iodinated contrast injection and administration of polyethylene glycol solution shows entero-enteric fistula between the descending colon and an adjacent ileal loop (arrows). Letter "A" indicates the coronal view of the CT-E image. Original figures by LMM and LL.

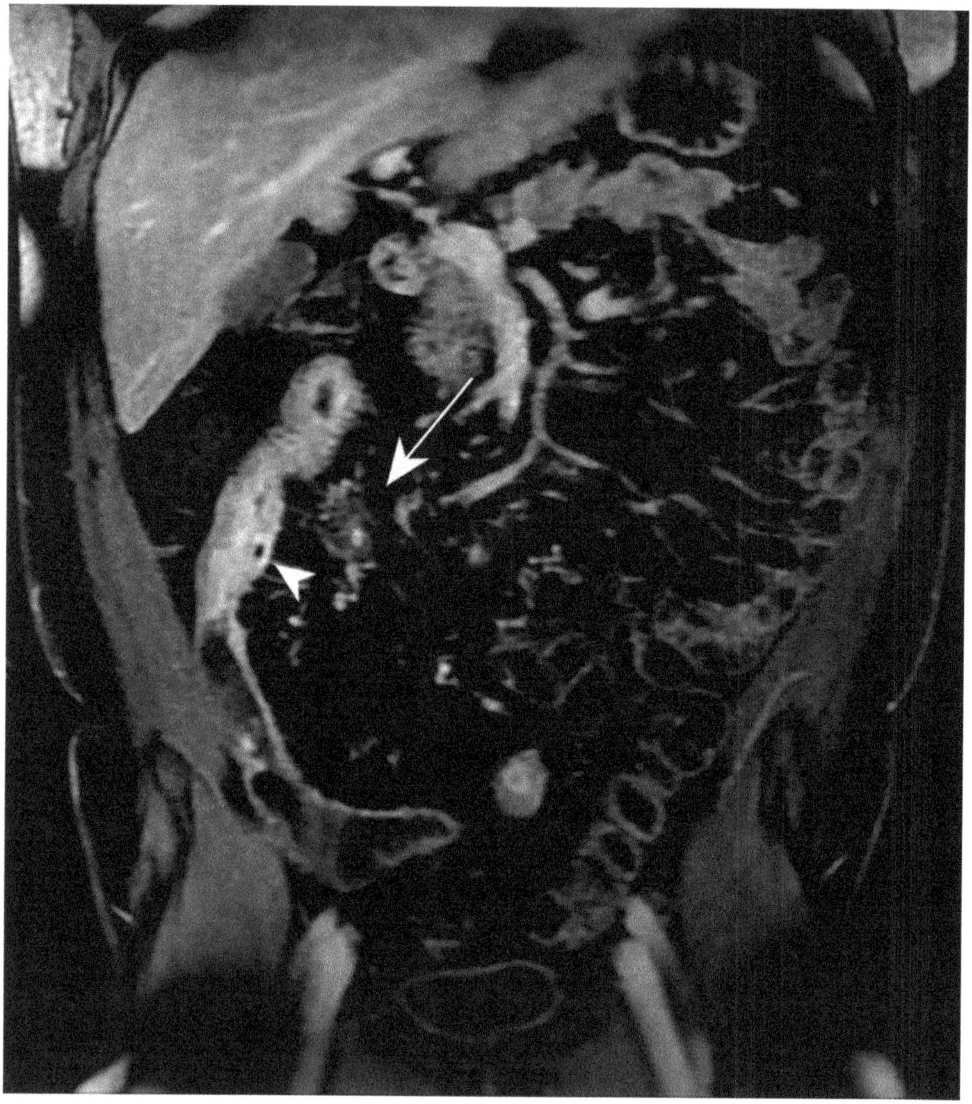

Figure 14. Intraparietal abscess and mesenteric inflammation. MR-E after gadolinium injection and administration of polyethylene glycol solution: axial image shows nodular formation with hypointense central core and hyperintense peripheral rim in the wall of a pathological loop (intraparietal abscess, arrowhead). In the adjacent mesentery, hyperintensity of the mesenteric fat is observed with local hypervascularization (hypertrophy of vasa recta, white arrow). Original figures by LMM and LL.

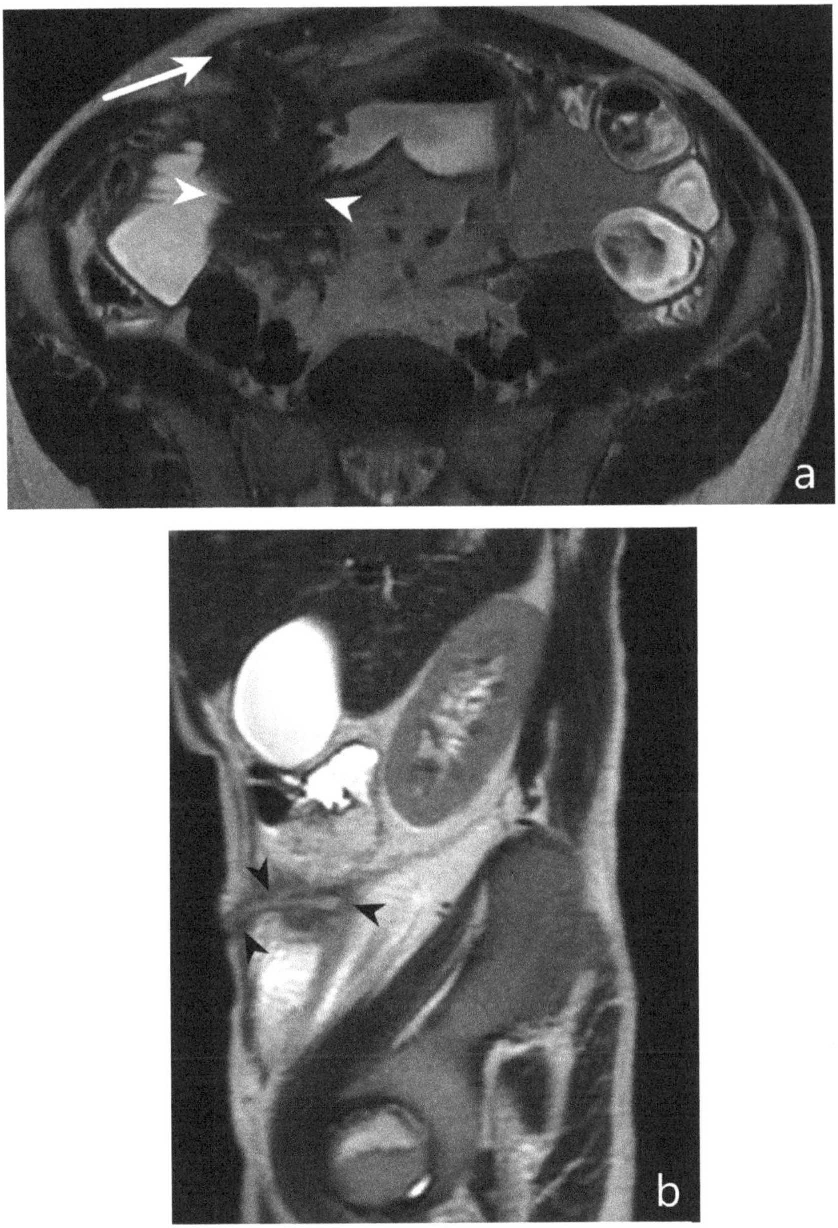

Figure 15. Entero-enteric fistula and entero-cutaneous fistula: MR-E after administration of polyethylene glycol solution. T2-weighted axial image (**a**) shows pathological loops with entero-enteric fistulas (white arrowheads). Further fistula with hyperintense T2 signal can be observed between the pathological loop and the anterior abdominal wall (arrow). T2-weighted sagittal image (**b**) shows the fistula between the pathological loop and the anterior abdominal wall; hyperintensity of signal in the lumen of fistula is present (black arrowheads). Original figures by LMM and LL.

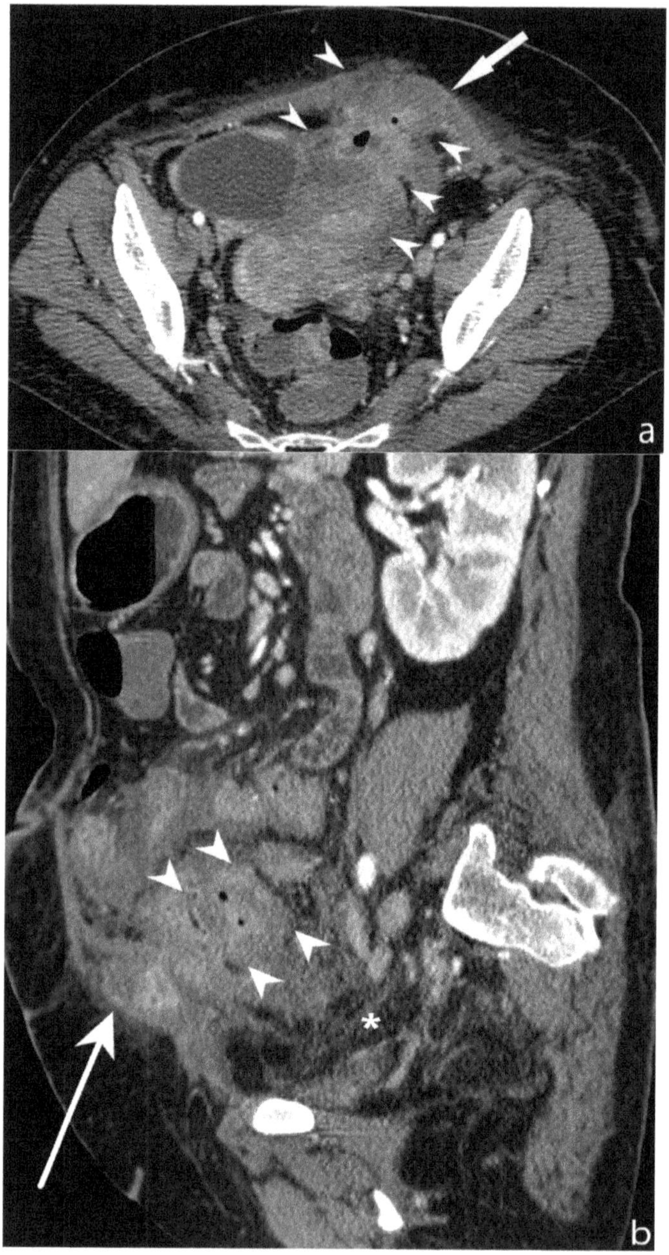

Figure 16. Abscess/phlegmon: CT-E after iodinated contrast injection and administration of polyethylene glycol solution. Axial image (**a**) shows an abscess/phlegmon (arrowheads) with extension to the wall of the left anterior rectus muscle (white arrow). Sagittal image (**b**) shows the extension of the abscess/phlegmon (arrowheads) to the wall of the left anterior rectus muscle (white arrow); perienteric fat stranding is present in pelvis (asterisk). Inhomogeneous hypodense tissue portion is present with anti-slope air components. Original figures by LMM and LL.

6. Is It Possible to Identify the Presence of Strictures and to Discriminate Inflammatory from Fibrotic Ones?

6.1. Definition of Stricture

Currently, there is no agreement in the literature concerning the radiological definition of stricture [37–43].

In 2019, Bettenworth et al. [37] performed a systematic review of radiology studies, showing great heterogeneity of the definitions adopted, which included one or more of the following features: pre-stenotic dilatation, wall thickening and/or luminal narrowing. The accuracy of cross-sectional imaging in the identification of strictures differs among studies, depending on the definition adopted—specifically, whether strictures are identified by the presence of the three abovementioned features, or just one or two. Chiorean et al. [38] used one item (bowel lumen narrowing) for stricture diagnosis in CT exams and found a sensitivity of 92% and specificity of 39%; on the contrary, another study with CT using two items (bowel lumen narrowing and increased wall thickness) found 100% sensitivity and 100% specificity [39]. Of four studies reporting the accuracy of MR-E, none provided an exact definition of stricture [40,41,44,45]. Example of stricture are shown in Figures 17 and 18.

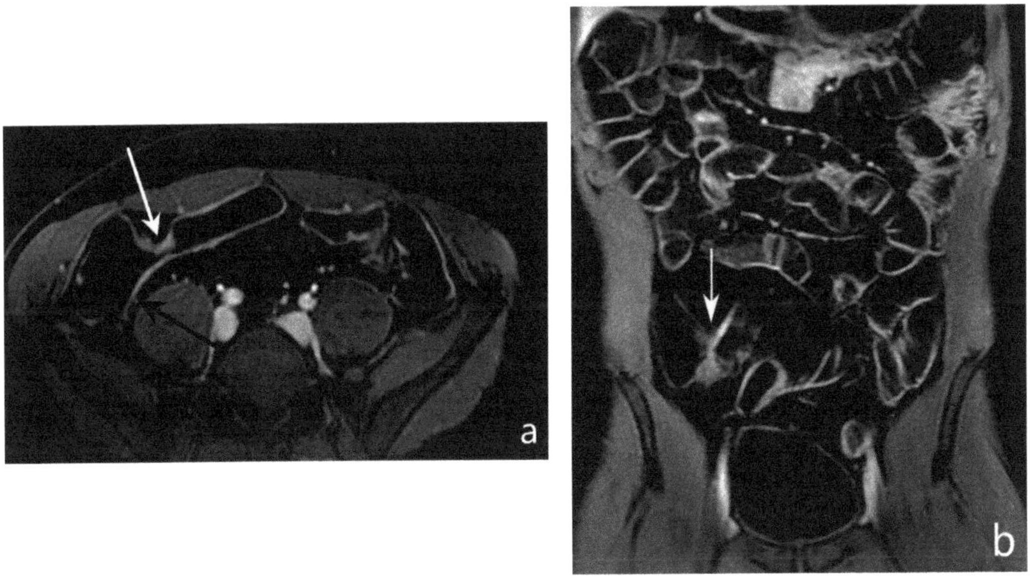

Figure 17. Fibro-stenotic subtype. MR-E after gadolinium injection and administration of polyethylene glycol solution; axial (**a**) and coronal (**b**) images show a homogeneous enhanced intestinal wall with narrowing of the terminal ileum (white arrow) and with dilation of the upstream small bowel loop (black arrow). Original figures by LMM and LL.

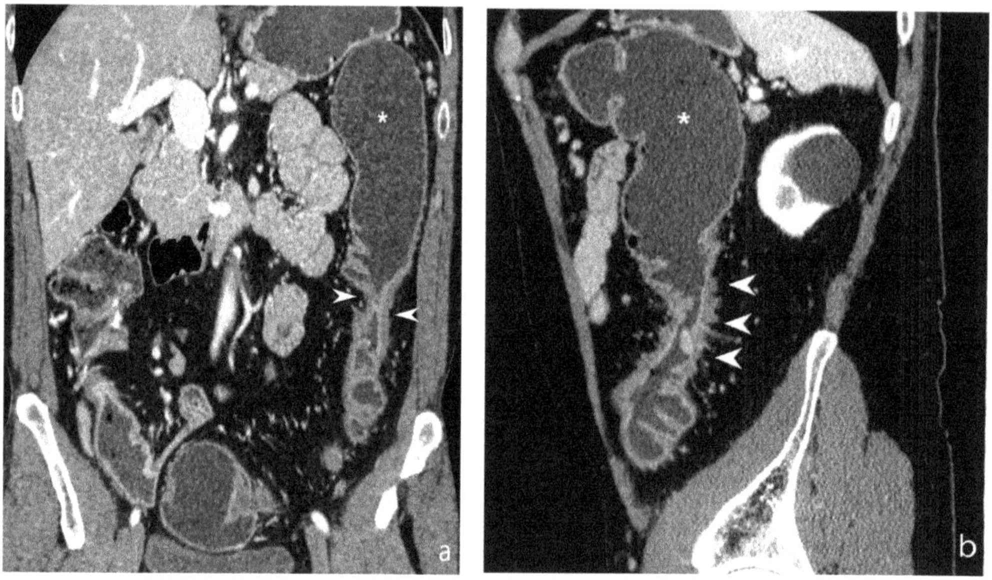

Figure 18. Intestinal stenosis: CT-E after iodinated contrast injection and administration of polyethylene glycol solution; coronal image (**a**) and sagittal image (**b**) show tight stenosis of the descendent colon (arrowheads), with stratified contrast enhancement; mild overdistention of the upstream descending colon (asterisk) is evident. Original figures by LMM and LL.

6.2. Differentiation between Fibrotic or Inflammatory Stenosis

Once the presence of stenosis has been established, radiologists are called upon to define whether it is fibrotic or inflammatory. To better characterize the implications of different radiological findings, several studies have assessed the correlation between CT or MR-E findings and pathological specimens in patients who underwent intestinal resection. Adler et al. [46] found significant correlations between CT-E findings and pathological specimens in detecting both inflammatory and fibrosis signs; in particular, CT-E findings of mesenteric hypervascularity, mucosal hyperenhancement, and mesenteric fat stranding predicted the presence of inflammatory features. Chiorean et al. [38] compared CT-E signs to histopathological specimens, using a four-grade scale for inflammation (none, mild, moderate and severe) and a three-grade scale for fibrosis (none, mild/moderate and severe): in their work, CT-E correctly detected inflammation and fibrosis with a sensitivity of 77% and 79%, respectively.

Moving to MRI, in 2011, Zappa et al. [34] found a positive association between histopathological inflammation and MR-E signs, such as wall thickness, degree of wall enhancement on the delayed phase, pattern of enhancement, relative mural hyperintensity on T2-weighted sequences, loco-regional hypervascularity, presence of a fistula and abscesses. Moreover, the authors found the presence of fibrosis to correlate well with active inflammation, indicating that both processes (i.e., acute inflammatory infiltrate and apposition of fibrotic tissue) might be contemporarily present: based on these findings, they suggest that the dichotomous distinction between 'inflammatory' and 'fibrotic' patients might not be relevant in clinical practice.

In 2014, Tielbeek and al. [47] compared the histological scores of acute inflammation and fibrosis with the following MR-E findings: intestinal mural thickness measured on T2-weighted fat-saturated images, T1 and T2 ratio, maximum contrast enhancement and slope of increase after contrast injection. Mural thickness and T1 ratio correlated with both inflammation and fibrosis, likely owing to their simultaneous presence in the same bowel segment. A higher T2 ratio was significantly associated with more severe inflammation as well as with mild fibro-stenotic disease; conversely, a lower T2 ratio correlated with low inflammation scores and severe fibro-stenosis. Maximum enhancement and initial slope of increase showed a good correlation with histopathology, confirming the importance of intravenously administered gadolinium to assess disease activity. The same authors also assessed the role of diffusion-weighted imaging (DWI), a new sequence performed with multiple *b* values (usually 0–800 s/mm^2 or 0–600 s/mm^2) and a measurement of the signal in a manually drawn region of interest (ROI) placed on the bowel wall on the apparent diffusion coefficient (ADC) map. Notably, they observed a significant correlation between ADC decrease and fibrosis.

In 2015, Rimola et al. [48] compared three-grade inflammatory and fibrosis histopathological scores with the following MR-E findings: wall thickening, oedema, ulcers, signal intensity of the submucosa after injection gadolinium contrast medium at 70 s and 7 min, stenosis and contrast enhancement pattern. The authors found a correlation between inflammation and the presence of T2 hyperintensity, enhancement of the mucosa, presence of ulcers and blurred margin; on the other hand, the percentage of enhancement gain, pattern of enhancement at 7 min and presence of stenosis correlated with fibrosis. Finally, the percentage of enhancement gain could differentiate between mild-to-moderate and severe fibrosis (sensitivity 94%, specificity 89%).

More recently, Wilkens et al. [49,50] evaluated if there was a correlation between small bowel wall perfusion measurements and histopathological scores for inflammation or fibrosis in CD, using both ultrasound (US) and MR-E. It emerged that intestinal wall thickness, assessed with either US or MR-E, was a valid marker of inflammation, but not of fibrosis. Moreover, a relative contrast enhancement in both techniques could not differentiate between acute inflammatory and fibrosis.

Finally, Cicero et al. [51] evaluated 59 patients, further divided into non-surgical (never undergone surgery) and surgical (at least one surgical operation for CD). Signal intensity in DWI images was measured at the highest b-value within pathologic intestinal walls and at lymph nodes, spleen and psoas muscle to calculate relative ratios (bowel/spleen, bowel/psoas and bowel/lymph node). In the non-surgical group, a positive correlation was found between endoscopic activity (assessed by the Simple Endoscopic Score for Crohn's Disease [50]) and all ratios; in the surgical group, endoscopic activity positively correlated only with the bowel/lymph node ratio and bowel/psoas ratio.

7. How Does Imaging Help Defining Disease Extension and Localization?

As previously reported, the length of the small bowel varies in relation to the age, sex, weight and height of the patient. Patients with CD seem to have a shorter small bowel than the general population; one of the explanations could be the presence of increased contractile activity of fibroblasts in the extracellular matrix in patients affected by stricturing CD [52,53].

Currently, the length of the small intestine is measured with MR-E or CT-E [54–57]. In 2014, Sinha et al. assessed the length of the small intestine with MR images using vascular imaging software, finding a good correlation between the MR-E and surgical measures [55].

Similar findings emerged in another study, in which the measures of 54 consecutive patients undergoing ileo-colic resection, calculated with CT-E or MR-E through 2D multiplanar (MPR) reconstructions, were compared with surgical results. The best correlation between the two measures emerged when the length of the pathological segments was less than or equal to 20 cm. For more extensive diseases, the imaging tends to overestimate the length of the pathological intestine [57].

In our department, we use postprocessing technologies, such as MPR, and specific post-processing 2D and 3D software (Vue PACS Carestream) to identify the small bowel and manually measure the pathological loops and residual normal bowel [54].

Measuring intestinal length is also useful in the presence of fistulas or stenosis: they can be precisely localized based on their distance from the ileocecal valve or from the Treitz ligament, thereby providing useful information to plan surgery or endoscopic dilation.

Examples of measurement are shown in Figures 19 and 20.

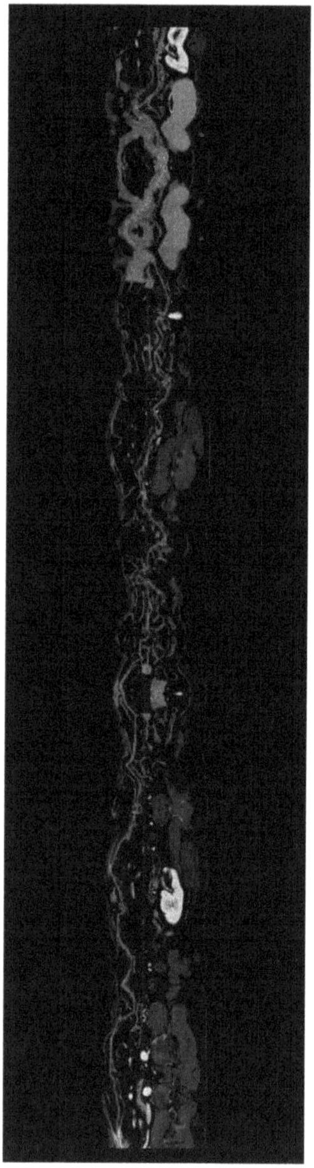

Figure 19. Calculation of the length of unaffected intestine using postprocessing software; a tubular view of the small bowel loops from MR-E is shown. The green line indicates the center of the bowel lumen. Original figures by LMM and LL.

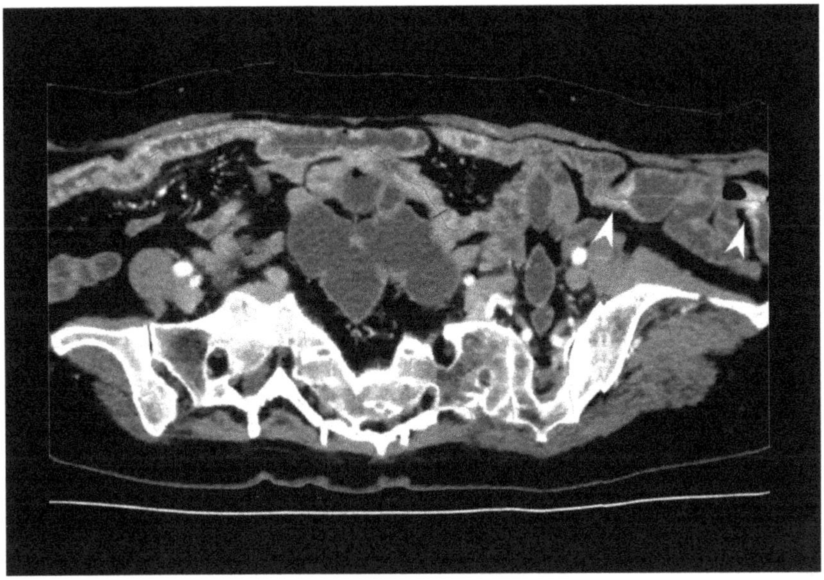

Figure 20. Calculation of the length of affected intestine using postprocessing software; a tubular view of the small bowel loops from CT-E is shown. There is evidence of two areas of pathological wall thickening on the right of the picture (arrowheads). The green line indicates the center of the bowel lumen. Original figures by LMM and LL.

8. Can Radiological Imaging Assess Disease Activity?

Clinical manifestations of CD are quite variable, and they do not always correlate with the severity of endoscopic lesions or radiologic involvement. The Crohn's Disease Activity Index (CDAI) is the most used clinical score in randomized controlled trials, but the complexity of its calculation, requiring a recall of 7 days, and the poor correlation with endoscopy limit its applicability in routine clinical practice [50]. The Harvey–Bradshaw Index represents an easier way to calculate clinical disease activity and has therefore been adopted in several real-world studies, but it has never been validated [50]. More recently, the Patient Reported Outcome (PRO)-2 score, including the two items of abdominal pain and stool frequency, is increasingly used in both clinical practice and clinical trials [58]. Biochemical parameters, mainly serum C-reactive protein and faecal calprotectin, are useful inflammatory markers for patient monitoring, and their normalization is currently considered an optimal target to pursue in the medium-term [59]. With regard to imaging, MR-E or CT-E are used to assess disease activity and also to evaluate how patients respond to medical therapy. Several scores have been developed so far to quantify the radiological activity of CD, showing a good correlation (Table 2) with clinical, laboratory and/or endoscopic parameters [31].

In a recent study comparing the MaRIA, Clermont and London indexes, the MaRIA index was shown to be the most accurate for the evaluation of disease activity and to grade its severity. The cut-offs established for the identification of active disease were 7 for the MaRIA, 8.4 for the Clermont index and 4.1 for the London index, while the cut-offs for severe inflammation were 11 for the MaRIA and 12.5 for the Clermont index [63].

Recently, Rimola et al. [64] evaluated the role of ADC values for the identification of bowel inflammation and therapeutic response in patients with CD treated with biologic therapy. The assessment of MaRIA score and the presence of endoscopic ulcers were determined at baseline and 46 weeks after starting therapy. Their findings did not support use of ADC rather than MaRIA scores for detecting the response to biologic therapy.

Table 2. (**a**) MEGS and CDMI. (**b**) MARIA Score and Clermont index.

(a)		
	MEGS Score (Score from 0 to 3)	**CDMI Score (Score from 0 to 3)**
Mural thickness of small bowel	0: <3 mm 1: >3–5 mm 2: >5–7 mm 3: >7 mm	0: <3 mm 1: >3–5 mm 2: >5–7 mm 3: >7 mm
Mural T2 signal compared to normal bowel wall	0: Equivalent to normal bowel wall 1: Minor increase in signal on fat-saturated images 2: Moderate increase in signal. 3: Marked increase in signal	0: Equivalent to normal bowel wall 1: Minor increase in signal on fat-saturated images 2: Moderate increase in signal. 3: Marked increase in signal
Perimural T2 signal	0: Equivalent to normal mesentery 1: Increase in mesenteric signal but no fluid 2: Small fluid rim (≤2 mm) 3: Larger fluid rim (>2 mm)	0: Equivalent to normal mesentery 1: Increase in mesenteric signal but no fluid 2: Small fluid rim (≤2 mm) 3: Larger fluid rim (>2 mm
T1 enhancement compared with nearest vessels	0: Equivalent to normal bowel wall 1: Minor enhancement of the bowel wall 2: Moderate enhancement but somewhat less than the nearby vascular structures 3: Moderate enhancement similar to the nearby vascular structures	0: Equivalent to normal bowel wall 1: Minor enhancement of the bowel wall 2: Moderate enhancement but somewhat less than the nearby vascular structures 3: Moderate enhancement similar to the nearby vascular structures
Mural enhancement pattern	0: Not available or homogeneous 1: Mucosal 2: Layered	0: Not available 1: Homogeneous 2: Mucosal 3: Layered
Haustral loss	0: None 1: <1/3 segment 2: 1/3 to 2/3 segment 3: >2/3 segment	
Multiplication factor per segment Length of disease segment	0–5 cm × 1 5–15 cm × 1.5 >15 cm × 2	
Additional score for extramural features	0–5	3 nodes greater than 1 cm
Lymph nodes (short diameter 1 cm or more)	Absent, present	0: absent 1: Cluster less than 1 cm 2: 1 node greater than 1 cm 3: 3 nodes greater than 1 cm
Engorged vasa recta	Absent, present	Absent, present
Abscess	Absent, present	
Fistulae	Absent, present	
Other		Lymph node enhancement compared to nearest vessel; Less than nearby vascular structure; Equivalent or greater to nearby vascular structure

Table 2. *Cont.*

(b)		
	MARIA Score	**Clermont Index**
Bowel mural thickness	>3 mm	>3 mm
Presence of mucosal ulcers (deep grooves in the mucosa)	No, yes	No, yes
Presence of wall oedema (hyperintensity on T2-weighted images of the bowel mural layers relative to the signal of the psoas muscle)	No, yes	No, yes
Wall signal intensity (WSI)	WSI was calculated in the areas with the predominant thickening and corresponded to the average of three WSI measurements	Not evaluated
Relative contrast enhancement (RCE)	RCE = ((WSI post-gadolinium − WSI pre-gadolinium)/(WSI pre-gadolinium)) × 100 × (standard deviation-SD noise pre-gadolinium/SD noise post-gadolinium).	Not evaluated
Fistulas, abscesses, enlarged (>8 mm) regional mesenteric lymph nodes, and fibrofatty proliferation.	Not evaluated	No, yes
DWI hyperintensity	Not evaluated	No, yes

MEGS Score = (Jejunal Score × Factor for Jejunum Involved Length) + (Proximal Ileum Score × Factor for Proximal Ileum Length) + (Terminal Ileum Score × Factor for Terminal Ileum Length) + (Caecum Score × Factor For Caecum Length) + (Ascending Score × Factor for Ascending Length) + (Transverse Score × Factor for Transverse Length) + (Descending Score × Factor for Descending Length) + (Sigmoid Score × Factor for Sigmoid Length) + (Rectum Score × Factor for Rectum Length) + Score for Abscess + Score for Fistula + Score for Adenopathy + Score for engorged vasa recta. No cut-off [60]. MRI index: 1.79 + 1.34 mural thickness (mm) + 0.94 mural T2 score; cut off = 4.1 [61]. MaRIA = 1.5 × mural thickness (mm) + 0.02 × relative contrast enhancement + 5 × oedema + 10 × ulcers. The total MaRIA score was calculated as the sum of the MaRIA in each intestinal tract. The cut-off points established for differentiating active from inactive disease is 7. A maria score > 11 is highly predictive of severe ileal CD [31]. Clermont score: −1.321 × ADC (mm^2/s) + 1.646 × mural thickening (mm) + 8.306 × ulcerations + 5.613 × oedema + 5.039. A Clermont score > 8.4 is highly predictive of ileal CD activity. A value of Clermont score ≥ 12.5 is highly predictive of severe ileal CD [62].

9. Is It Possible to Assess Post-Operative Recurrence?

About 20% of patients affected by CD undergo surgery in the first five years following the diagnosis and most of them experience post-operative recurrence (POR) [65]. Smoking habits, fistulising disease at index surgery, history of previous intestinal surgery and perianal disease are considered the main risk factors of POR. In the case of POR, endoscopic lesions usually precede the onset of symptoms [66]. Accordingly, in clinical practice, tight control with an endoscopy at 6–9 months after surgery and a stepwise treatment in the case of POR is routinely performed [67]. Currently, the endoscopic Rutgeerts score [50], albeit not validated, represents the reference standard scoring system in post-operative settings.

Several radiological studies have explored the role of MR-E or CT-E (± water enema) in comparison to endoscopy for detecting POR [68–74].

In particular, MR-E performed similarly to ileocolonoscopy for predicting clinical recurrence and to faecal calprotectin for predicting endoscopic recurrence [72]. Djelouah et al. [71] compared the diagnostic capabilities of MR-E using contrast-enhanced sequences to DWI, with endoscopy as the reference standard, and found that DWI-MRE has diagnostic capabilities similar to those of CE-MRE for the diagnosis of anastomotic POR. Schaefer et al. [68] developed and validated a MR imaging-based index (MONITOR index) to predict clinical POR and found that it was an efficient and reliable tool that can be used in clinical practice.

Choi et al. [70] evaluated the diagnostic yield and accuracy of CT-E and found that it can represent a viable option for early (<12 months) surveillance of anastomotic recurrence. Furthermore, the addition of a water enema provided a good distension of both sides of ileocolic anastomoses, allowing for the detection of recurrence [69].

10. Conclusions

CD is characterized by transmural inflammation potentially involving any tract of the digestive tube; the progression of disease can induce the development of complications and irreparable bowel damage. Imaging has a key role in clinical practice for assessing disease activity and extension and characterizing the disease pattern (i.e., inflammatory, fibrotic or fistulizing/penetrating). All these aspects have a meaningful impact on patient management, especially in those situations requiring a precise risk–benefit assessment between medical and surgical approaches. Moreover, imaging can be used for detecting POR, even though endoscopy still represents the reference standard. CT and MRI can both answer the abovementioned questions, but MRI should be preferred, owing to its greater sensitivity and specificity for assessing disease activity and to the lack of ionizing radiation. Regardless of the technique employed, adequate distension of the small bowel is essential to maximize its diagnostic performance, while the distention of the colon, via rectal enemas, should be adopted only in special situations.

In conclusion, radiologists are essential healthcare professionals to be involved in multidisciplinary teams for the management of CD patients, and strict collaboration is required among specialists to obtain the necessary answers for clinically relevant questions.

Our review aimed to be as pragmatic as possible by answering clinical questions that are posed daily in the management of CD, and it has provided a synthesis of the available data on these topics; however, a systematic review was not performed, and this review might suffer from subjectivity in the determination of which studies to include, the way the studies were analysed and the conclusions drawn.

Despite providing some useful indications regarding the role of radiology in the management of patients with CD, further research and systematic reviews are undoubtedly needed.

Author Contributions: Conceptualization, L.M.M. and D.P.; software, L.L. (Luigi Larosa); validation, B.B., D.P. and L.C.; formal analysis, F.B.D.; data curation, F.B.D.; writing—original draft preparation, L.M.M.; writing—review and editing, D.P.; visualization, G.P.; supervision, A.P., L.L. (Lucrezia Laterza) and F.S. All authors have read and agreed to the published version of the manuscript.

Funding: This research received no external funding.

Institutional Review Board Statement: Not applicable.

Informed Consent Statement: Informed consent was obtained from all subjects involved in the study.

Data Availability Statement: No new data were created.

Conflicts of Interest: The authors declare no conflict of interest.

References

1. Chang, J.T. Pathophysiology of Inflammatory Bowel Diseases. *N. Engl. J. Med.* **2020**, *383*, 2652–2664. [CrossRef] [PubMed]
2. Kaplan, G.G.; Windsor, J.W. The Four Epidemiological Stages in the Global Evolution of Inflammatory Bowel Disease. *Nat. Rev. Gastroenterol. Hepatol.* **2020**, *18*, 56–66. [CrossRef] [PubMed]
3. Le Berre, C.; Honap, S.; Peyrin-Biroulet, L. Ulcerative Colitis. *Lancet* **2023**, *402*, 571–584. [CrossRef] [PubMed]
4. Dolinger, M.; Torres, J.; Vermeire, S. Crohn's Disease. *Lancet* **2024**, *403*, 1177–1191. [CrossRef] [PubMed]

5. Maaser, C.; Sturm, A.; Vavricka, S.R.; Kucharzik, T.; Fiorino, G.; Annese, V.; Calabrese, E.; Baumgart, D.C.; Bettenworth, D.; Borralho Nunes, P.; et al. ECCO-ESGAR Guideline for Diagnostic Assessment in IBD Part 1: Initial Diagnosis, Monitoring of Known IBD, Detection of Complications. *J. Crohns Colitis* **2019**, *13*, 144–164. [CrossRef] [PubMed]
6. Rieder, F.; Zimmermann, E.M.; Remzi, F.H.; Sandborn, W.J. Crohn's Disease Complicated by Strictures: A Systematic Review. *Gut* **2013**, *62*, 1072–1084. [CrossRef] [PubMed]
7. Minordi, L.M.; Bevere, A.; Papa, A.; Larosa, L.; Manfredi, R. CT and MRI Evaluations in Crohn's Complications: A Guide for the Radiologist. *Acad. Radiol.* **2022**, *29*, 1206–1227. [CrossRef]
8. Minordi, L.M.; Vecchioli, A.; Mirk, P.; Bonomo, L. CT Enterography with Polyethylene Glycol Solution vs CT Enteroclysis in Small Bowel Disease. *Br. J. Radiol.* **2011**, *84*, 112–119. [CrossRef]
9. Pierro, A.; Minordi, L.M.; Larosa, L.; Guerri, G.; Grimaldi, A.; Quinto, F.; Rotondi, F.; Marcellino, A.; Bevere, T.; Basilico, R.; et al. Small Bowel Imaging from Stepchild of Roentgenology to MR Enterography, Part I: Guidance in Performing and Observing Normal and Abnormal Imaging Findings. *Life* **2023**, *13*, 1691. [CrossRef]
10. Schmidt, S.A.; Baumann, J.A.; Stanescu-Siegmund, N.; Froehlich, E.; Brambs, H.J.; Juchems, M.S. Oral Distension Methods for Small Bowel MRI: Comparison of Different Agents to Optimize Bowel Distension. *Acta Radiol.* **2016**, *57*, 1460–1467. [CrossRef]
11. Sinha, R.; Rawat, S. MRI Enterography with Divided Dose Oral Preparation: Effect on Bowel Distension and Diagnostic Quality. *Indian J. Radiol. Imaging* **2013**, *23*, 86–91. [CrossRef]
12. Masselli, G.; Casciani, E.; Polettini, E.; Gualdi, G. Comparison of MR Enteroclysis with MR Enterography and Conventional Enteroclysis in Patients with Crohn's Disease. *Eur. Radiol.* **2008**, *18*, 438–447. [CrossRef] [PubMed]
13. Schreyer, A.G.; Geissler, A.; Albrich, H.; Schölmerich, J.; Feuerbach, S.; Rogler, G.; Völk, M.; Herfarth, H. Abdominal MRI after Enteroclysis or with Oral Contrast in Patients with Suspected or Proven Crohn's Disease. *Clin. Gastroenterol. Hepatol.* **2004**, *2*, 491–497. [CrossRef]
14. Negaard, A.; Paulsen, V.; Sandvik, L.; Berstad, A.E.; Borthne, A.; Try, K.; Lygren, I.; Storaas, T.; Klow, N.E. A Prospective Randomized Comparison between Two MRI Studies of the Small Bowel in Crohn's Disease, the Oral Contrast Method and MR Enteroclysis. *Eur. Radiol.* **2007**, *17*, 2294–2301. [CrossRef]
15. Masselli, G. Small Bowel Imaging: Clinical Applications of the Different Imaging Modalities—A Comprehensive Review. *Int. Sch. Res. Not.* **2013**, *2013*, 419542. [CrossRef]
16. Panés, J.; Bouzas, R.; Chaparro, M.; García-Sánchez, V.; Gisbert, J.P.; Martínez De Guereñu, B.; Mendoza, J.L.; Paredes, J.M.; Quiroga, S.; Ripollés, T.; et al. Systematic Review: The Use of Ultrasonography, Computed Tomography and Magnetic Resonance Imaging for the Diagnosis, Assessment of Activity and Abdominal Complications of Crohn's Disease. *Aliment. Pharmacol. Ther.* **2011**, *34*, 125–145. [CrossRef] [PubMed]
17. Engin, G. Computed Tomography Enteroclysis in the Diagnosis of Intestinal Diseases. *J. Comput. Assist. Tomogr.* **2008**, *32*, 9–16. [CrossRef]
18. Minordi, L.M.; Scaldaferri, F.; Larosa, L.; Marra, R.; Giordano, F.; Laterza, L.; Scoleri, I.; Poscia, A.; Gerardi, V.; Bruno, G.; et al. Comparison between clinical and radiological evaluation before and after medical therapy in patients with Crohn's disease: New prospective roles of CT enterography. *Radiol. Med.* **2015**, *120*, 449–457. [CrossRef] [PubMed]
19. Maglinte, D.D.T.; Sandrasegaran, K.; Lappas, J.C.; Chiorean, M. CT Enteroclysis. *Radiology* **2007**, *245*, 661–671. [CrossRef]
20. Deepak, P.; Axelrad, J.E.; Ananthakrishnan, A.N. The Role of the Radiologist in Determining Disease Severity in Inflammatory Bowel Diseases. *Gastrointest. Endosc. Clin. N. Am.* **2019**, *29*, 447–470. [CrossRef]
21. Pierro, A.; Minordi, L.M.; Larosa, L.; Cipri, C.; Guerri, G.; Quinto, F.; Rotondi, F.; Marcellino, A.; Basilico, R.; Iezzi, R.; et al. Small Bowel Imaging from Stepchild of Roentgenology to MR Enterography, Part II: The Reliable Disclosure of Crohn's Disease and Non-Inflammatory Small Bowel Disorder Plot through MRI Findings. *Life* **2023**, *13*, 1836. [CrossRef] [PubMed]
22. Chatu, S.; Subramanian, V.; Pollok, R.C.G. Meta-Analysis: Diagnostic Medical Radiation Exposure in Inflammatory Bowel Disease. *Aliment. Pharmacol. Ther.* **2012**, *35*, 529–539. [CrossRef] [PubMed]
23. Kalra, M.K.; Rizzo, S.M.R.; Novelline, R.A. Reducing Radiation Dose in Emergency Computed Tomography with Automatic Exposure Control Techniques. *Emerg. Radiol.* **2005**, *11*, 267–274. [CrossRef] [PubMed]
24. Kielar, A.Z.; Tao, H.; Thipphavong, S. Modified Small Bowel CT (MBCT) for Evaluating Sub-Acute and Chronic Conditions Affecting the Small Bowel: A Low Radiation-Dose, Unenhanced CT Protocol. *Insights Imaging* **2011**, *2*, 539–542. [CrossRef] [PubMed]
25. Craig, O.; O'Neill, S.; O'Neill, F.; McLaughlin, P.; McGarrigle, A.M.; McWilliams, S.; O'Connor, O.; Desmond, A.; Walsh, E.K.; Ryan, M.; et al. Diagnostic Accuracy of Computed Tomography Using Lower Doses of Radiation for Patients With Crohn's Disease. *Clin. Gastroenterol. Hepatol.* **2012**, *10*, 886–892. [CrossRef] [PubMed]
26. Taylor, S.A.; Avni, F.; Cronin, C.G.; Hoeffel, C.; Kim, S.H.; Laghi, A.; Napolitano, M.; Petit, P.; Rimola, J.; Tolan, D.J.; et al. The First Joint ESGAR/ESPR Consensus Statement on the Technical Performance of Cross-Sectional Small Bowel and Colonic Imaging. *Eur. Radiol.* **2017**, *27*, 2570–2582. [CrossRef] [PubMed]
27. Minordi, L.M.; Scaldaferri, F.; Marra, R.S.; Pecere, S.; Larosa, L.; Poscia, A.; Gasbarrini, A.; Vecchioli, A.; Bonomo, L. Enterography CT without and with Water Enema in Patients with Crohn's Disease: Results from a Comparative Observational Study in Comparison with Endoscopy. *Eur. J. Radiol.* **2016**, *85*, 404–413. [CrossRef] [PubMed]
28. Ajaj, W.; Veit, P.; Kuehle, C.; Joekel, M.; Lauenstein, T.C.; Herborn, C.U. Digital Subtraction Dark-Lumen MR Colonography: Initial Experience. *J. Magn. Reson. Imaging* **2005**, *21*, 841–844. [CrossRef]

29. Tkalčić, L.; Matana Kaštelan, Z.; Grubešić, T.; Mijandrušić Sinčić, B.; Milić, S.; Miletić, D. MR Enterocolonography in Patients with Crohn's Disease and Healthy Volunteers—Do We Achieve Diagnostic Bowel Distension? *Eur. J. Radiol.* **2020**, *129*, 109100. [CrossRef]
30. Maglinte, D.D.T.; Heitkamp, D.E.; Howard, T.J.; Kelvin, F.M.; Lappas, J.C. Current Concepts in Imaging of Small Bowel Obstruction. *Radiol. Clin. N. Am.* **2003**, *41*, 263–283. [CrossRef]
31. Rimola, J.; Rodriguez, S.; García-Bosch, O.; Ordás, I.; Ayala, E.; Aceituno, M.; Pellisé, M.; Ayuso, C.; Ricart, E.; Donoso, L.; et al. Magnetic Resonance for Assessment of Disease Activity and Severity in Ileocolonic Crohn's Disease. *Gut* **2009**, *58*, 1113–1120. [CrossRef]
32. Taylor, S.A.; Punwani, S.; Rodriguez-Justo, M.; Bainbridge, A.; Greenhalgh, R.; De Vita, E.; Forbes, A.; Cohen, R.; Windsor, A.; Obichere, A.; et al. Mural Crohn Disease: Correlation of Dynamic Contrast-Enhanced MR Imaging Findings with Angiogenesis and Inflammation at Histologic Examination—Pilot Study. *Radiology* **2009**, *251*, 369–379. [CrossRef] [PubMed]
33. Bruining, D.H.; Zimmermann, E.M.; Loftus, E.V.; Sandborn, W.J.; Sauer, C.G.; Strong, S.A.; Fletcher, J.G. Consensus Recommendations for Evaluation, Interpretation, and Utilization of Computed Tomography and Magnetic Resonance Enterography in Patients with Small Bowel Crohn's Disease. *Radiology* **2018**, *286*, 776–799. [CrossRef]
34. Zappa, M.; Stefanescu, C.; Cazals-Hatem, D.; Bretagnol, F.; Deschamps, L.; Attar, A.; Larroque, B.; Tréton, X.; Panis, Y.; Vilgrain, V.; et al. Which Magnetic Resonance Imaging Findings Accurately Evaluate Inflammation in Small Bowel Crohn's Disease? A Retrospective Comparison with Surgical Pathologic Analysis. *Inflamm. Bowel Dis.* **2011**, *17*, 984–993. [CrossRef]
35. Rodriguez, P.; Mendez, R.; Matute, F.; Hernandez, P.; Mendoza, J.L. Imaging Crohn Disease: MR Enterography. *J. Comput. Assist. Tomogr.* **2014**, *38*, 219–227. [CrossRef] [PubMed]
36. Minordi, L.M.; Larosa, L.; Papa, A.; Cimino, G.; Bevere, A.; Brizi, M.G.; Manfredi, R. A Review of Magnetic Resonance Enterography Classification and Quantitative Evaluation of Active Disease in Patients with Crohn's Disease. *Clin. Imaging* **2021**, *69*, 50–62. [CrossRef] [PubMed]
37. Bettenworth, D.; Bokemeyer, A.; Baker, M.; Mao, R.; Parker, C.E.; Nguyen, T.; Ma, C.; Panés, J.; Rimola, J.; Fletcher, J.G.; et al. Assessment of Crohn's Disease-Associated Small Bowel Strictures and Fibrosis on Cross-Sectional Imaging: A Systematic Review. *Gut* **2019**, *68*, 1115–1126. [CrossRef]
38. Chiorean, M.V.; Sandrasegaran, K.; Saxena, R.; Maglinte, D.D.; Nakeeb, A.; Johnson, C.S. Correlation of CT Enteroclysis with Surgical Pathology in Crohn's Disease. *Am. J. Gastroenterol.* **2007**, *102*, 2541–2550. [CrossRef]
39. Vogel, J.; Da Luz Moreira, A.; Baker, M.; Hammel, J.; Einstein, D.; Stocchi, L.; Fazio, V. CT Enterography for Crohn's Disease: Accurate Preoperative Diagnostic Imaging. *Dis. Colon Rectum* **2007**, *50*, 1761–1769. [CrossRef]
40. Sinha, R.; Murphy, P.; Sanders, S.; Ramachandran, I.; Hawker, P.; Rawat, S.; Roberts, S. Diagnostic Accuracy of High-Resolution MR Enterography in Crohn's Disease: Comparison with Surgical and Pathological Specimen. *Clin. Radiol.* **2013**, *68*, 917–927. [CrossRef]
41. Kumar, S.; Hakim, A.; Alexakis, C.; Chhaya, V.; Tzias, D.; Pilcher, J.; Vlahos, J.; Pollok, R. Small Intestinal Contrast Ultrasonography for the Detection of Small Bowel Complications in Crohn's Disease: Correlation with Intraoperative Findings and Magnetic Resonance Enterography. *J. Gastroenterol. Hepatol.* **2015**, *30*, 86–91. [CrossRef] [PubMed]
42. Guglielmo, F.F.; Anupindi, S.A.; Fletcher, J.G.; Al-Hawary, M.M.; Dillman, J.R.; Grand, D.J.; Bruining, D.H.; Chatterji, M.; Darge, K.; Fidler, J.L.; et al. Small Bowel Crohn Disease at CT and MR Enterography: Imaging Atlas and Glossary of Terms. *Radiographics* **2020**, *40*, 354–375. [CrossRef] [PubMed]
43. Minordi, L.M.; Larosa, L.; Bevere, A.; D'Angelo, F.B.; Pierro, A.; Cilla, S.; Del Ciello, A.; Scaldaferri, F.; Barbaro, B. Imaging of Strictures in Crohn's Disease. *Life* **2023**, *13*, 2283. [CrossRef] [PubMed]
44. Pous-Serrano, S.; Frasson, M.; Palasí Giménez, R.; Sanchez-Jordá, G.; Pamies-Guilabert, J.; Llavador Ros, M.; Nos Mateu, P.; Garcia-Granero, E. Accuracy of Magnetic Resonance Enterography in the Preoperative Assessment of Patients with Crohn's Disease of the Small Bowel. *Color. Dis.* **2017**, *19*, O126–O133. [CrossRef]
45. Pellino, G.; Nicolai, E.; Catalano, O.A.; Campione, S.; D'Armiento, F.P.; Salvatore, M.; Cuocolo, A.; Selvaggi, F. PET/MR Versus PET/CT Imaging: Impact on the Clinical Management of Small-Bowel Crohn's Disease. *J. Crohns Colitis* **2016**, *10*, 277–285. [CrossRef] [PubMed]
46. Adler, J.; Punglia, D.R.; Dillman, J.R.; Polydorides, A.D.; Dave, M.; Al-Hawary, M.M.; Platt, J.F.; McKenna, B.J.; Zimmermann, E.M. Computed Tomography Enterography Findings Correlate with Tissue Inflammation, Not Fibrosis in Resected Small Bowel Crohn's Disease. *Inflamm. Bowel Dis.* **2012**, *18*, 849–856. [CrossRef] [PubMed]
47. Tielbeek, J.A.W.; Ziech, M.L.W.; Li, Z.; Lavini, C.; Bipat, S.; Bemelman, W.A.; Roelofs, J.J.T.H.; Ponsioen, C.Y.; Vos, F.M.; Stoker, J. Evaluation of Conventional, Dynamic Contrast Enhanced and Diffusion Weighted MRI for Quantitative Crohn's Disease Assessment with Histopathology of Surgical Specimens. *Eur. Radiol.* **2014**, *24*, 619–629. [CrossRef] [PubMed]
48. Rimola, J.; Planell, N.; Rodríguez, S.; Delgado, S.; Ordás, I.; Ramírez-Morros, A.; Ayuso, C.; Aceituno, M.; Ricart, E.; Jauregui-Amezaga, A.; et al. Characterization of Inflammation and Fibrosis in Crohn's Disease Lesions by Magnetic Resonance Imaging. *Am. J. Gastroenterol.* **2015**, *110*, 432–440. [CrossRef] [PubMed]
49. Wilkens, R.; Hagemann-Madsen, R.H.; Peters, D.A.; Nielsen, A.H.; Nørager, C.B.; Glerup, H.; Krogh, K. Validity of Contrast-Enhanced Ultrasonography and Dynamic Contrast-Enhanced MR Enterography in the Assessment of Transmural Activity and Fibrosis in Crohn's Disease. *J. Crohns Colitis* **2018**, *12*, 48–56. [CrossRef]

50. Sturm, A.; Maaser, C.; Calabrese, E.; Annese, V.; Fiorino, G.; Kucharzik, T.; Vavricka, S.R.; Verstockt, B.; Van Rheenen, P.; Tolan, D.; et al. Ecco-Esgar Guideline for Diagnostic Assessment in Ibd Part 2: Ibd Scores and General Principles and Technical Aspects. *J. Crohns Colitis* **2019**, *13*, 273–284. [CrossRef]
51. Cicero, G.; Alibrandi, A.; Blandino, A.; Ascenti, V.; Fries, W.; Viola, A.; Mazziotti, S. DWI Ratios: New Indexes for Crohn's Disease Activity at Magnetic Resonance Enterography? *Radiol. Med.* **2023**, *128*, 16–26. [CrossRef]
52. Glehen, O.; Lifante, J.C.; Vignal, J.; Francois, Y.; Gilly, F.N.; Flourié, B.; Descos, L.; Chung, R.J.H.; Mithieux, F. Small Bowel Length in Crohn's Disease. *Int. J. Color. Dis.* **2003**, *18*, 423–427. [CrossRef]
53. Shatari, T.; Clark, M.A.; Lee, J.R.; Keighley, M.R.B. Reliability of Radiographic Measurement of Small Intestinal Length. *Color. Dis.* **2004**, *6*, 327–329. [CrossRef]
54. Minordi, L.M.; Larosa, L.; Brizi, M.G.; Armuzzi, A.; Manfredi, R. Length of the Healthy and Pathological Small Intestine in Patients with Crohn's Disease: Calculations Using Computed Tomography and Magnetic Resonance Enterography. *Diagn. Interv. Radiol.* **2023**, *29*, 24–28. [CrossRef] [PubMed]
55. Sinha, R.; Trivedi, D.; Murphy, P.D.; Fallis, S. Small-Intestinal Length Measurement on MR Enterography: Comparison with in vivo surgical measurement. *AJR Am. J. Roentgenol.* **2014**, *203*, W274–W279. [CrossRef] [PubMed]
56. Wilson, N.A.; Park, H.S.; Lee, K.S.; Barron, L.K.; Warner, B.W. A Novel Approach to Calculating Small Intestine Length Based on Magnetic Resonance Enterography. *J. Am. Coll. Surg.* **2017**, *225*, 266–273. [CrossRef]
57. Brouquet, A.; Rangheard, A.S.; Ifergan, J.; Lazure, T.; Carbonnel, F.; Penna, C.; Benoist, S. The Accuracy of Preoperative Imaging in Measuring the Length of the Ileocolic Segment Affected by Crohn's Disease: A Prospective Cohort Study. *Color. Dis.* **2017**, *19*, 437–445. [CrossRef] [PubMed]
58. Khanna, R.; Zou, G.; D'Haens, G.; Feagan, B.G.; Sandborn, W.J.; Vandervoort, M.K.; Rolleri, R.L.; Bortey, E.; Paterson, C.; Forbes, W.P.; et al. A Retrospective Analysis: The Development of Patient Reported Outcome Measures for the Assessment of Crohn's Disease Activity. *Aliment. Pharmacol. Ther.* **2015**, *41*, 77–86. [CrossRef]
59. Turner, D.; Ricciuto, A.; Lewis, A.; D'Amico, F.; Dhaliwal, J.; Griffiths, A.M.; Bettenworth, D.; Sandborn, W.J.; Sands, B.E.; Reinisch, W.; et al. STRIDE-II: An Update on the Selecting Therapeutic Targets in Inflammatory Bowel Disease (STRIDE) Initiative of the International Organization for the Study of IBD (IOIBD): Determining Therapeutic Goals for Treat-to-Target Strategies in IBD. *Gastroenterology* **2020**, *160*, 1570–1583. [CrossRef]
60. Makanyanga, J.C.; Pendsé, D.; Dikaios, N.; Bloom, S.; McCartney, S.; Helbren, E.; Atkins, E.; Cuthbertson, T.; Punwani, S.; Forbes, A.; et al. Evaluation of Crohn's Disease Activity: Initial Validation of a Magnetic Resonance Enterography Global Score (MEGS) against Faecal Calprotectin. *Eur. Radiol.* **2014**, *24*, 277–287. [CrossRef]
61. Steward, M.J.; Punwani, S.; Proctor, I.; Adjei-Gyamfi, Y.; Chatterjee, F.; Bloom, S.; Novelli, M.; Halligan, S.; Rodriguez-Justo, M.; Taylor, S.A. Non-Perforating Small Bowel Crohn's Disease Assessed by MRI Enterography: Derivation and Histopathological Validation of an MR-Based Activity Index. *Eur. J. Radiol.* **2012**, *81*, 2080–2088. [CrossRef] [PubMed]
62. Hordonneau, C.; Buisson, A.; Scanzi, J.; Goutorbe, F.; Pereira, B.; Borderon, C.; Da Ines, D.; Montoriol, P.F.; Garcier, J.M.; Boyer, L.; et al. Diffusion-Weighted Magnetic Resonance Imaging in Ileocolonic Crohn's Disease: Validation of Quantitative Index of Activity. *Am. J. Gastroenterol.* **2014**, *109*, 89–98. [CrossRef] [PubMed]
63. Rimola, J.; Alvarez-Cofiño, A.; Pérez-Jeldres, T.; Ayuso, C.; Alfaro, I.; Rodríguez, S.; Ricart, E.; Ordás, I.; Panés, J. Comparison of Three Magnetic Resonance Enterography Indices for Grading Activity in Crohn's Disease. *J. Gastroenterol.* **2017**, *52*, 585–593. [CrossRef] [PubMed]
64. Rimola, J.; Fernandez-Clotet, A.; Capozzi, N.; Caballol, B.; Rodríguez, S.; Gallego, M.; Masamunt, M.C.; Panés, J.; Ricart, E.; Ordás, I. ADC Values for Detecting Bowel Inflammation and Biologic Therapy Response in Patients With Crohn Disease: A Post Hoc Prospective Trial Analysis. *AJR Am. J. Roentgenol.* **2024**, *222*, e2329639. [CrossRef] [PubMed]
65. Pariente, B.; Cosnes, J.; Danese, S.; Sandborn, W.J.; Lewin, M.; Fletcher, J.G.; Chowers, Y.; D'Haens, G.; Feagan, B.G.; Hibi, T.; et al. Development of the Crohn's Disease Digestive Damage Score, the Lémann Score. *Inflamm. Bowel Dis.* **2011**, *17*, 1415. [CrossRef] [PubMed]
66. Lichtenstein, G.R.; Loftus, E.V.; Isaacs, K.L.; Regueiro, M.D.; Gerson, L.B.; Sands, B.E. ACG Clinical Guideline: Management of Crohn's Disease in Adults. *Am. J. Gastroenterol.* **2018**, *113*, 481–517. [CrossRef] [PubMed]
67. De Cruz, P.; Kamm, M.A.; Hamilton, A.L.; Ritchie, K.J.; Krejany, E.O.; Gorelik, A.; Liew, D.; Prideaux, L.; Lawrance, I.C.; Andrews, J.M.; et al. Crohn's Disease Management after Intestinal Resection: A Randomised Trial. *Lancet* **2015**, *385*, 1406–1417. [CrossRef]
68. Schaefer, M.; Laurent, V.; Grandmougin, A.; Vuitton, L.; Bourreille, A.; Luc, A.; Clerc-Urmes, I.; Orry, X.; Frampas, E.; De Billy, M.; et al. A Magnetic Resonance Imaging Index to Predict Crohn's Disease Postoperative Recurrence: The MONITOR Index. *Clin. Gastroenterol. Hepatol.* **2022**, *20*, e1040–e1049. [CrossRef]
69. Paparo, F.; Revelli, M.; Puppo, C.; Bacigalupo, L.; Garello, I.; Garlaschi, A.; Biscaldi, E.; Rollandi, L.; Binda, G.A.; Rollandi, G.A. Crohn's Disease Recurrence in Patients with Ileocolic Anastomosis: Value of Computed Tomography Enterography with Water Enema. *Eur. J. Radiol.* **2013**, *82*, e434–e440. [CrossRef]
70. Choi, I.Y.; Park, S.H.; Park, S.H.; Yu, C.S.; Yoon, Y.S.; Lee, J.L.; Ye, B.D.; Kim, A.Y.; Yang, S.K. CT Enterography for Surveillance of Anastomotic Recurrence within 12 Months of Bowel Resection in Patients with Crohn's Disease: An Observational Study Using an 8-Year Registry. *Korean J. Radiol.* **2017**, *18*, 906–914. [CrossRef]

71. Djelouah, M.; Marical, V.; Kanagaratnam, L.; Kianmanesh, R.; Biron, A.; Cadiot, G.; Hoeffel, C. Diagnosis of Postoperative Recurrence of Crohn Disease with MR-Enterography: Value of Diffusion-Weighted Imaging. *Diagn. Interv. Imaging* **2021**, *102*, 743–751. [CrossRef] [PubMed]
72. Baillet, P.; Cadiot, G.; Goutte, M.; Goutorbe, F.; Brixi, H.; Hoeffel, C.; Allimant, C.; Reymond, M.; Obritin-Guilhen, H.; Magnin, B.; et al. Faecal Calprotectin and Magnetic Resonance Imaging in Detecting Crohn's Disease Endoscopic Postoperative Recurrence. *World J. Gastroenterol.* **2018**, *24*, 641. [CrossRef] [PubMed]
73. Koilakou, S.; Sailer, J.; Peloschek, P.; Ferlitsch, A.; Vogelsang, H.; Miehsler, W.; Fletcher, J.; Turetschek, K.; Schima, W.; Reinisch, W. Endoscopy and MR Enteroclysis: Equivalent Tools in Predicting Clinical Recurrence in Patients with Crohn's Disease after Ileocolic Resection. *Inflamm. Bowel Dis.* **2010**, *16*, 198–203. [CrossRef] [PubMed]
74. Chavoshi, M.; Zamani, S.; Kolahdoozan, S.; Radmard, A.R. Diagnostic Value of MR and CT Enterography in Post-Operative Recurrence of Crohn's Disease: A Systematic Review and Meta-Analysis. *Abdom. Radiol.* **2024**, 1–12. [CrossRef] [PubMed]

Journal of
Clinical Medicine

MDPI

Review

Endoscopic Management of Strictures in Crohn's Disease: An Unsolved Case

Gaetano Coppola [1,2,*], Chiara Principessa [2], Federica Di Vincenzo [1,2], Pierluigi Puca [1,2], Angelo Del Gaudio [1,2], Ivan Capobianco [1,2], Bianca Bartocci [1,2], Alfredo Papa [1,2], Giovanni Cammarota [1,2], Loris Riccardo Lopetuso [1,2,3] and Franco Scaldaferri [1,2]

1 CEMAD—IBD Unit, Fondazione Policlinico Universitario Agostino Gemelli IRCCS, 00168 Rome, Italy; capobianco_ivan@yahoo.it (I.C.)
2 Dipartimento Universitario di Medicina e Chirurgia Traslazionale, Università Cattolica del Sacro Cuore, 00168 Rome, Italy; chiara99princ@gmail.com
3 Dipartimento di Medicina e Scienze dell'Invecchiamento, Università degli Studi "G. D'Annunzio", 66100 Chieti, Italy
* Correspondence: gaetano.coppola@guest.policlinicogemelli.it

Abstract: Crohn's disease (CD) is a chronic inflammatory disease associated with a significant burden in terms of quality of life and health care costs. It is frequently associated with several complications, including the development of intestinal strictures. Stricturing CD requires a careful multidisciplinary approach involving medical therapy and surgery, still posing a continuous management challenge; in this context, endoscopic treatment represents a valuable, in-between opportunity as a minimally invasive strategy endorsed by extensive yet heterogeneous evidence and evolving research and techniques. This review summarizes current knowledge on the role of therapeutic endoscopy in stricturing CD, focusing on evidence gaps, recent updates, and novel techniques intended for optimizing efficacy, safety, and tailoring of this approach in the view of precision endoscopy.

Keywords: Crohn's disease; Crohn; stricture; balloon dilation; EBD; stricturotomy; intestinal stent; fibrosis; nanoparticles

1. Introduction

Crohn's disease (CD) is a chronic inflammatory condition that can affect all gastrointestinal tract segments, with an intermittent and chronic course and increasing incidence [1]. Intestinal strictures represent one of the most frequent complications of CD, resulting from sustained transmural inflammation and abnormal extracellular matrix deposition and affecting approximately one-third of CD patients [2]. Two types of stricture can be identified: primary (de novo) and secondary (post-operative, anastomotic) strictures: primary strictures can develop in all segments affected by the disease, with the ileum being the most frequent site of onset, given the higher prevalence of disease-related inflammation in this segment and its smaller diameter compared to the colon [3,4].

Prompt multidisciplinary management of stricturing CD is required, considering the risk of bowel obstruction, the neoplastic potential [5], and the need to monitor upstream disease activity hidden proximally to the stricture. In this scenario, advanced therapy with biologics and small molecules may delay or reduce the need for repeated surgery in an bowel-sparing perspective [6]. Endoscopy stands out between medical therapy and surgery as a feasible, minimally invasive tool in selected cases, with an established role and still growing evidence in managing stricturing CD. Endoscopic balloon dilation (EBD) is the most extensively employed endoscopic procedure, being associated with a technical success rate exceeding 90% in most studies and a favorable safety profile for the treatment of short intestinal strictures [7]. Beyond EBD, in the last two decades, a wide range of alternative procedures have been gathering attention [8], with still limited data and a lack of standardization both in techniques and study designs [9]. In the era of precision endoscopy in inflammatory bowel disease (IBD), there is growing interest in advanced imaging techniques and artificial intelligence tools. These innovations aid in the detection of inflammation and dysplasia, as well as the identifications of molecular patterns for targeted interventions [10,11]. Both established and emerging therapeutic endoscopic tools hold promise for the management of persistent Crohn's disease (CD) through increasingly microinvasive and personalized approaches. However, several challenges remain and there are many breakthrough opportunities to be explored.

Our review aims to build on established knowledge of endoscopic treatment of CD-associated strictures, identify evidence gaps, and highlight the latest advancements in the most intriguing techniques in development (Figure 1).

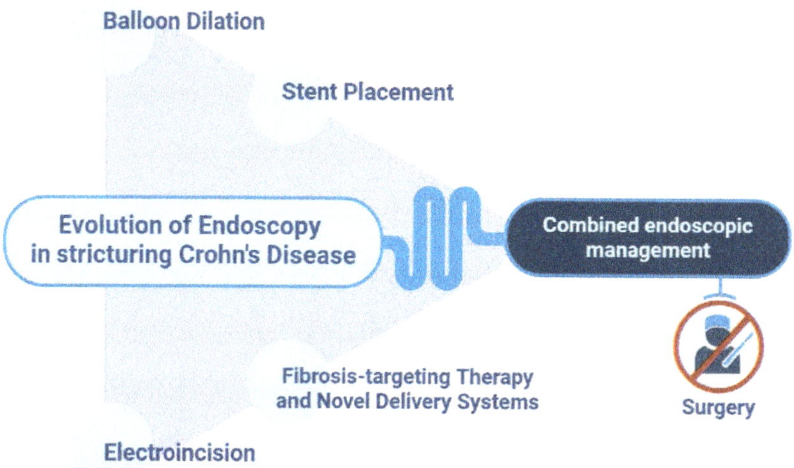

Figure 1. Evolution of endoscopy in stricturing Crohn's Disease. The improvement of the known techniques alongside with the development of new technologies paves the way for an increasingly less invasive, combined endoscopic approach, with a view to tailored management, bowel-sparing strategy, and better quality of life.

2. Methods

A bibliographic search was conducted using electronic databases including PubMed, Scopus, Embase and ClinicalTrials.gov. Search terms used included 'Crohn's disease', 'IBD', 'stricture' combined with 'EBD', 'balloon dilation', 'stricturotomy', 'strictureplasty', 'electroincision', 'intestinal stent', 'nanomedicine', and 'fibrosis'. Additional search terms for comparative studies included 'comparison', 'outcome', 'efficacy', 'safety', 'long-term results', 'clinical trials', 'meta-analysis' and 'randomized controlled trials'. Bibliographies of relevant articles were searched manually; individual authors reviewed the titles and abstracts of the articles to assess their relevance to the study. Special attention was given to identifying comparative studies that directly evaluated the outcomes of EBD compared to other techniques in clinical trials and clinical practice for the treatment of CD-associated strictures. We ensured that the selected comparative studies provided robust data and clear results on regarding efficacy, safety, and long-term outcomes. This approach allowed us to gather relevant information to support the conclusions of our work.

3. Endoscopic Balloon Dilation

3.1. Endoscopic Balloon Dilation as the Standard Endoscopic Procedure for Short Strictures in Crohn's Disease

EBD is the first described endoscopic treatment for intestinal strictures [12]. Since 1986, EBD has been applied for a wide range of gastrointestinal strictures and has been shown to be a straightforward, effective, and safe procedure, rapidly developing into the most used endoscopic treatment in stricturing CD upon proper selection of the patient, setting, and stricture type. Although extensive data are available, the heterogeneity of techniques and study designs made the adequate standardization and generalization of results challenging.

The definition of the efficacy outcomes and the procedure technique widely vary both in study settings and clinical practice. According to the recent practical guidelines on endoscopic management of stricturing CD [9], a standardization of efficacy outcomes is advisable, in particular technical success (post-procedural resistance-free passage of the endoscope through the stricture, specifying the type of endoscope used), clinical efficacy (relief from occlusive symptoms at 6 months), and long-term efficacy (surgery-free survival at 1-year follow up). However, symptoms of CD-associated strictures may not reflect objective findings and the threshold for surgical intervention varies based on the patient and the surgeon's preferences; moreover, the severity of the stricture and the persistence of symptoms might influence the need for an additional EBD [9]. The procedure technique is also not precisely defined and varies widely in the available studies. Currently, graded inflation is recommended over one-step inflation, as it allows proper inspection of the dilated tract after each controlled expansion and reduces the risk of bleeding and intestinal perforation [13]. Balloon sizes range from 12 to 20 mm and each dilation step varying from 20 s to 3 min in the available studies [12]. In a pooled analysis by Reutemann et al., no association between balloon size and surgery-free survival was found. Notably, patients undergoing dilations greater than 18 mm had an increased risk of surgery compared with 14 to 18 mm sizes, possibly due to the refractoriness of the disease in patients treated with larger balloons [14]. Whether all strictures can tolerate the same degree of dilation in a single episode, or instead, if features exist to stratify the dilation capacity of individual stenoses, remains to be clarified. In a systematic review including 33 studies from 1991 to 2013, with 1463 CD patients who underwent 3213 EBD procedures (62% anastomotic, 38% de novo strictures), a length < 5 cm was associated with a longer surgery-free interval after EBD; the rate of technical success was 89.1% and EBD resulted in clinical efficacy (remission of obstructive symptoms) in 80.9% of all patients, with no statistical difference between anastomotic and de novo strictures. However, at 2-year follow-up, 73.5% and 42.9% of patients underwent redilation and resective surgery respectively. A stricture length of <5 cm was associated with a surgery-free outcome with (HR 2.5; 95% CI 1.4–4.4; $p = 0.002$) and without (HR 2.4; 95% CI 1.3–4.2; $p = 0.003$) correction for stricture location, type of strictures, balloon caliber, steroid injection, and accessory endoscopic therapy. A cut-off for stricture length of <5 cm also showed a strong tendency to be associated with a redilation-free outcome ($p = 0.06$); however, no specific cut-off value for balloon size could be definitively recommended, although a larger balloon diameter was identified as a predictive factor for greater technical success [15]. Major complications, like perforation, bleeding, or surgery after dilation, occurred in 2.8% per procedure and 6.2% per patient. It remains unclear whether the efficacy and the complication rate may differ based on a different dilation strategy and technique (single-session versus multiple-session dilation, one-step versus graded dilation). The optimal dilation method for different types of strictures remains unclear. The number of dilations, the interval between dilations, and the length of follow-up highly varied widely between and, in some cases, within the included studies. Moreover, some patients may have undergone dilation in the absence of overt obstruction, which may limit the reliability and stratification of the results. Overall, EBD is indicated in CD patients with symptoms of bowel obstruction and non-complicated, non-angulated strictures shorter than 5 cm (Figure 2) [9]; graded dilation with balloons up to a maximum size of 18–20 mm is recommended [9]. Currently, there is no full agreement on whether or not to perform endoscopic dilation in asymptomatic patients; the patient's symptoms do not necessarily correlate with the functional impairment caused by the stenosis, whereas the endoscopic treatment could delay or prevent symptoms and complication risk. Notably, symptomatic patients who undergo EBD typically have a poorer response to treatment and are at a higher risk of subsequent surgery compared to asymptomatic patients [9]; Similarly, pre-stenotic dilatation is associated with poor response to EBD and increased risk of bowel obstruction and surgery [16] despite representing the setting of the highest potential benefit of the endoscopic strategy when effective [17].

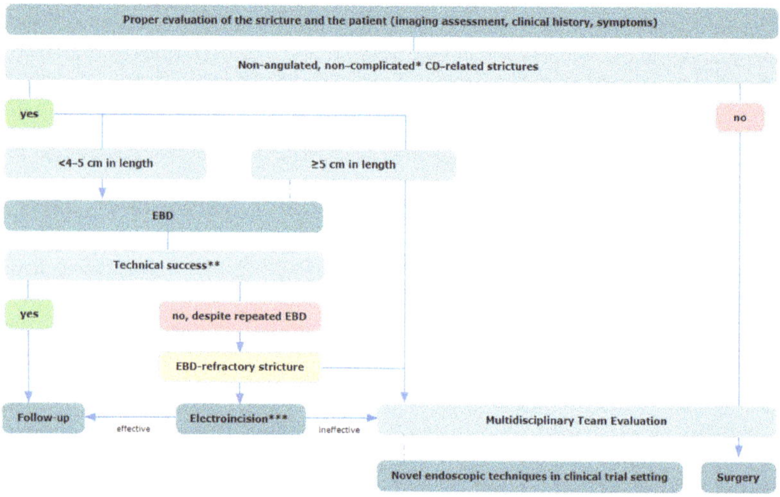

Figure 2. Endoscopic management of strictures in Crohn's Disease based on the practice guidelines on endoscopic treatment for Crohn's disease strictures [9]. CD, Crohn's Disease; EBD, endoscopic balloon dilation. * No adjacent fistulae or abscesses; ** technical success in defined as post-procedural resistance-free passage of the endoscope through the stricture; *** only in centers with specific expertise.

Beyond the many details to be clarified for proper standardization, recent comparative studies (Table 1) and ongoing trials promise to give new insights into the therapeutic role of EBD in CD. For instance, a prospective multicenter observational study is underway to evaluate the role of EBD in ameliorating mucosal and transmural inflammation of the prestenotic intestinal tract. Improved fecal flow and clearance of inflammatory mediators and microbiota could enhance the local gut microenvironment and reduce upstream inflammation (NCT04803916).

Table 1. Comparative studies currently available on the management of CD-associated strictures.

	Study Design	Strictures Location	Treatment and No of Pts	Technical Success Rate	Long-Term Outcomes (Years fu)	Adverse Events, %
[17] 2017	Retrospective	Ileocolic anastomosis	176 EBD 131 surgery	-	average time to surgery/re-surgery delayed by 6.45 years in EBD group	1.1 (perforation) 8.8 (~infection)
[18] 2024	Retrospective	Duodenal	30 EBD 18 surgery	-	2.96 years recurrence-free 6.31 years recurrence-free, $p = 0.01$	0.74 16.67

Table 1. *Cont.*

	Study Design	Strictures Location	Treatment and No of Pts	Technical Success Rate	Long-Term Outcomes (Years fu)	Adverse Events, %
[19] 2018	Retrospective	Anastomosis (85.7% ileocolic)	21 ES 164 EBD	100% 89.5%	9.5% surgery (0.8) 33.5% re-surgery (4)	8.8 (bleeding) 1.1 (perforation)
[20] 2019	Retrospective	Ileocolic anastomosis	35 ES 147 ICR	-	11.3% surgery (0.8) 10.2% re-surgery (2.2), $p = 0.83$	10.2 (~bleeding) 31.9 (~ileus)
[21] 2020	Retrospective	Distal ileum, ileocecal valve	13 ES 32 ICR	100% 100%	15.4% surgery (1.8) 18.8% re-surgery (1.5), $p = 0.79$	6,9 (perforation) 25 (~infection)
[22] 2022	Randomized trial	-	41 EBD 39 FCSEMS	-	80% no re-intervention (1) 51% no re-intervention (1), $p = 0.0061$	2 (perforation) 3 (perforation)

ES, endoscopic electroincision; EBD, endoscopic balloon dilation; FCSEMS, fully-covered self-expandable metallic stents; fu, follow-up ICR, ileocolic resection; *p*, *p*-value; pts, patients; ~, most frequent.

3.2. Intralesional Corticosteroid Injection

The role of intralesional corticosteroid injection following EBD remains unclear, aso two outdated prospective, randomized clinical trials have yielded conflicting results. East et al. compared local quadrantic injection of 40 mg of triamcinolone after EBD of short ileocolic anastomotic CD strictures (<5 cm) to saline placebo [23]; 1 in 6 patients in the placebo group required redilation compared to 5 in 7 in the steroid group, with a statistical trend towards a difference in time to repeat dilation, which was worse in the steroid group (p 0.06, HR 6.1). In a similar setting, Di Nardo et al. enrolled 29 pediatric CD patients with both de novo (17) and anastomotic (12) short strictures to receive or not intralesional quadrantic injection of 40 mg triamcinolone after EBD. In the placebo group, 5 and 4 of 14 patients required redilation and surgery at 12-month follow-up, respectively; in the experimental group only 1 out of 15 patients required redilation, and none required surgery. The groups differed significantly in time without re-dilation ($p = 0.04$) and surgery ($p = 0.02$) [24]. The results of these two trials are quite contrasting despite using similar injection techniques. However, a proper comparison between the two studies is limited by small sample sizes, different populations, and different stricture locations. In 2022, Feleshtynsky et al. displayed a new perspective on this issue, evaluating the efficacy of intralesional prednisolone injection after EBD compared to EBD alone in 64 CD patients [25]. The stricture recurrence risk in the combination arm was 4.5 times lower than in the EBD-alone arm at the 12-month follow-up, with clinical remission maintained in 90.7% of patients in the combination arm compared to 65.7% in the EBD_alone arm. In addition, the redilation rate was lower in the combination arm (1.1 ± 0.3 versus 1.44 ± 0.66). Notably, the combination arm observed a better epithelial structure and decreased cellular infiltration and fibrotic deposition at the histological level. No significant difference was reported in terms of perforation and bleeding risk; however, no data concerning stricture location was shown. As a result, the true benefits or harms of intralesional steroid injections after EBD remain unknown, and this technique is not recommended in clinical practice, still representing a missed chance in stricturing CD management.

3.3. Endoscopic Balloon Dilation in the Upper Gastrointestinal Tract

Available data on endoscopic management of strictures of upper gastrointestinal tract is still limited, in part due to the lower prevalence of upper gastrointestinal localization and the higher incidence of complex disease in this region, which often requires surgical intervention. Most studies do not provide a separate analysis on the use of EBD for CD-associated strictures of the upper gastrointestinal tract. However, Betterworth et al. analyzed data from multicenter cohort studies involving 94 CD patients who underwent EBD for upper gastrointestinal strictures (107 in the duodenum, 30 in the stomach, 4 in both).

Technical and clinical success rates were 100% and 87% respectively. Major complications occurred in 2.9% per procedure, and patients with small-bowel disease location had a higher risk of symptom recurrence and need for redilation. Long-term outcomes were not significantly different fromileocecal stricturesat 24 months (70.5% vs. 75.9% symptom recurrence, 59.6% vs. 73.5% need for redilation, and 30.8% vs. 42.9% surgery) [16]. A recent single-center experience study (2002–2018) investigated the outcomes of 86 patients with benign duodenal stenosis treated with EBD, including 19 patients with CD. This cohort study reported high technical and clinical success rates, which was higher for repeated EBD in CD patients (91.7%)compared to the clinical success rate of repeated EBD for all other aetiologies (74.3%). There were two cases of bleeding (2.3%) and no perforations [26]. Furthermore, patients who underwent aggressive initial dilation were less likely to repeat dilation compared to non-aggressive initial dilation (mean 5.39 versus 4.07 mm more than the estimated caliber of the stricture, p 0.07). However, among the 19 patients with CD, 6 still required surgical intervention.

Despite limited evidence available, EBD is gaining traction for duodenal disease [18], demonstrating its potential use in the upper gastrointestinal tract as well. Overall, EBD is considered comparably effective in the short term for both the upper and lower gastrointestinal tract, although its impact on long-term outcomes remains to be evaluated.

3.4. Focus on Dilation during Enteroscopy, a Stand-Alone Situation?

CD-related deep small bowel strictures require access through device-assisted enteroscopy, including balloon-assisted enteroscopy (BAE), with outcomes similar to those for strictures reachable by ileocolonoscopy [5,27–29]. In a recent meta-analysis of 463 CD patients who underwent EBD for deep small bowel strictures, the overall technical success rate was 94.9%, with a short-term clinical efficacy of 82.3%. During follow-up (median time 25.5 months, IQR 6–53 months), 48.3% of patients reported a recurrence of symptoms, 38.8% were re-dilated, and 27.4% underwent surgery [13]. A nationwide, multicenter, retrospective Japanese study reported surgical conversion rates of 26.0%, 45.6%, and 55.7% at 1, 5, and 10 years post-EBD, respectively [30]; however, this study is based on a large population of patients undergoing dilation with enteroscopy over dilation of the lower gastrointestinal tract (181 over 305), with no differential analysis on deep small bowel strictures. Another prospective, multicenter, Japanese study analyzed EBD through BAE in 95 CD patients, reporting clinical success in 69.5% of the patients, associated with a larger balloon diameter (15.20 $\pm$ 1.70 vs. 13.65 $\pm$ 2.59 mm, $p = 0.03$) and with a good safety profile (5%, all conservatively managed complications) [27]. Furthermore, a systematic review concluded that dilation of 15 mm or more is a risk factor for perforation [31]; consequently, the generally recommended final target diameter is 12–15 mm in this setting, despite heterogeneous data [32]. Focusing on complications, a systematic review reported incidence rates of severe bleeding and complications requiring surgery between 1.82% and 3.21%, while the incidence rate of perforation ranged from 0–10% in several observational studies [13,27,33]. Possibly due to the increased difficulty and invasiveness of the procedure, higher complication rates have been observed after enteroscopic EBD compared to EBD for ileocecal and gastroduodenal stenosis [15,16].

Overall, due to the lack of specific and comparative evidence on EBD efficacy stratified by stricture localization, these data allow us to affirm that EBD during BAE is comparable to EBD performed in locations achievable by colonoscopy in terms of short-term safety and efficacy. This suggests that EBD has a similar efficacy regardless of stricture location. However, lacking location-specific data, it is still not possible to speculate further, especially on long-term effectiveness and surgery rates.

4. Endoscopic Electroincision: Stricturotomy and Strictureplasty

In recent years, there has been increasing interest in stricturotomy (ESt) and strictureplasty (ESTx) as alternatives to EBD in the endoscopic management of stricturing CD. Similar to EBD, these procedures lack standardization in technique and outcome terminology, possibly delaying their exact placement in the IBD landscape. In 2020, the Global Interventional Inflammatory Bowel Disease Group provided detailed guidance and suggested the use of 'endoscopic electroincision (ES)' as a unique term for techniques utilizing electrocautery to cut strictured tissue. Electroincision to widen the stenotic lumen (ESt) can be performed using different needle-knives in radial, horizontal, or circumferential orientations, with the possibility of endoscopic clipping after the incision to consolidate the cut with a secondary closure, keeping the lumen wider (ESx) [9]. Endoscopic electroincision is commonly used for papillotomy in endoscopic retrograde cholangiopancreatography, with recent data on esophageal and, more recently, biliopancreatic strictures [34–36].

In 2011, Nal et al. published the first case series describing 10 IBD patients with long, fibrotic ileal-pouch strictures refractory to EBD who were treated with ES [37]; the same group from the Cleveland Clinic retrospectively evaluated the efficacy and safety of ES in treating primary and secondary strictures in IBD patients, comparing it with EBD and ileocolic resection [19–21,38]. The retrospective study included 50 UC patients with ileal-pouch anastomosis strictures and 35 CD patients (mostly ileocolic anastomosis), with a total of 127 strictures treated with ES, demonstrating a 100% technical success of the procedure [38]. In a median follow-up of 0.9 years, 60.6% of strictures required multiple treatments after the first ES, mostly a subsequent ES (44.9%), an EBD (22.8%), or both combined (11.0%). The cumulative 3-year surgery-free survival rate was 62.0%. Only one patient (0.4% per procedure) experienced perforation, and nine patients (3.3% per procedure) had postprocedural bleeding. The study comparing ES with EBD included CD patients with anastomotic strictures (85.7% ileocolic). It showed a technical success rate of 100% in the 21 patients treated with ES and 89.5% in the 164 patients treated with EBD ($p = 0.25$) [19]. No significant difference in the need for additional endoscopic treatment was found between the two groups ($p = 0.85$). Only two patients (9.5%) in the ES group required subsequent surgery, compared to 55 (33.5%) in the EBD group ($p = 0.03$). It should be noted that the follow-up varied between the two groups, with a median of 0.8 years (IQR: 0.1–1.6) for the ES group and 4.0 years (IQR: 0.8–6.9) for the EBD group ($p < 0.0001$). ES showed a lower risk of perforation than EBD (0% vs. 1.1%), although there were major concerns about bleeding (8.8% vs. 0%). When compared with ileocolic resection (ICR), ES showed comparable surgery-free survival in two different retrospective studies. In the first study on ileocolic anastomosis strictures, 4 out of 35 patients (11.3%) in the ES group and 15 out of 147 patients (10.2%) in the ICR group required subsequent surgery ($p = 0.83$), with a median follow-up duration of 0.8 years for the ES group and 2.2 years for the ICR group ($p < 0.001$) [20]. In the second study on primary distal ileal and ileocecal valve strictures, 2 out of 13 patients (15.4%) in the ES group and 6 out of 32 patients (18.8%) in the ICR group required subsequent surgery ($p = 0.79$) [21]. In this case, the median follow-up duration was comparable: 1.8 years for the ES group and 1.5 years for the ICR group ($p = 0.84$). In both studies, ES showed a lower incidence of major adverse events compared to ICR. Nevertheless, the two groups differed significantly in stricture complexity, with the ICR group having statistically longer and more symptomatic strictures. Even if the majority of the strictures treated with ES in the published studies were located in the ileocolic anastomosis, ES was found to be feasible and safe also for refractory rectal anastomotic strictures [39].

In the IBD setting, low data on ES efficacy is available. Recently, 24 patients with endoscopic non-traversable anorectal/anopouch strictures (18 CD and 4 UC patients) were treated with ES, with a technical success of 100%. However, the mean time to endoscopic reintervention with subsequent ES of 5.3 months. Over a 12.8-month follow-up, two patients (8%) required surgical intervention for refractory stricture disease. No 30-day post-procedure adverse events were reported [40]. ES has been used for deep small bowel strictures in CD (including both the ileum and the jejunum). A multicenter cohort study evaluated the efficacy and safety of BAE-assisted ES for treating these strictures in 28 CD patients with 58 non-passable deep small bowel strictures, resulting in a technical success of 96% and a 1-year cumulative surgery-free rate of 74.8% [41]. Finally, ES is a feasible option for CD-associated anorectal strictures, although evidence is still limited [9].

Overall, ES is a promising procedure for the endoscopic management of stricturing CD, although a slow learning curve could hinder the widespread use of these techniques. Two randomized clinical trials (BEST-CD and DESTRESS) are currently underway to compare EBD and ES in terms of clinical success, need for surgery, and safety with 1-year follow-up in patients with short CD-associated strictures (NCT05521867, NCT05009212).

5. The Graveyard of Endoscopic Techniques: Is There Room for a Second Chance?

The history of the endoscopic treatment of stricturing CD has seen the development of several techniques, eventually failing to emerge from the overgrowth into clinical practice for several reasons, including inconsistent clinical trial results, technical difficulties, invasiveness to the patient, poor reproducibility, limited large-scale applicability, and cost. Among the most explored, local injection therapy with anti-tumor necrosis factor (anti-TNF) and endoscopic stents have shown promising results, as well as ongoing novel attempts of improvement to access the IBD treatment landscape.

5.1. Anti-TNF Intralesional Injection

Anti-TNF injection has shown promise, although this approach has been nearly abandoned also in the trial setting. In 2008, a pilot study involving 3 CD patients investigated local injections of infliximab (IFX) (90–120 mg) into colonic strictures, resulting in clinical efficacy at 5–8 months in all patients. One patient unresponsive to IFX therapy saw the complete resolution of the stricture after the first local injection and remained symptom-free for 5 months after a second injection. Another patient required additional stricture dilation, while the third one needed five injections every four months [42]. Similarly, another exploratory study from 2014 assessed the efficacy of intralesional injections of 40 mg of infliximab combined with EBD in EBD-refractory small bowel strictures (either primary or anastomotic) in 6 CD patients. Five out of 6 patients underwent serial EBD at 0, 2, and 6 weeks, receiving intralesional infliximab injections after each session. All patients showed a decrease of modified Simple Endoscopic Score for Crohn's Disease (mSES-CD) by an average of 3 points (reduction in ulcer size, ulcerated surface area, and disease-affected surface area of the distal visible part of the narrowed tract) and improved symptoms, with no adverse effects observed at 6-month follow-up [43]. However, although the authors specify that all enrolled patients had not been previously exposed to infliximab, they do not provide information on any concomitant medical therapies the patients might have been receiving.

A larger, multicenter, randomized, controlled trial on the efficacy of injecting adalimumab into intestinal CD strictures is displayed on trialgov, but it was eventually not published (NCT01986127). While local anti-TNF therapy seems well tolerated, more extended follow-up and larger randomized controlled clinical trials would be necessary to establish its potential benefits. The effectiveness could be significant, moving from a one-time therapy to repeated injection, with anticipated issues concerning quality of life, invasiveness, and health care costs [42,44].

5.2. Self-Expanding Metal Stents

Self-expandable metallic stents (SEMS) constitute an effective, non-surgical treatment for neoplastic intestinal obstruction, both as a palliative measure and as a bridge to surgery [45]. SEMS must be fully or partially covered with a plastic film, which prevents colonization by the intestinal mucosa and allows a smooth, delayed extraction. Loras et al. conducted an extensive literature review, describing 19 studies for a total of 65 patients. They identified SEMS as a safe and effective alternative to EBD and surgery for the treatment of short stenosis in CD patients, with possible advantages for complex or longer (>5 cm) strictures [45]. A retrospective study by the same group, involving 17 CD patients treated with SEMS for symptomatic refractory colonic and ileocolic anastomosis strictures, reported a clinical efficacy rate of 64.7%, with patients remaining free of symptoms for an average follow-up period of 67 weeks [46]. Migration occurred in 52% of patients, and there were 4 cases of impaction, with one patient requiring surgery due to proximal stent migration. Another retrospective cohort study involving five patients with anastomotic strictures, where uncovered SEMS were placed for an average of 9.7 months, reported an 80% clinical efficacy rate at a mean follow-up of 28 months [47]. The complication rate was 20% (n = 1), and the four patients who did not require re-intervention showed an average long-term luminal patency of 34.8 months [47]. A prospective cohort study involving 11 patients who received SEMS showed a 60% clinical success rate, with an adverse event rate of 73% (8/11), of which two patients required surgery related to the procedure, and six patients experienced stent migration after an average time of 3 days. As a result, it was concluded that the risk of complications was too high to recommend the routine use of endoscopic metal stents for CD strictures [48]. In a recent study with 21 CD patients, SEMS placement and following removal on day 7 resulted in clinical remission in 88% (14 of 16) of patients during follow-up (3–50 months) [49], with an adverse event rate of 21%, including abdominal pain and asymptomatic stent migration. In a comparative study, 80 CD patients with symptomatic strictures (60% shorter than 4 cm) were randomized to fully-covered SEMS (39) or EBD (41). Despite a similar safety profile, the stent group had a significantly higher proportion of patients requiring new therapeutic intervention at one-year follow-up due to symptoms recurrence (49% vs. 20%) [22]. Notably, the difference in efficacy between EBD and fully-covered SEMS was not significant for strictures over 3 cm (both treatments achieving nearly 65% success) and primary stenosis (respectively 60% and 70%), with a high migration rate representing a potential limiting factor. Given the high rate of stent migration, Branche et al. investigated the Hanarostent stent, a partly covered SEMS with an antimigratory design and an early removal protocol. Following promising results of an exploratory study in 7 CD patients [50], they conducted a larger national study with the same device in 46 CD patients (73.9% with anastomotic stricture, median length of 3.1 ± 1.7 cm). The study observed clinical efficacy in 58.7% of the patients at 26 months follow-up, with no perforations and only three stent migrations reported (6.5%) [51]. Comparative research is ongoing with a randomized clinical trial comparing EBD followed by SEMS placement versus surgical intervention in CD patients with de novo and primary symptomatic stenosis less than 10 cm long [52].

5.3. Lumen-Apposing Metal Stents

Lumen-apposing metal stents (LAMS) are short, fully covered metal stents with large flanges at each end to anchor the stent and minimize migration risk [53,54]. Initially designed for draining pancreatic fluid collections, LAMS has been used off-label to manage short-segment luminal strictures [55,56], with several studies showing promising outcomes. Regarding CD patients, evidence is limited: In the light of two case reports on anastomotic strictures showing short-term clinical efficacy and no post-procedural complications [57,58], Hedjoudje et al. evaluated LAMS for lower gastrointestinal anastomotic strictures in 28 patients, including 18 with CD-associated anastomotic strictures. Technical success was achieved in all patients, with clinical efficacy at the last follow-up visit in 85.7% (24/28) of patients. Among the three patients experiencing adverse events, one patient missing his 3-month CT scan experienced failed stent extraction 7 months post-placement and subsequently required surgical resection. Spontaneous asymptomatic stent migration occurred in 47% (13/28) of patients without recurrent symptoms or significant complications [59]. Unfortunately, the authors did not provide a separate analysis for the subgroup of patients with IBD.

5.4. Biodegradable Stents

Considering the high migration rates and the need for follow-up endoscopy for the removal of SEMS, biodegradable stents (BDS) have been developed and primarily evaluated for esophageal strictures, yielding promising outcomes [60–62]. However, they are not approved for bowel strictures. BDS exert a constant radial force for approximately 4–5 weeks to treat the underlying esophageal disease, while progressive hydrolysis-mediated self-degradation prevents tissue overgrowth and leads to dissolving within 12 weeks [63]. A prospective study evaluated polydioxanone monofilament stents, which provide 6–8 weeks of radial force before degradation, in a cohort of 11 patients with benign small and large intestinal stenosis naïve to EBD [64]. The study showed a technical success rate of 91%, with no adverse events other than early stent migration in three patients. However, few studies, mainly case reports and series, have investigated BDS in stricturing CD. Rejchrt et al. reported successful BDS insertion for small and large bowel stenosis in 10 out of 11 CD patients, with early stent migration (2 days to 8 weeks) observed in three patients [64]. Karstensen et al. documented the case of a 52-year-old man with CD, successfully treated with a custom-made biodegradable polydioxanone monofilament stent (15 cm) for a 12 cm small bowel stricture, remaining symptom-free at 3-month follow-up [65]. However, a subsequent study by the same group involving six CD patients with intestinal stenosis at various locations (duodenal bulb, ileocolic anastomosis, afferent limb of a J-pouch, and sigmoid colon) refractory to EBD and treated with biodegradable stents, reported clinical success in only one patient. Failures were attributed to mucosal overgrowth in two patients, stent migration in one patient, and stent collapse in another [66].

6. New Techniques and Future Scenarios for Stenosis and Fibrosis Treatment in IBD Involving Pathogenesis and Molecular Pathways

Future scenarios for stenosis treatment in IBD are likely to involve a combination of minimally invasive procedures and targeted therapies. As we improve our knowledge of fibrosis pathogenesis and stenosis development in IBD, novel therapeutic opportunities are emerging, combining the identification of new molecular targets with the development of innovative local delivery systems.

The advent of single-cell transcriptomics has better defined the transcriptional profile of fibroblasts in CD and ulcerative colitis (UC) [67,68]. Targeting fibroblasts at a cellular and molecular level has been a promising subject of investigation. For instance, when adding pirfenidone, an agent approved for treating idiopathic pulmonary fibrosis, to fibroblasts isolated from patients with stricturing CD, their function and proliferation are inhibited via downregulation of the transforming growth factor beta 1 (TGFβ1) pathway [69]. Parallelly, several small experimental molecules have been tested as potential inhibitors of the main molecular pattern of fibrosis, with still inconclusive and inconsistent results [70,71]. Moreover, stem cell manipulation and administration offer a promising scenario with a constantly increasing body of evidence. Human adipose-derived mesenchymal stem cells, pretreated in vivo with interferon (IFN)γ and kynurenic acid, ameliorate intestinal injury in a fibrosis rat model [72]. Both prophylactic and therapeutic treatment with bone marrow-derived mesenchymal stem cells improve fibrosis and reduce collagen deposition, via interleukin(IL)-1beta, IL-6, and IL-13 downregulation, and IL-10 upregulation [73]. In experimental colitis mice, mesenchymal stem cells can reduce the thickness of submucosa/muscularis propria, as well as collagen deposition. Furthermore, in human primary intestinal myofibroblasts mesenchymal stem cells reduce the TGF-β1-induced fibrogenic activation [74]. Antibodies targeting proteins involved in collagen remodeling have been identified as a possible therapeutic strategy as well; the inhibition of matrix metalloproteinase-9 (MMP-9), a type IV collagenase overexpressed in fistulizing and stricturing CD, led to reduced collagen deposition in heterotopic xenograft models of intestinal fibrosis [75]. Among other unexplored therapeutic targets is teduglutide, already approved for the treatment of short bowel syndrome. Teduglutide has shown a reduction in fibrogenesis and improved fibrinolysis from the first week after surgery in a murine model of ileal resection and anastomosis [76,77]. More recently, the anti-fibrogenic effects of glucagon-like peptide 2 (GLP2) have also been demonstrated in the liver of a murine model of cholangitis [78].

Novel biomarkers and pharmacological agents will play a crucial role in enhancing treatment outcomes, possibly involving novel local delivery systems to allow tissue-targeted therapy and minimize side effects. Over the past two decades, there was a slow but consistent understory of research and development of a large number of nanoparticles (NPs) in IBDs. NPs are polymeric fine units with at least one dimension up to 100 nm, which can be built to reach an intended target, be detected with a molecular imaging technique and further engineered to locally deploy a certain agent. They employ several mechanisms of activation, including charge-mediated targeting, micro-environment–triggered release targeting, and ligand-mediated targeting [79,80]. Nanomedicine combined with endoscopy has built up a solid background in ex vivo and in vivo preclinical settings, with minimal preliminary clinical data concerning esophageal and biliary cancers [79,81,82]. However, there has been no significant impact on clinical practice, partly due to safety concerns, heterogeneity of NPs, practical application issues, and variability in study designs. The dual potential of NPs as drug-eluting and detectable nano vehicles represents an exciting perspective in IBD, potentially leading to dose-controlled and selective insite bioavailability of a drug or a therapeutic intervention targeting inflamed mucosa [83], eventually within strictures. Among intestinal delivery systems, another remarkable product recently developed is a biocompatible hydrogel amenable to endoscopic application (CoverGel), showing intriguing preclinical data. In experimental colitis mice, when comparing CoverGel + IFX versus subcutaneous IFX alone, similar efficacy on inflammation was observed, with significantly lower levels of antibodies to infliximab in the CoverGel group [84].

7. Conclusions

In the last decades, endoscopy has been engaging stricturing CD as a minimally invasive approach aiming to delay and prevent surgery and promote a superior quality of life. Although EBD is indeed the standard of care for short strictures, the extensive data available is burdened by wide variability in dilation technique and study settings, leaving several unsolved issues mostly concerning long-term outcomes. In this scenario, novel endoscopic techniques are emerging, with still preliminary conflicting results and active research ongoing. Moreover, the new insight into the molecular patterns of fibrosis paves the way for future developments, possibly aided by new endoscopic local drug-eluting systems.

More long-term, head-to-head prospective studies are essential to eventually move endoscopic management out of the gray area between a bridge to surgery and a bowel-sparing technique.

Author Contributions: C.P., F.D.V., P.P., A.D.G., I.C. and B.B. revised the literature and wrote the manuscript; G.C. (Gaetano Coppola) developed the concept, revised the literature, and wrote the manuscript; A.P., G.C. (Giovanni Cammarota) and L.R.L. supervised the research and revised the manuscript; F.S. developed the concept, supervised the research, and revised the manuscript. All investigators participated in data interpretation and contributed to the revision of the final version of the manuscript. All authors have read and agreed to the published version of the manuscript.

Funding: This research received no external funding.

Institutional Review Board Statement: Not applicable.

Informed Consent Statement: Not applicable.

Data Availability Statement: Not applicable.

Acknowledgments: Figure 1 was created with BioRender.com.

Conflicts of Interest: The authors declare no conflict of interest.

References

1. Torres, J.; Mehandru, S.; Colombel, J.-F.; Peyrin-Biroulet, L. Crohn's disease. *Lancet* **2017**, *389*, 1741–1755. [CrossRef] [PubMed]
2. Rieder, F.; Zimmermann, E.M.; Remzi, F.H.; Sandborn, W.J. Crohn's disease complicated by strictures: A systematic review. *Gut* **2013**, *62*, 1072–1084. [CrossRef]

3. Gasche, C.; Scholmerich, J.; Brynskov, J.; D'Haens, G.; Hanauer, S.B.; Irvine, J.E.; Jewell, D.P.; Rachmilewitz, D.; Sachar, D.B.; Sandborn, W.J.; et al. A simple classification of Crohn's disease: Report of the working party for the world congresses of gastroenterology, vienna 1998. *Inflamm. Bowel Dis.* **2000**, *6*, 8–15. [CrossRef] [PubMed]
4. Nikolaus, S.; Schreiber, S. Diagnostics of inflammatory bowel disease. *Gastroenterology* **2007**, *133*, 1670–1689. [CrossRef] [PubMed]
5. Rieder, F.; Latella, G.; Magro, F.; Yuksel, E.S.; Higgins, P.D.R.; Di Sabatino, A.; de Bruyn, J.R.; Rimola, J.; Brito, J.; Bettenworth, D.; et al. European Crohn's and Colitis organisation topical review on prediction, diagnosis and management of fibrostenosing crohn's disease. *J. Crohn's Colitis* **2016**, *10*, 873–885. [CrossRef]
6. Maaser, C.; Sturm, A.; Vavricka, S.R.; Kucharzik, T.; Fiorino, G.; Annese, V.; Calabrese, E.; Baumgart, D.C.; Bettenworth, D.; Borralho Nunes, P.; et al. ECCO-ESGAR Guideline for Diagnostic Assessment in IBD Part 1: Initial diagnosis, monitoring of known IBD, detection of complications. *J. Crohn's Colitis* **2019**, *13*, 144–164. [CrossRef]
7. Lopes, S.; Rodrigues-Pinto, E.; Andrade, P.; Afonso, J.; Baron, T.H.; Magro, F.; Macedo, G. Endoscopic balloon dilation of Crohn's disease strictures-safety, efficacy and clinical impact. *World J. Gastroenterol.* **2017**, *23*, 7397–7406. [CrossRef]
8. Pokala, A.; Shen, B. Update of endoscopic management of Crohn's disease strictures. *Intest. Res.* **2020**, *18*, 1–10. [CrossRef]
9. Shen, B.; Kochhar, G.; Navaneethan, U.; Farraye, F.A.; Schwartz, D.A.; Iacucci, M.; Bernstein, C.N.; Dryden, G.; Cross, R.; Bruining, D.H.; et al. Practical guidelines on endoscopic treatment for Crohn's disease strictures: A consensus statement from the Global Interventional Inflammatory Bowel Disease Group. *Lancet Gastroenterol. Hepatol.* **2020**, *5*, 393–405. [CrossRef]
10. Nardone, O.M.; Cannatelli, R.; Zardo, D.; Ghosh, S.; Iacucci, M. Can advanced endoscopic techniques for assessment of mucosal inflammation and healing approximate histology in inflammatory bowel disease? *Ther. Adv. Gastroenterol.* **2019**, *12*, 1756284819863015. [CrossRef]
11. Santacroce, G.; Zammarchi, I.; Tan, C.K.; Coppola, G.; Varley, R.; Ghosh, S.; Iacucci, M. Present and future of endoscopy precision for inflammatory bowel disease. *Dig. Endosc.* **2024**, *36*, 292–304. [CrossRef] [PubMed]
12. Klag, T.; Wehkamp, J.; Goetz, M. Endoscopic Balloon Dilation for Crohn's Disease-Associated Strictures. *Clin. Endosc.* **2017**, *50*, 429–436. [CrossRef] [PubMed]
13. Bettenworth, D.; Bokemeyer, A.; Kou, L.; Lopez, R.; Bena, J.F.; El Ouali, S.; Mao, R.; Kurada, S.; Bhatt, A.; Beyna, T.; et al. Systematic review with meta-analysis: Efficacy of balloon-assisted enteroscopy for dilation of small bowel Crohn's disease strictures. *Aliment. Pharmacol. Ther.* **2020**, *52*, 1104–1116. [CrossRef]
14. Reutemann, B.A.; Turkeltaub, J.A.; Al-Hawary, M.; Waljee, A.K.; Higgins, P.D.R.; Stidham, R.W. Endoscopic balloon dilation size and avoidance of surgery in stricturing crohn's disease. *Inflamm. Bowel Dis.* **2017**, *23*, 1803–1809. [CrossRef]
15. Bettenworth, D.; Gustavsson, A.; Atreja, A.; Lopez, R.; Tysk, C.; van Assche, G.; Rieder, F. A Pooled Analysis of Efficacy, Safety, and Long-term Outcome of Endoscopic Balloon Dilation Therapy for Patients with Stricturing Crohn's Disease. *Inflamm. Bowel Dis.* **2017**, *23*, 133–142. [CrossRef] [PubMed]
16. Bettenworth, D.; Mücke, M.M.; Lopez, R.; Singh, A.; Zhu, W.; Guo, F.; Matsui, T.; James, T.W.; Herfarth, H.; Goetz, M.; et al. Efficacy of Endoscopic Dilation of Gastroduodenal Crohn's Disease Strictures: A Systematic Review and Meta-Analysis of Individual Patient Data. *Clin. Gastroenterol. Hepatol.* **2019**, *17*, 2514–2522.e8. [CrossRef]
17. Lian, L.; Stocchi, L.; Remzi, F.H.; Shen, B. Comparison of endoscopic dilation vs surgery for anastomotic stricture in patients with crohn's disease following ileocolonic resection. *Clin. Gastroenterol. Hepatol.* **2017**, *15*, 1226–1231. [CrossRef] [PubMed]
18. Chen, Y.; Sun, Z.; Li, Z.; Duan, M.; Zhou, Y.; Li, Y.; Zhu, W.; Guo, Z. Comparison of endoscopic balloon dilation and surgery for duodenal stricture in patients with Crohn's disease. *Scand. J. Gastroenterol.* **2024**, *59*, 39–45. [CrossRef] [PubMed]
19. Lan, N.; Shen, B. Endoscopic stricturotomy versus balloon dilation in the treatment of anastomotic strictures in crohn's disease. *Inflamm. Bowel Dis.* **2018**, *24*, 897–907. [CrossRef]
20. Lan, N.; Stocchi, L.; Delaney, C.P.; Hull, T.L.; Shen, B. Endoscopic stricturotomy versus ileocolonic resection in the treatment of ileocolonic anastomotic strictures in Crohn's disease. *Gastrointest. Endosc.* **2019**, *90*, 259–268. [CrossRef]
21. Lan, N.; Hull, T.L.; Shen, B. Endoscopic stricturotomy and ileo-colonic resection in patients with primary Crohn's disease-related distal ileum strictures. *Gastroenterol. Rep.* **2020**, *8*, 312–318. [CrossRef] [PubMed]
22. Loras, C.; Andújar, X.; Gornals, J.B.; Sanchiz, V.; Brullet, E.; Sicilia, B.; Martín-Arranz, M.D.; Naranjo, A.; Barrio, J.; Dueñas, C.; et al. Self-expandable metal stents versus endoscopic balloon dilation for the treatment of strictures in Crohn's disease (ProtDilat study): An open-label, multicentre, randomised trial. *Lancet Gastroenterol. Hepatol.* **2022**, *7*, 332–341. [CrossRef]
23. East, J.E.; Brooker, J.C.; Rutter, M.D.; Saunders, B.P. A pilot study of intrastricture steroid versus placebo injection after balloon dilatation of Crohn's strictures. *Clin. Gastroenterol. Hepatol.* **2007**, *5*, 1065–1069. [CrossRef]
24. Di Nardo, G.; Oliva, S.; Passariello, M.; Pallotta, N.; Civitelli, F.; Frediani, S.; Gualdi, G.; Gandullia, P.; Mallardo, S.; Cucchiara, S. Intralesional steroid injection after endoscopic balloon dilation in pediatric Crohn's disease with stricture: A prospective, randomized, double-blind, controlled trial. *Gastrointest. Endosc.* **2010**, *72*, 1201–1208. [CrossRef]
25. Feleshtynskiy, Y.; Mylianovska, A.; Pirogovsky, V.; Dyadyk, O. Evaluation of the endoscopic treatment with topical prednisolone administration for intestinal strictures in Crohn's disease. *Pol. Przegl. Chir.* **2021**, *94*, 28–33. [CrossRef] [PubMed]
26. Chittajallu, V.; Omar, Y.A.; Simons-Linares, C.R.; Chahal, P. Endoscopic balloon dilation management for benign duodenal stenosis. *Surg. Endosc.* **2023**, *37*, 3610–3618. [CrossRef]
27. Hirai, F.; Andoh, A.; Ueno, F.; Watanabe, K.; Ohmiya, N.; Nakase, H.; Kato, S.; Esaki, M.; Endo, Y.; Yamamoto, H.; et al. Efficacy of Endoscopic Balloon Dilation for Small Bowel Strictures in Patients with Crohn's Disease: A Nationwide, Multi-centre, Open-label, Prospective Cohort Study. *J. Crohn's Colitis* **2018**, *12*, 394–401. [CrossRef]

28. Gionchetti, P.; Dignass, A.; Danese, S.; Magro Dias, F.J.; Rogler, G.; Lakatos, P.L.; Adamina, M.; Ardizzone, S.; Buskens, C.J.; Sebastian, S.; et al. 3rd European Evidence-based Consensus on the Diagnosis and Management of Crohn's Disease 2016: Part 2: Surgical Management and Special Situations. *J. Crohn's Colitis* **2017**, *11*, 135–149. [CrossRef] [PubMed]
29. Adamina, M.; Bonovas, S.; Raine, T.; Spinelli, A.; Warusavitarne, J.; Armuzzi, A.; Bachmann, O.; Bager, P.; Biancone, L.; Bokemeyer, B.; et al. ECCO guidelines on therapeutics in crohn's disease: Surgical treatment. *J. Crohn's Colitis* **2020**, *14*, 155–168. [CrossRef]
30. Bamba, S.; Sakemi, R.; Fujii, T.; Takeda, T.; Fujioka, S.; Takenaka, K.; Kitamoto, H.; Umezawa, S.; Sakuraba, H.; Inokuchi, T.; et al. A nationwide, multi-center, retrospective study of symptomatic small bowel stricture in patients with Crohn's disease. *J. Gastroenterol.* **2020**, *55*, 615–626. [CrossRef]
31. Baars, J.E.; Theyventhiran, R.; Aepli, P.; Saxena, P.; Kaffes, A.J. Double-balloon enteroscopy-assisted dilatation avoids surgery for small bowel strictures: A systematic review. *World J. Gastroenterol.* **2017**, *23*, 8073–8081. [CrossRef] [PubMed]
32. Yamamoto, H.; Yano, T.; Araki, A.; Esaki, M.; Ohtsuka, K.; Ohmiya, N.; Oka, S.; Nakase, H.; Bamba, S.; Hirai, F.; et al. Guidelines for endoscopic balloon dilation in treating Crohn's disease-associated small intestinal strictures (supplement to the Clinical Practice Guidelines for Enteroscopy). *Dig. Endosc.* **2022**, *34*, 1278–1296. [CrossRef] [PubMed]
33. Fukumoto, A.; Tanaka, S.; Yamamoto, H.; Yao, T.; Matsui, T.; Iida, M.; Goto, H.; Sakamoto, C.; Chiba, T.; Sugano, K. Diagnosis and treatment of small-bowel stricture by double balloon endoscopy. *Gastrointest. Endosc.* **2007**, *66*, S108–S112. [CrossRef] [PubMed]
34. Fukatsu, H.; Kawamoto, H.; Harada, R.; Tsutsumi, K.; Fujii, M.; Kato, H.; Hirao, K.; Nakanishi, T.; Mizuno, O.; Ogawa, T.; et al. Quantitative assessment of technical proficiency in performing needle-knife precut papillotomy. *Surg. Endosc.* **2009**, *23*, 2066–2072. [CrossRef] [PubMed]
35. Simmons, D.T.; Baron, T.H. Electroincision of refractory esophagogastric anastomotic strictures. *Dis. Esophagus* **2006**, *19*, 410–414. [CrossRef] [PubMed]
36. Tringali, A.; Milluzzo, S.M.; Perri, V.; Schepis, T.; Bove, V.; Costamagna, G. Endoscopic electroincision of challenging benign biliopancreatic strictures. *Endosc. Int. Open* **2022**, *10*, E1297–E1301. [CrossRef] [PubMed]
37. Shen, B.; Lian, L.; Kiran, R.P.; Queener, E.; Lavery, I.C.; Fazio, V.W.; Remzi, F.H. Efficacy and safety of endoscopic treatment of ileal pouch strictures. *Inflamm. Bowel Dis.* **2011**, *17*, 2527–2535. [CrossRef] [PubMed]
38. Lan, N.; Shen, B. Endoscopic Stricturotomy with Needle Knife in the Treatment of Strictures from Inflammatory Bowel Disease. *Inflamm. Bowel Dis.* **2017**, *23*, 502–513. [CrossRef] [PubMed]
39. Kouladouros, K.; Reissfelder, C.; Kähler, G. Endoscopic Stricturoplasty with Linear Stapler: An Efficient Alternative for the Refractory Rectal Anastomotic Stricture. *Dig. Dis. Sci.* **2023**, *68*, 4432–4438. [CrossRef]
40. Herman, K.; Kiran, R.P.; Shen, B. Insulated tip/needle-knife endoscopic stricturotomy is safe and effective for treatment of non-traversable anorectal strictures. *Endosc. Int. Open* **2024**, *12*, E231–E236. [CrossRef]
41. Ning, S.-B.; Yang, H.; Li, B.; Zhang, Y.; Huang, S.; Peng, B.; Lin, H.; Kurban, M.; Li, M.; Guo, Q. Balloon-assisted enteroscopy-based endoscopic stricturotomy for deep small bowel strictures from Crohn's disease: First cohort study of a novel approach. *Dig. Liver Dis.* **2023**, *55*, 1397–1402. [CrossRef] [PubMed]
42. Swaminath, A.; Lichtiger, S. Dilation of colonic strictures by intralesional injection of infliximab in patients with Crohn's colitis. *Inflamm. Bowel Dis.* **2008**, *14*, 213–216. [CrossRef] [PubMed]
43. Hendel, J.; Karstensen, J.G.; Vilmann, P. Serial intralesional injections of infliximab in small bowel Crohn's strictures are feasible and might lower inflammation. *United Eur. Gastroenterol. J.* **2014**, *2*, 406–412. [CrossRef] [PubMed]
44. Sorrentino, D.; Avellini, C.; Beltrami, C.A.; Pasqual, E.; Zearo, E. Selective effect of infliximab on the inflammatory component of a colonic stricture in Crohn's disease. *Int. J. Color. Dis.* **2006**, *21*, 276–281. [CrossRef] [PubMed]
45. Loras Alastruey, C.; Andújar Murcia, X.; Esteve Comas, M. The role of stents in the treatment of Crohn's disease strictures. *Endosc. Int. Open* **2016**, *4*, E301–E308. [CrossRef] [PubMed]
46. Loras, C.; Pérez-Roldan, F.; Gornals, J.B.; Barrio, J.; Igea, F.; González-Huix, F.; González-Carro, P.; Pérez-Miranda, M.; Espinós, J.C.; Fernández-Bañares, F.; et al. Endoscopic treatment with self-expanding metal stents for Crohn's disease strictures. *Aliment. Pharmacol. Ther.* **2012**, *36*, 833–839. [CrossRef] [PubMed]
47. Levine, R.A.; Wasvary, H.; Kadro, O. Endoprosthetic management of refractory ileocolonic anastomotic strictures after resection for Crohn's disease: Report of nine-year follow-up and review of the literature. *Inflamm. Bowel Dis.* **2012**, *18*, 506–512. [CrossRef]
48. Attar, A.; Maunoury, V.; Vahedi, K.; Vernier-Massouille, G.; Vida, S.; Bulois, P.; Colombel, J.F.; Bouhnik, Y. GETAID Safety and efficacy of extractible self-expandable metal stents in the treatment of Crohn's disease intestinal strictures: A prospective pilot study. *Inflamm. Bowel Dis.* **2012**, *18*, 1849–1854. [CrossRef] [PubMed]
49. Das, R.; Singh, R.; Din, S.; Lund, J.; Krishnamoorthy, R.; Hearing, S.; Norton, B.; Williams, J.; Fraser, C.; Goddard, A.; et al. Therapeutic resolution of focal, predominantly anastomotic Crohn's disease strictures using removable stents: Outcomes from a single-center case series in the United Kingdom. *Gastrointest. Endosc.* **2020**, *92*, 344–352. [CrossRef]
50. Branche, J.; Attar, A.; Vernier-Massouille, G.; Bulois, P.; Colombel, J.F.; Bouhnik, Y.; Maunoury, V. Extractible self-expandable metal stent in the treatment of Crohn's disease anastomotic strictures. *Endoscopy* **2012**, *44* (Suppl. S2), E325–E326. [CrossRef]
51. Attar, A.; Branche, J.; Coron, E.; Privat, J.; Caillo, L.; Chevaux, J.-B.; Vuitton, L.; Amiot, A.; Belkhodja, H.; Dray, X.; et al. An Anti-migration Self-expandable and Removable Metal Stent for Crohn's Disease Strictures: A Nationwide Study From GETAID and SFED. *J. Crohn's Colitis* **2021**, *15*, 521–528. [CrossRef]

52. Loras, C.; Ruiz-Ramirez, P.; Romero, J.; Andújar, X.; Bargallo, J.; Bernardos, E.; Boscá-Watts, M.M.; Brugiotti, C.; Brunet, E.; Busquets, D.; et al. Endoscopic treatment (endoscopic balloon dilation/self-expandable metal stent) vs surgical resection for the treatment of de novo stenosis in Crohn's disease (ENDOCIR study): An open-label, multicentre, randomized trial. *Trials* **2023**, *24*, 432. [CrossRef]
53. van Boeckel, P.G.A.; Siersema, P.D. Refractory esophageal strictures: What to do when dilation fails. *Curr. Treat. Opt. Gastroenterol.* **2015**, *13*, 47–58. [CrossRef] [PubMed]
54. Hallac, A.; Srikureja, W.; Liu, E.; Dhumal, P.; Thatte, A.; Puri, N. Economical effect of lumen apposing metal stents for treating benign foregut strictures. *World J. Gastrointest. Endosc.* **2018**, *10*, 294–300. [CrossRef]
55. Adler, D.G. Lumen-Apposing Metal Stents for the Treatment of Refractory Benign Esophageal Strictures. *Am. J. Gastroenterol.* **2017**, *112*, 516–517. [CrossRef] [PubMed]
56. Mirchin, R.B.; Mahmood, S.K. Lumen-Apposing Metal Stent Used to Treat Malignant Esophageal Stricture. *ACG Case Rep. J.* **2020**, *7*, e00362. [CrossRef]
57. Axelrad, J.E.; Lichtiger, S.; Sethi, A. Treatment of Crohn's Disease Anastomotic Stricture with a Lumen-apposing Metal Stent. *Clin. Gastroenterol. Hepatol.* **2018**, *16*, A25–A26. [CrossRef] [PubMed]
58. Marcellier, G.; Lorenzo, D.; Hedjoudje, A.; Jais, B.; Bouhnik, Y.; Prat, F. First treatment of Crohn's disease refractory anastomotic stricture with a lumen-apposing metallic stent suitable for colonoscopy. *Endoscopy* **2022**, *54*, E409–E410. [CrossRef]
59. Hedjoudje, A.; Jais, B.; Stefanescu, C.; Lorenzo, D.; Aubert, A.; Badurdeen, D.; Bouhnik, Y.; Prat, F. Clinical Efficacy of Lumen-Apposing Metallic Stents for Lower Gastrointestinal Anastomotic Strictures. *J. Gastrointest. Surg.* **2023**, *27*, 1458–1460. [CrossRef] [PubMed]
60. Griffiths, E.A.; Gregory, C.J.; Pursnani, K.G.; Ward, J.B.; Stockwell, R.C. The use of biodegradable (SX-ELLA) oesophageal stents to treat dysphagia due to benign and malignant oesophageal disease. *Surg. Endosc.* **2012**, *26*, 2367–2375. [CrossRef]
61. Saito, Y.; Tanaka, T.; Andoh, A.; Minematsu, H.; Hata, K.; Tsujikawa, T.; Nitta, N.; Murata, K.; Fujiyama, Y. Usefulness of biodegradable stents constructed of poly-l-lactic acid monofilaments in patients with benign esophageal stenosis. *World J. Gastroenterol.* **2007**, *13*, 3977–3980. [CrossRef] [PubMed]
62. Krokidis, M.; Burke, C.; Spiliopoulos, S.; Gkoutzios, P.; Hynes, O.; Ahmed, I.; Dourado, R.; Sabharwal, T.; Mason, R.; Adam, A. The use of biodegradable stents in malignant oesophageal strictures for the treatment of dysphagia before neoadjuvant treatment or radical radiotherapy: A feasibility study. *Cardiovasc. Intervent. Radiol.* **2013**, *36*, 1047–1054. [CrossRef] [PubMed]
63. Lorenzo-Zúñiga, V.; Moreno-de-Vega, V.; Marín, I.; Boix, J. Biodegradable stents in gastrointestinal endoscopy. *World J. Gastroenterol.* **2014**, *20*, 2212–2217. [CrossRef] [PubMed]
64. Rejchrt, S.; Kopacova, M.; Brozik, J.; Bures, J. Biodegradable stents for the treatment of benign stenoses of the small and large intestines. *Endoscopy* **2011**, *43*, 911–917. [CrossRef] [PubMed]
65. Karstensen, J.G.; Vilmann, P.; Hendel, J. Successful endoscopic treatment of a 12-cm small-bowel Crohn stricture with a custom-made biodegradable stent. *Endoscopy* **2014**, *46* (Suppl. S1.), E227–E228. [CrossRef] [PubMed]
66. Karstensen, J.G.; Christensen, K.R.; Brynskov, J.; Rønholt, C.; Vilmann, P.; Hendel, J. Biodegradable stents for the treatment of bowel strictures in Crohn's disease: Technical results and challenges. *Endosc. Int. Open* **2016**, *4*, E296–E300. [CrossRef] [PubMed]
67. Martin, J.C.; Chang, C.; Boschetti, G.; Ungaro, R.; Giri, M.; Grout, J.A.; Gettler, K.; Chuang, L.-S.; Nayar, S.; Greenstein, A.J.; et al. Single-Cell Analysis of Crohn's Disease Lesions Identifies a Pathogenic Cellular Module Associated with Resistance to Anti-TNF Therapy. *Cell* **2019**, *178*, 1493–1508.20. [CrossRef] [PubMed]
68. Corridoni, D.; Antanaviciute, A.; Gupta, T.; Fawkner-Corbett, D.; Aulicino, A.; Jagielowicz, M.; Parikh, K.; Repapi, E.; Taylor, S.; Ishikawa, D.; et al. Single-cell atlas of colonic $CD8^+$ T cells in ulcerative colitis. *Nat. Med.* **2020**, *26*, 1480–1490. [CrossRef] [PubMed]
69. Kurahara, L.H.; Hiraishi, K.; Hu, Y.; Koga, K.; Onitsuka, M.; Doi, M.; Aoyagi, K.; Takedatsu, H.; Kojima, D.; Fujihara, Y.; et al. Activation of myofibroblast TRPA1 by steroids and pirfenidone ameliorates fibrosis in experimental crohn's disease. *Cell. Mol. Gastroenterol. Hepatol.* **2018**, *5*, 299–318. [CrossRef]
70. Li, X.; Yu, M.; Zhao, Q.; Yu, Y. Prospective therapeutics for intestinal and hepatic fibrosis. *Bioeng. Transl. Med.* **2023**, *8*, e10579. [CrossRef]
71. Solitano, V.; Jairath, V.; Ungaro, F.; Peyrin-Biroulet, L.; Danese, S. TL1A inhibition for inflammatory bowel disease treatment: From inflammation to fibrosis. *MED* **2024**, *5*, 386–400. [CrossRef] [PubMed]
72. Ye, Y.; Zhang, X.; Su, D.; Ren, Y.; Cheng, F.; Yao, Y.; Shi, G.; Ji, Y.; Chen, S.; Shi, P.; et al. Therapeutic efficacy of human adipose mesenchymal stem cells in Crohn's colon fibrosis is improved by IFN-γ and kynurenic acid priming through indoleamine 2,3-dioxygenase-1 signaling. *Stem Cell Res. Ther.* **2022**, *13*, 465. [CrossRef] [PubMed]
73. Lian, L.; Huang, Q.; Zhang, L.; Qin, H.; He, X.; He, X.; Ke, J.; Xie, M.; Lan, P. Anti-fibrogenic Potential of Mesenchymal Stromal Cells in Treating Fibrosis in Crohn's Disease. *Dig. Dis. Sci.* **2018**, *63*, 1821–1834. [CrossRef] [PubMed]
74. Choi, Y.J.; Kim, W.R.; Kim, D.H.; Kim, J.H.; Yoo, J.H. Human umbilical cord/placenta mesenchymal stem cell conditioned medium attenuates intestinal fibrosis in vivo and in vitro. *Stem Cell Res. Ther.* **2024**, *15*, 69. [CrossRef] [PubMed]
75. Goffin, L.; Fagagnini, S.; Vicari, A.; Mamie, C.; Melhem, H.; Weder, B.; Lutz, C.; Lang, S.; Scharl, M.; Rogler, G.; et al. Anti-MMP-9 Antibody: A Promising Therapeutic Strategy for Treatment of Inflammatory Bowel Disease Complications with Fibrosis. *Inflamm. Bowel Dis.* **2016**, *22*, 2041–2057. [CrossRef] [PubMed]

76. Pizzoferrato, M.; Puca, P.; Ennas, S.; Cammarota, G.; Guidi, L. Glucagon-like peptide-2 analogues for Crohn's disease patients with short bowel syndrome and intestinal failure. *World J. Gastroenterol.* **2022**, *28*, 6258–6270. [CrossRef] [PubMed]
77. Costa, B.P.; Gonçalves, A.C.; Abrantes, A.M.; Matafome, P.; Seiça, R.; Sarmento-Ribeiro, A.B.; Botelho, M.F.; Castro-Sousa, F. Teduglutide effects on gene regulation of fibrogenesis on an animal model of intestinal anastomosis. *J. Surg. Res.* **2017**, *216*, 87–98. [CrossRef]
78. Fuchs, C.D.; Claudel, T.; Mlitz, V.; Riva, A.; Menz, M.; Brusilovskaya, K.; Haller, F.; Baumgartner, M.; Königshofer, P.; Unger, L.W.; et al. GLP-2 Improves Hepatic Inflammation and Fibrosis in Mdr2$^{-/-}$ Mice via Activation of NR4a1/Nur77 in Hepatic Stellate Cells and Intestinal FXR Signaling. *Cell. Mol. Gastroenterol. Hepatol.* **2023**, *16*, 847–856. [CrossRef]
79. Nassani, N.; Alsheikh, M.; Carroll, B.; Nguyen, D.; Carroll, R.E. Theranostic gastrointestinal endoscopy: Bringing healing light to the lumen. *Clin. Transl. Gastroenterol.* **2020**, *11*, e00119. [CrossRef] [PubMed]
80. Chen, F.; Liu, Q.; Xiong, Y.; Xu, L. Current Strategies and Potential Prospects of Nanomedicine-Mediated Therapy in Inflammatory Bowel Disease. *Int. J. Nanomed.* **2021**, *16*, 4225–4237. [CrossRef]
81. Nishida, T.; Takeno, S.; Nakashima, K.; Kariya, M.; Inatsu, H.; Kitamura, K.; Nanashima, A. Salvage photodynamic therapy accompanied by extended lymphadenectomy for advanced esophageal carcinoma: A case report. *Int. J. Surg. Case Rep.* **2017**, *36*, 155–160. [CrossRef] [PubMed]
82. Ertan, A.; Zaheer, I.; Correa, A.M.; Thosani, N.; Blackmon, S.H. Photodynamic therapy vs radiofrequency ablation for Barrett's dysplasia: Efficacy, safety and cost-comparison. *World J. Gastroenterol.* **2013**, *19*, 7106–7113. [CrossRef] [PubMed]
83. Hartwig, O.; Shetab Boushehri, M.A.; Shalaby, K.S.; Loretz, B.; Lamprecht, A.; Lehr, C.-M. Drug delivery to the inflamed intestinal mucosa-targeting technologies and human cell culture models for better therapies of IBD. *Adv. Drug Deliv. Rev.* **2021**, *175*, 113828. [CrossRef] [PubMed]
84. Bon, I.; Cano-Sarabia, M.; de la Ossa, N.; Bartolí, R.; Lorenzo-Zúñiga, V. Development and Characterization of a New Endoscopic Drug-Eluting Platform with Proven Efficacy in Acute and Chronic Experimental Colitis. *Front. Med.* **2020**, *7*, 415. [CrossRef] [PubMed]

Journal of
Clinical Medicine

MDPI

Article

Biomarkers for Monitoring of Changes in Disease Activity in Ulcerative Colitis

Yoshihiro Tatsumi [1], Kazuki Kakimoto [1,2,*], Azusa Hara [1,2], Noboru Mizuta [1], Keijiro Numa [1], Naohiko Kinoshita [1], Kei Nakazawa [1], Ryoji Koshiba [1], Yuki Hirata [1,2], Kazuhiro Ota [1], Takako Miyazaki [1,2], Shiro Nakamura [1], Kayoko Sakagami [2], Shoko Arimitsu [2], Hiroaki Ito [2] and Hiroki Nishikawa [1]

1 2nd Department of Internal Medicine, Osaka Medical and Pharmaceutical University, Takatsuki City 569-8686, Japan; t_cop_doradora@yahoo.co.jp (Y.T.); wakayamakisyu@yahoo.co.jp (A.H.); noboru.mizuta@ompu.ac.jp (N.M.); jeni_like_0902@yahoo.co.jp (K.N.); naohiko.kinoshita@ompu.ac.jp (N.K.); kei.nakazawa@ompu.ac.jp (K.N.); ryouji.koshiba@ompu.ac.jp (R.K.); yuki.hirata.ln@ompu.ac.jp (Y.H.); clash_kaz@yahoo.co.jp (K.O.); takako.miyazaki@ompu.ac.jp (T.M.); saab460@gmail.com (S.N.); hiroki.nishikawa@ompu.ac.jp (H.N.)

2 Kinshukai Infusion Clinic, Osaka-shi 530-0011, Japan; office@kic-clinic.jp (K.S.); aripikari@ares.eonet.ne.jp (S.A.); lovemagicflute@yahoo.co.jp (H.I.)

* Correspondence: kazuki.kakimoto@ompu.ac.jp

Abstract: Background: In recent years, various biomarkers of ulcerative colitis (UC) have emerged; however, few studies have simultaneously examined the utility of multiple biomarkers for monitoring disease activity. Additionally, serum leucine-rich alpha-2 glycoprotein (LRG), a new biomarker, may show a blunt response to anti-TNF antibody therapy. This prospective study explored effective biomarkers that could monitor disease activity changes in patients with UC. In addition, we examined the effect of anti-TNF antibody therapy on changes in LRG. Methods: Blood and stool samples were collected twice from patients with UC: at baseline and at least 8 weeks later. Changes in serum LRG, interleukin (IL)-6, prealbumin (pre-Alb), high-sensitivity C-reactive protein (hs-CRP), CRP, and fecal calprotectin (FC) were measured and correlated with changes in disease activity. The relationship between anti-TNF antibody therapy and LRG levels was also examined in patients with the same disease activity. Results: Forty-eight patients with UC (96 samples) were analyzed. ΔLRG and ΔIL-6 correlated strongly with the change in the partial Mayo (pMayo) score between the two time points (ΔpMayo) (r = 0.686, 0.635, respectively). In contrast, FC and IL-6 were particularly accurate predictors of clinical remission, and their area under the curves (AUCs) were significantly higher than that of CRP (AUC: 0.81, 0.76 vs. 0.50; $p = 0.001, 0.005$). No association was found between the administration of anti-TNF antibody preparations and the LRG values. Conclusions: Correlations were found between changes in UC disease activity and LRG, IL-6, pre-Alb, hs-CRP, CRP, and FC. LRG reflects disease activity during anti-TNF antibody therapy.

Keywords: ulcerative colitis; biomarkers; LRG (leucine-rich alpha-2-glycoprotein); fecal calprotectin; anti-TNF antibody therapy

1. Introduction

Ulcerative colitis (UC) is a chronic inflammatory bowel disease of unknown etiology that affects the large intestine. In recent years, various biomarkers of UC have emerged, making it possible to objectively evaluate disease activity. In the clinical setting of UC, the measurement of biomarkers has various implications, including estimation of the grade and severity of mucosal inflammation, measurement of response to therapy, and surveillance of relapse after induced remission [1]. It is known that individual variations exist in biomarker levels, even within groups of patients with the same level of disease activity [2]. Therefore, aside from measuring biomarker levels at baseline and during treatment, it is also important to measure the changes of these biomarkers during the clinical course of the disease [2]; this is especially valuable when monitoring for relapse and treatment response. Even so, no prospective studies have been conducted to simultaneously track multiple biomarkers in relation to changes in disease activity. It is clinically important to understand the correlation of disease activity with biomarkers in monitoring the changes in disease activity; however, such information is currently lacking. For example, the fecal calprotectin (FC) is an excellent biomarker for determining mucosal healing; however, it has large numerical variability and may not accurately reflect treatment-induced changes in disease activity [3,4].

Various biomarkers have been reported to correlate with disease activity in UC. Calprotectin is an inflammation-associated protein that is primarily localized within neutrophilic cytoplasm, and its presence in stool indicates neutrophil migration into the gastrointestinal tract during inflammation [5,6]. FC can predict endoscopic activity with high sensitivity [7]. However, it is challenging to utilize this biomarker as a measure of treatment response since the change in FC levels after treatment initiation is highly variable between individuals [8,9]. Leucine-rich alpha-2 glycoprotein (LRG) is a plasma glycoprotein containing a repeating sequence of leucine-rich motifs [10]. Inflammatory cytokines, such as tumor necrosis factor (TNF)-α, interleukin (IL)-1β, and IL-6, induce LRG production in the hepatocytes, neutrophils, and macrophages [11,12]. In recent years, LRG has attracted considerable attention because of their marked correlation with disease activity in inflammatory bowel disease (IBD), particularly in UC [13]. IL-6 is a multifaceted mediator that modulates the intestinal immune system through classical IL-6 signaling or IL-6 trans-signaling [14,15]. Serum IL-6 levels are markedly elevated in patients with active IBD and have been shown to be positively correlated with disease activity [16,17]. C-reactive protein (CRP) is an acute-phase protein produced by hepatocytes upon IL-6 stimulation; it is also the most well-studied inflammatory parameter in patients with IBD [7,18]. However, the sensitivity of CRP to endoscopic activity in patients with IBD is low [8]. CRP levels are also associated with high-sensitivity CRP (hs-CRP) and prealbumin (pre-Alb) levels. The hs-CRP assay can measure values below the detection limit of CRP, and its results are correlated with disease activity in patients with UC [19,20]. Furthermore, pre-Alb levels are inversely correlated with disease activity in patients with IBD [21,22]. Although studies have reported various useful biomarkers in UC, few have simultaneously analyzed their correlation with disease activity.

Another factor that has to be taken into consideration is the interaction between biomarkers. For example, CRP is less likely to be elevated under anti-IL-6 receptor antibody therapy in patients with rheumatoid arthritis since the release of CRP is affected by IL-6; therefore, it is not useful for assessing disease activity [23]. Similarly, LRG is induced by stimuli such as TNFα [12]; therefore, under the administration of anti-TNFα antibody preparations, which are typical biologics for the treatment of refractory UC, the reactivity of LRG may be slowed down with a decrease in TNFα. However, there have been no reports on LRG reactivity in patients with UC receiving anti-TNFα antibody agents.

This prospective study aimed to investigate the correlation of six biomarkers (FC, serum LRG, IL-6, pre-Alb, hs-CRP, and CRP) with the changes in disease activity in patients with UC. As a secondary endpoint, we also examined whether serum LRG accurately reflects disease activity in patients with UC receiving anti-TNFα antibody preparations.

2. Materials and Methods

2.1. Patients

Patients attending the Kinshukai Infusion Clinic between May 2020 and April 2021 were prospectively enrolled. The diagnosis of UC was based on a combination of clinical presentation, endoscopic findings, histology, and the exclusion of alternative diagnoses. Biomarker measurements were carried out at two time points; once at baseline and once at least 8 weeks after the first examination. At each measurement, patients provided blood and stool samples at the same time. LRG, IL-6, pre-Alb, hs-CRP, and CRP levels were measured in two blood samples, and FC was measured using two stool samples from the same patient. Demographic data, current medications, clinical disease activity, and laboratory blood data were recorded at the two time points when the samples were collected. Partial Mayo (pMayo) scores were used to assess clinical disease activity, excluding the endoscopic subscores [24]. Clinical remission was defined as a pMayo score ≤ 2 with each subscore ≤ 1.

2.2. Study Endpoints

The primary endpoint was the correlation between the change in clinical activity and the change in each biomarker at the two time points. The main secondary endpoint was the diagnostic accuracy of each biomarker for clinical remission. Another secondary endpoint was the change in serum LRG reactivity with anti-TNF antibody therapy. We compared LRG values between patients with and without anti-TNF antibody therapy who had the same level of disease activity.

2.3. Biomarker Measurements

Serum LRG, IL-6, pre-Alb, hs-CRP, and FC levels were analyzed at the laboratory of LSI MEDIENCE Co., Ltd., Osaka, Japan. Serum LRG levels were measured using a NANOPIA LRG kit based on the latex turbidimetric method (SEKISUI MEDICAL Co., Ltd., Tokyo, Japan). Serum IL-6 levels were measured by chemiluminescent enzyme immunoassay (CLEIA) using the Quanti Glo Human IL-6 Immunoassay kit (R&D Systems Inc., Minneapolis, MN, USA). Serum pre-Alb levels were measured by a turbidimetric immunoassay (TIA) using the N-assay TIA Prealbumin Nittobo (NITTOBO MEDICAL Co., Ltd., Tokyo, Japan). Serum hs-CRP levels were measured using nephelometry (N-latex CRPII; Siemens Healthineers, Osaka, Japan). FC was measured by fluorescence enzyme immunoassay (FEIA) using Elia Calprotectin 2 (Thermo Fisher Scientific, Tokyo, Japan). Serum CRP levels were analyzed by an in-hospital laboratory using CHM-4120 (NIHON KOHDEN Co., Tokyo, Japan).

2.4. Statistical Analysis

Quantitative data were summarized using medians and interquartile ranges (IQR), while categorical variables were presented as frequencies and percentages. We used the Wilcoxon signed-rank test to compare non-parametric paired values. To evaluate the predictive performance of each biomarker for clinical remission, the receiver operating characteristic (ROC) curves were plotted to calculate the area under the ROC curve. Pearson's test was performed to analyze the correlation between the biomarkers and activity indices. Statistical significance was set as $p < 0.05$ (two-sided test). The sample size was based on previous studies where the correlation between biomarkers and pMayo scores were assessed [25]. Using a two-sided hypothesis with $\alpha = 0.05$, we estimated that 46 patients would be required, providing 80% power to detect a moderate correlation ($r = 0.4$) between biomarkers and pMayo scores [26]. To be conservative, we planned to enroll 48 patients in case of protocol violations or technical difficulties associated with blood sampling. All statistical analyses were performed using JMP®, Version 15.2.1, SAS Institute, Inc., Cary, NC, 1989-2021, USA.

3. Results

3.1. Patients' Characteristics

There were 48 patients (24 men and 24 women) with a median age of 43.5 years, a median disease duration of 12.5 years, and an extent of disease as follows: 30 cases of total colitis type and 18 cases of left-sided colon type (Table 1). At the first measurement, treatments included the use of 5ASA preparations in 87.5% of patients, corticosteroids in 2.1%, azathioprine in 14.6%, and molecularly targeted drugs in 52.1%. At the second measurement, patients were receiving the same treatments, with the exception of molecularly targeted drugs, which were used in 50% of patients (vs. 52.1% at the previous measurement). The median pMayo was one (0–3) at the first measurement and one (0–2.3) at the second measurement. Clinical remission was observed in 35 patients (72.9%) at the first measurement and 36 patients (75%) at the second measurement. The median interval between the two measurements was 60.5 (56–82.5) days.

Table 1. Baseline Demographics and Clinical Characteristics.

Number of Patients	*n* = 48
Male/Female, *n*	24/24
Age, year, median (IQR)	43.5 (32.8–52.3)
Duration of disease, year, median (IQR)	12.5 (7–18.3)
UC location; Left side/Extensive, *n*	30/18
Medications for UC	
Aminosalicylates, *n* (%)	42 (87.5)
Azathioprine, *n* (%)	7 (14.6)
Corticosteroids, *n* (%)	1 (2.1)
Anti-TNF-α agents, *n* (%)	17 (35.4%)
(infliximab, adalimumab, golimumab, *n* (%))	(10/4/3 (20.8/8.3/6.3))
Vedolizumab, *n* (%)	4(8.3)
Ustekinumab, *n* (%)	1(2.1)
Tofacitinib, *n* (%)	2(4.2)
Partial Mayo score, median (IQR)	1 (0–3)
Clinical remission/non-remission	35/13
WBC, /μL, median (IQR)	6300 (5050–7300)
Hb, g/dL, median (IQR)	13.8 (13.0–15.5)
Albumin, g/dL, median (IQR)	4.5 (4.3–4.6)
CRP, mg/L, median (IQR)	0.05 (0–0.14)

IQR, interquartile range; UC, ulcerative colitis; WBC, white blood cell; Hb, hemoglobin, CRP, C-reactive protein.

3.2. Comparison of Various Biomarkers in Clinical Remission and Non-Remission

A total of 96 samples were used to compare the levels of each biomarker in patients with clinical remission and non-remission of UC. As shown in Figure 1, three biomarkers had significantly higher medians in patients with active disease than those in remission: FC (522 [224–1650] vs. 65.8 [24.6–228.5] μg/g, respectively), LRG (14.2 [10.9–17] vs. 11.1 [9.5–13.4] μg/mL, respectively), and IL-6 (1.29 [1.02–2.09] vs. 0.79 [0.59–1.16] pg/dL). In contrast, pre-Alb had a significantly lower median in patients with active disease (21.9 [19.5–26] vs. 25 [21.9–29] mg/dL, respectively). The two remaining biomarkers were not statistically different between patients with active disease and those with remission: CRP (0.04 [0–0.22] vs. 0.09 [0–0.11] mg/dL, respectively) and hs-CRP (0.076 [0.023–0.283] vs. 0.035 [0.013–0.087] mg/dL, respectively).

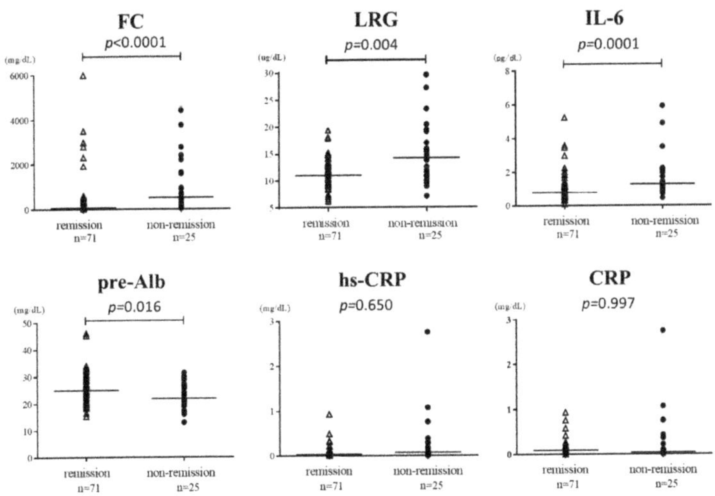

Figure 1. Comparison of each biomarker in patients in clinical remission and those not in remission. FC, fecal calprotectin; LRG, leucine-rich alpha-2 glycoprotein; IL-6, interleukin-6; pre-Alb, prealbumin; hs-CRP, high-sensitivity C-reactive protein.

3.3. Diagnostic Accuracy of Each Biomarker for Clinical Remission

Subsequently, the diagnostic accuracy of each biomarker for the clinical remission of UC was examined by calculating the optimal cutoff value, sensitivity, and specificity of each biomarker using ROC curves and comparing the area under the curve (AUC). The cut-off value of FC was 184 μg/g, with a sensitivity of 84.0% and specificity of 70.4%, while that of LRG was 13.8 μg/mL, with a sensitivity of 56.0% and specificity of 78.9% (Figure 2).

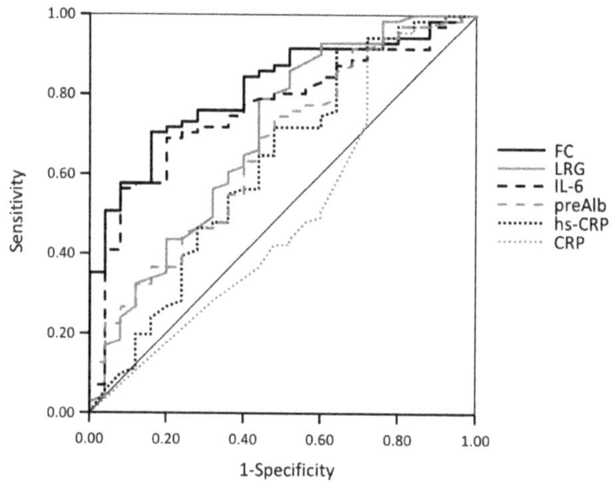

Figure 2. Receiver operating characteristic curve of the respective biomarkers for predicting clinical remission. FC, fecal calprotectin; LRG, leucine-rich alpha-2 glycoprotein; IL-6, interleukin-6; pre-Alb, prealbumin; hs-CRP, high-sensitivity C-reactive protein.

Only the AUCs for FC and IL-6 were significantly higher than the AUC for CRP. (AUC:0.81, 0.76 vs. 0.50; $p = 0.001, 0.005$) (Table 2). In contrast, LRG had moderate accuracy (AUC = 0.70), which was higher than the AUC of CRP but not significantly ($p = 0.105$). The AUCs for pre-Alb and hs-CRP were low and did not differ significantly from those for CRP (AUC:0.66, 0.63 vs. 0.50; $p = 0.141, 0.333$).

Table 2. Analysis by receiver operating characteristic curve of the respective biomarkers for clinical remission ($n = 96$).

Variables	AUC (95%CI)	*p*-Value (vs. CRP)
CRP	0.50 (0.36–0.64)	
FC	0.81 (0.72–0.90)	0.001
IL-6	0.76 (0.66–0.86)	0.005
LRG	0.70 (0.57–0.83)	0.105
pre-Alb	0.66 (0.54–0.79)	0.141
hs-CRP	0.63 (0.49–0.76)	0.333

AUC, area under the curve; CRP, C-reactive protein; FC, fecal calprotectin; IL-6, interleukin-6; LRG, leucine-rich alpha-2 glycoprotein; pre-Alb, prealbumin; hs-CRP, high-sensitivity CRP.

3.4. Correlation between Clinical Activity and Each Biomarker

We examined the correlation between the clinical activity of UC and each biomarker using a total of 96 samples (Table 3) and found that LRG and IL-6 were significantly correlated with pMayo (r = 0.442 and 0.405, respectively). Levels of hs-CRP, FC, CRP and pre-Alb showed relatively weak correlations (r = 0.361, 0.354, 0.310, and −0.231, respectively).

Table 3. Correlation between clinical activity and each biomarker (n = 96).

Variables	r	p
FC	0.354	0.0004
LRG	0.442	<0.0001
IL-6	0.405	<0.0001
pre-Alb	−0.231	0.0238
hs-CRP	0.361	0.0003
CRP	0.310	0.0021

FC, fecal calprotectin; LRG, leucine-rich alpha-2 glycoprotein; IL-6, interleukin-6; pre-Alb, prealbumin; hs-CRP, high-sensitivity C-reactive protein.

3.5. Correlation between Changes in pMayo Scores at Two Time Points and Change in Each Biomarker

We examined the correlation between changes in clinical activity and changes in each biomarker at two time points in the same patients (Figure 3). The pMayo at the second measurement was lower than that at the first measurement in 12 patients, higher in 8 patients, and unchanged in 28 patients. ΔLRG and ΔIL-6 correlated strongly with the change in pMayo (ΔpMayo) (r = 0.686, $p < 0.0001$ and 0.635, $p < 0.0001$, respectively). ΔFC, Δpre-Alb, Δhs-CRP, and ΔCRP were also correlated with ΔpMayo but not strongly (r = 0.487, −0.368, 0.483, and 0.407, respectively; $p < 0.01$). When the correlation coefficient of ΔCRP was compared with those of the other biomarkers, those of ΔLRG and ΔIL-6 were significantly higher than that of ΔCRP (p = 0.005, 0.029). In contrast, the correlation coefficients of ΔFC, Δpre-Alb, and Δhs-CRP were not significantly different from that of ΔCRP (p = 0.497, 0.787, and 0.497, respectively). These results suggest that LRG and IL-6 in particular are useful biomarkers for the sensitive detection of changes in disease activity in UC.

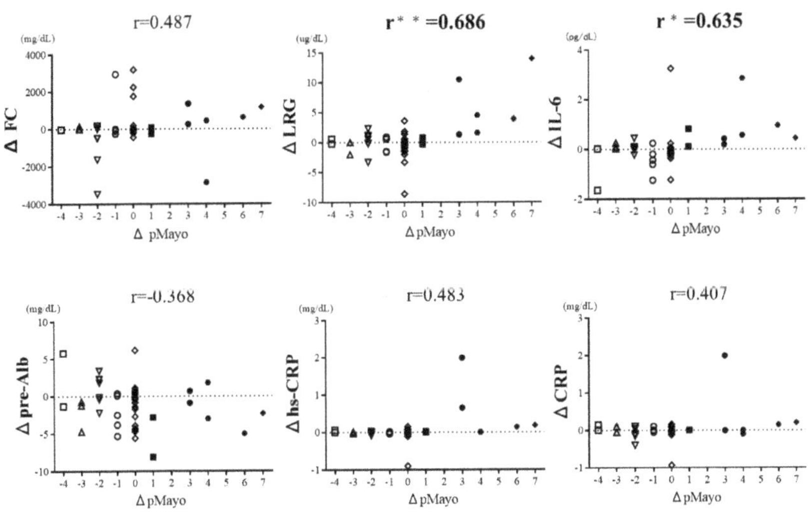

Figure 3. Correlation between pMayo change and change in each biomarker at two time points. When the correlation coefficient of ΔCRP was compared with those of the other biomarkers, those of ΔLRG and ΔIL-6 were significantly higher than that of ΔCRP: ** $p < 0.01$, * $p < 0.05$. FC, fecal calprotectin; LRG, leucine-rich alpha-2 glycoprotein; IL-6, interleukin-6; pre-Alb, prealbumin; hs-CRP, high-sensitivity C-reactive protein. The shape of the symbols in the graphs is represented by a different shape for each ΔpMayo value.

3.6. Association between Anti-TNF Antibody Preparations and LRG

To examine whether LRG reactivity was blunted in patients with UC receiving anti-TNF antibody preparations, we compared LRG values between patients with and without anti-TNF antibody preparations; this comparison was only made between patients with the same clinical disease activity (pMayo: 0, 1–2, and ≥3). No association was observed between LRG and the administration of anti-TNF antibody preparations in any of the disease activity groups (Figure 4).

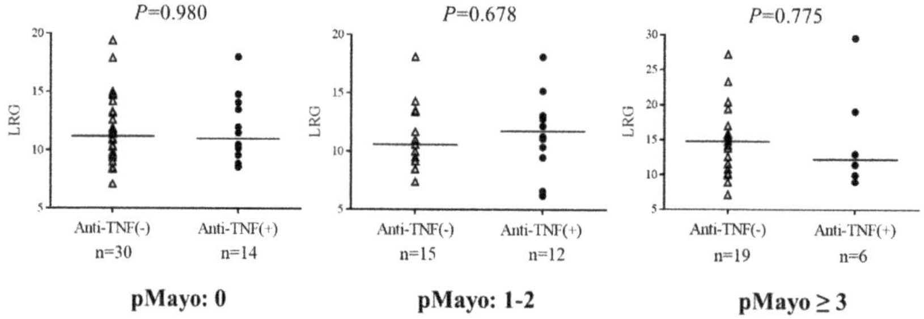

Figure 4. Comparison of LRG values between patients receiving anti-TNF antibodies and those not receiving anti-TNF antibodies according to the grade of clinical disease activity. LRG, leucine-rich alpha-2 glycoprotein; pMayo, partial Mayo score.

In addition, the correlation coefficients between LRG and other biomarkers were examined to determine whether the presence or absence of anti-TNF agents was associated with LRG (Table 4). pMayo and FC did not change with anti-TNF antibody administration (pMayo; anti-TNF (−): 0.470 vs. anti-TNF (+): 0.393, $p = 0.66$, FC; anti-TNF (−): 0.380 vs. anti-TNF (+): 0.384, $p = 1$). These results suggested that the administration of anti-TNF antibody preparations had no apparent effect on LRG reactivity. In contrast, the correlation coefficient between hs-CRP and LRG was significantly higher in patients receiving anti-TNF agents than in those not receiving anti-TNF agents (hs-CRP; anti-TNF (−): 0.593 vs. anti-TNF (+): 0.825, $p = 0.034$). The correlation coefficient between CRP and LRG also tended to be higher in patients receiving anti-TNF antibody agents (CRP; anti-TNF (−):0.620 vs. anti-TNF (+):0.827, $p = 0.057$).

Table 4. The correlation coefficients between LRG and other biomarkers with and without anti-TNF antibody preparations.

	Total (n = 96)		Anti-TNF (-) (N = 64)		Anti-TNF (+) (n = 32)		Anti-TNF(-) vs. (+)
	r	p	r	p	r	p	p
pMayo	0.442	<0.0001	**0.470**	<0.0001	**0.393**	0.026	**0.660**
FC	0.324	0.001	**0.380**	0.002	**0.384**	0.03	**1**
IL-6	0.257	0.012	**0.302**	0.015	**0.156**	0.393	**N/A**
pre-Alb	−0.474	<0.0001	**−0.394**	0.001	**−0.584**	0.001	**0.271**
hs-CRP	0.657	<0.0001	**0.593**	<0.0001	**0.825**	<0.0001	**0.034**
CRP	0.681	<0.0001	**0.620**	<0.0001	**0.827**	<0.0001	**0.057**

LRG, leucine-rich alpha-2 glycoprotein; pMayo, partial Mayo score; FC, fecal calprotectin; IL-6, interleukin-6; pre-Alb, prealbumin; hs-CRP, high-sensitivity C-reactive protein; anti-TNF, anti-TNF antibody preparation.

4. Discussion

In this study, we searched for biomarkers that could accurately monitor changes in disease activity in UC. When six biomarkers were prospectively and simultaneously assessed, LRG and IL-6 were particularly strongly associated with changes in disease activity. The correlation with changes in disease was stronger for these two biomarkers compared with CRP. In recent years, the value of using biomarkers to objectively assess disease activity in inflammatory bowel disease has gained recognition. LRG is a biomarker that has recently received attention and has the advantage of being easily measurable in serum [14]. This is the first prospective study to simultaneously analyze the sensitivity of various biomarkers including LRG to changes in disease activity. The results of this study suggest that LRG levels acutely reflect changes in disease activity.

It has been reported that FC values tend to correlate positively with endoscopic inflammation in patients with clinically remitted UC and are considered useful for monitoring relapse during clinical remission because of their high sensitivity to microinflammation [8,27–29]. The present study suggested that FC was able to distinguish clinical remission and non-remission very accurately; however, it was not very sensitive to changes in disease activity. Therefore, different biomarkers should be utilized to serve different clinical purposes.

Certain biomarkers may be undetectable in patients treated with biological agents. It is known that serum CRP, which is induced by IL-6, is less likely to be elevated in patients with rheumatoid arthritis who are being treated with anti-IL-6 receptor antibody preparations [23]. Similarly, since LRG is induced by stimulation from inflammatory cytokines such as TNFα, IL-1β, and IL-6, this study examined whether LRG is less likely to be detected in patients with UC receiving anti-TNF antibody preparations. No particular change in LRG reactivity was observed in these patients. These results suggest that LRG is a useful marker of disease activity even in patients receiving anti-TNF antibody preparations.

Interestingly, LRG was strongly correlated with CRP and hs-CRP, and the correlation was even stronger in patients receiving anti-TNF antibody preparations. Since the expression of TNFα is presumably reduced in patients treated with anti-TNF antibodies, and the correlation between IL-6 and LRG was very weak, these two cytokines (TNFα was and IL-6) should have a low effect on LRG. IL-6 is the major proinflammatory cytokine that induces CRP, although IL-1β is also involved [30,31]. These findings suggest that the reason for the strong correlation between LRG and CRP levels is that IL-1β is the main inflammatory cytokine that induces LRG following anti-TNF antibody treatment.

This study has a few limitations. First, colonoscopy was not performed, thus, the association between endoscopic activity and each biomarker could not be examined. One of the major benefits of biomarkers in UC is that they can be used to estimate mucosal inflammation without colonoscopy. Clinical disease activity cannot accurately reflect the disease state on its own; however, since mucosal inflammation was not assessed in this study, only clinical disease activity was taken into consideration when assessing biomarkers. Second, due to the small number of cases, it was not possible to compare the diagnostic accuracy between biomarkers and investigate which biomarkers are more useful. Third, of the 48 patients enrolled, pMayo changed in only 20 patients. The presence of many unchanged cases may have weakened the correlation analyses; however, we also included the unchanged cases in the analysis, bearing in mind that the biomarker values varied slightly, even in cases where pMayo did not change. Fourth, this was a cross-sectional study of patients with UC in an outpatient setting, and patients with active disease who required hospitalization were not enrolled. Fifth, the study cohort consisted of patients regardless of their treatment timing. Sixth, biomarkers are expensive to measure, and their use in routine practice may be limited.

5. Conclusions

Correlations were found between changes in UC disease activity and LRG, IL-6, pre-Alb, hs-CRP, CRP, and FC. The LRG reflects disease activity in patients with UC receiving anti-TNF antibody agents.

Author Contributions: Y.T., A.H., and S.A. collected data. K.K. interpreted the data and drafted the manuscript. H.I. designed the study. All other authors have contributed to data collection and interpretation and have critically reviewed the manuscript. All authors have read and agreed to the published version of the manuscript.

Funding: This research was funded by The Osaka Medical Research Foundation for Intractable Diseases, grant number 26-2-35.

Institutional Review Board Statement: This study was conducted in accordance with the principles of the Declaration of Helsinki. The study protocol was approved by the Ethics Committee of Hanwasumiyoshi General Hospital (No. 26-2-35, 13 May 2020). Written informed consent was obtained from all patients included in the study.

Informed Consent Statement: Written informed consent was obtained from the patients to publish this paper.

Data Availability Statement: The data are not publicly available because there is no appropriate site for uploading at present. The data underlying this article will be shared upon reasonable request to the corresponding author.

Acknowledgments: We are grateful to Akiyoshi Inaba, Med-Link Consulting (mlconsulting.jp) for her help in conducting the statistical analysis.

Conflicts of Interest: Shiro Nakamura reports receiving speaking fees from AbbVie GK, EA Pharma Co., Ltd., Mitsubishi Tanabe Pharma Corporation., Mochida Pharmaceutical Co., Ltd., Takeda Pharmaceutical Co., Ltd., and Janssen Pharmaceutical K.K. Dr.

References

1. Jones, J.; Loftus, E.V.; Panaccione, R.; Chen, L.; Peterson, S.; Mcconnell, J.; Baudhuin, L.; Hanson, K.; Feagan, B.G.; Harmsen, S.W.; et al. Relationships between disease activity and serum and fecal biomarkers in patients with Crohn's disease. *Clin. Gastroenterol. Hepatol.* **2008**, *6*, 1218–1224. [CrossRef]
2. Plevris, N.; Lees, C.W. Disease Monitoring in Inflammatory Bowel Disease: Evolving Principles and Possibilities. *Gastroenterology* **2022**, *162*, 1456–1475.e1. [CrossRef]
3. Kolho, K.-L.; Raivio, T.; Lindahl, H.; Savilahti, E. Fecal calprotectin remains high during glucocorticoid therapy in children with inflammatory bowel disease. *Scand. J. Gastroenterol.* **2006**, *41*, 720–725. [CrossRef]
4. Sipponen, T.; Björkesten, C.-G.A.; Färkkilä, M.; Nuutinen, H.; Savilahti, E.; Kolho, K.-L. Faecal calprotectin and lactoferrin are reliable surrogate markers of endoscopic response during Crohn's disease treatment. *Scand. J. Gastroenterol.* **2010**, *45*, 325–331. [CrossRef] [PubMed]
5. Smith, L.A.; Gaya, D.R. Utility of faecal calprotectin analysis in adult inflammatory bowel disease. *World J. Gastroenterol.* **2012**, *18*, 6782–6789. [CrossRef] [PubMed]
6. Vermeire, S.; Van Assche, G.; Rutgeerts, P. Laboratory markers in IBD: Useful, magic, or unnecessary toys? *Gut* **2006**, *55*, 426–431. [CrossRef]
7. Mosli, M.H.; Zou, G.; Garg, S.K.; Feagan, S.G.; MacDonald, J.K.; Chande, N.; Sandborn, W.J.; Feagan, B.G. C-Reactive Protein, Fecal Calprotectin, and Stool Lactoferrin for Detection of Endoscopic Activity in Symptomatic Inflammatory Bowel Disease Patients: A Systematic Review and Meta-Analysis. *Am. J. Gastroenterol.* **2015**, *110*, 802–819. [CrossRef] [PubMed]
8. Regueiro, M.; Kip, K.E.; Schraut, W.; Baidoo, L.; Sepulveda, A.R.; Pesci, M.; El-Hachem, S.; Harrison, J.; Binion, D. Crohn's disease activity index does not correlate with endoscopic recurrence one year after ileocolonic resection. *Inflamm. Bowel Dis.* **2011**, *17*, 118–126. [CrossRef]
9. Sorrentino, D.; Paviotti, A.; Terrosu, G.; Avellini, C.; Geraci, M.; Zarifi, D. Low-dose maintenance therapy with infliximab prevents postsurgical recurrence of Crohn's disease. *Clin. Gastroenterol. Hepatol.* **2010**, *8*, 591–599. [CrossRef]
10. Takahashi, N.; Takahashi, Y.; Putnam, F.W. Periodicity of leucine and tandem repetition of a 24-amino acid segment in the primary structure of leucine-rich alpha 2-glycoprotein of human serum. *Proc. Natl. Acad. Sci. USA* **1985**, *82*, 1906–1910. [CrossRef]
11. Shirai, R.; Hirano, F.; Ohkura, N.; Ikeda, K.; Inoue, S. Up-regulation of the expression of leucine-rich alpha(2)-glycoprotein in hepatocytes by the mediators of acute-phase response. *Biochem. Biophys. Res. Commun.* **2009**, *382*, 776–779. [CrossRef]
12. O'Donnell, L.C.; Druhan, L.J.; Avalos, B.R. Molecular characterization and expression analysis of leucine-rich alpha2-glycoprotein, a novel marker of granulocytic differentiation. *J. Leukoc. Biol.* **2002**, *72*, 478–485. [CrossRef] [PubMed]
13. Serada, S.; Fujimoto, M.; Terabe, F.; Iijima, H.; Shinzaki, S.; Matsuzaki, S.; Ohkawara, T.; Nezu, R.; Nakajima, S.; Kobayashi, T.; et al. Serum leucine-rich alpha-2 glycoprotein is a disease activity biomarker in ulcerative colitis. *Inflamm. Bowel Dis.* **2012**, *18*, 2169–2179. [CrossRef] [PubMed]
14. Scheller, J.; Garbers, C.; Rose-John, S. Interleukin-6: From basic biology to selective blockade of pro-inflammatory activities. *Semin. Immunol.* **2014**, *26*, 2–12. [CrossRef] [PubMed]
15. Mavropoulou, E.; Mechie, N.-C.; Knoop, R.; Petzold, G.; Ellenrieder, V.; Kunsch, S.; Pilavakis, Y.; Amanzada, A. Association of serum interleukin-6 and soluble interleukin-2-receptor levels with disease activity status in patients with inflammatory bowel disease: A prospective observational study. *PLoS ONE* **2020**, *15*, e0233811. [CrossRef]
16. Napetschnig, J.; Wu, H. Molecular basis of NF-κB signaling. *Annu. Rev. Biophys.* **2013**, *42*, 443–468. [CrossRef]

17. Lochhead, P.; Khalili, H.; Ananthakrishnan, A.N.; Richter, J.M.; Chan, A.T. Association Between Circulating Levels of C-reactive Protein and Interleukin-6 and Risk of Inflammatory Bowel Disease. *Clin. Gastroenterol. Hepatol.* **2016**, *14*, 818–824. [CrossRef]
18. Darlington, G.J.; Wilson, D.R.; Lachman, L.B. Monocyte-conditioned medium, interleukin-1, and tumor necrosis factor stimulate the acute phase response in human hepatoma cells in vitro. *J. Cell Biol.* **1986**, *103*, 787–793. [CrossRef]
19. Mańkowska-Wierzbicka, D.; Karczewski, J.; Poniedziałek, B.; Grzymisławska, M.; Staszewski, R.; Królczyk, A.; Dobrowolska, A.; Grzymisławski, M. C-reactive protein as a diagnostic and prognostic factor in inflammatory bowel diseases. *Adv. Hyg. Exp. Med.* **2016**, *70*, 1124–1130. [CrossRef]
20. Zilberman, L.; Maharshak, N.; Arbel, Y.; Rogowski, O.; Rozenblat, M.; Shapira, I.; Berliner, S.; Arber, N.; Dotan, I. Correlated expression of high-sensitivity C-reactive protein in relation to disease activity in inflammatory bowel disease: Lack of differences between Crohn's disease and ulcerative colitis. *Digestion* **2006**, *73*, 205–209. [CrossRef]
21. Buckell, N.A.; Lennard-Jones, J.E.; Hernandez, M.A.; Kohn, J.; Riches, P.G.; Wadsworth, J. Measurement of serum proteins during attacks of ulcerative colitis as a guide to patient management. *Gut* **1979**, *20*, 22–27. [CrossRef]
22. Marner, I.L.; Friborg, S.; Simonsen, E. Disease activity and serum proteins in ulcerative colitis. Immunochemical quantitation. *Scand. J. Gastroenterol.* **1975**, *10*, 537–544. [CrossRef]
23. Naka, T.; Fujimoto, M. LRG is a novel inflammatory marker clinically useful for the evaluation of disease activity in rheumatoid arthritis and inflammatory bowel disease. *Immunol. Med.* **2018**, *41*, 62–67. [CrossRef]
24. Lewis, J.D.; Chuai, S.; Nessel, L.; Lichtenstein, G.R.; Aberra, F.N.; Ellenberg, J.H. Use of the noninvasive components of the Mayo score to assess clinical response in ulcerative colitis. *Inflamm. Bowel Dis.* **2008**, *14*, 1660–1666. [CrossRef]
25. Shinzaki, S.; Matsuoka, K.; Tanaka, H.; Takeshima, F.; Kato, S.; Torisu, T.; Ohta, Y.; Watanabe, K.; Nakamura, S.; Yoshimura, N.; et al. Leucine-rich alpha-2 glycoprotein is a potential biomarker to monitor disease activity in inflammatory bowel disease receiving adalimumab: PLANET study. *J. Gastroenterol.* **2021**, *56*, 560–569. [CrossRef]
26. Machin, D.; Campbell, M.J.; Fayers, P.; Pinol, A. (Eds.) *Sample Size Tables for Clinical Studies*, 2nd ed.; Blackwell Science: Hoboken, NJ, USA, 1997; 315p.
27. Walkiewicz, D.; Werlin, S.L.; Fish, D.; Scanlon, M.; Hanaway, P.; Kugathasan, S. Fecal calprotectin is useful in predicting disease relapse in pediatric inflammatory bowel disease. *Inflamm. Bowel Dis.* **2008**, *14*, 669–673. [CrossRef] [PubMed]
28. D'haens, G.; Ferrante, M.; Vermeire, S.; Baert, F.; Noman, M.; Moortgat, L.; Geens, P.; Iwens, D.; Aerden, I.; Van Assche, G.; et al. Fecal calprotectin is a surrogate marker for endoscopic lesions in inflammatory bowel disease. *Inflamm. Bowel Dis.* **2012**, *18*, 2218–2224. [CrossRef] [PubMed]
29. Chang, S.; Malter, L.; Hudesman, D. Disease monitoring in inflammatory bowel disease. *World J. Gastroenterol.* **2015**, *21*, 11246–11259. [CrossRef]
30. Ullah, N.; Wu, Y. Regulation of Conformational Changes in C-reactive Protein Alters its Bioactivity. *Cell Biochem. Biophys.* **2022**, *80*, 595–608. [CrossRef] [PubMed]
31. Ain, Q.U.; Sarfraz, M.; Prasesti, G.K.; Dewi, T.I.; Kurniati, N.F. Confounders in Identification and Analysis of Inflammatory Biomarkers in Cardiovascular Diseases. *Biomolecules* **2021**, *11*, 1464. [CrossRef]

Journal of
Clinical Medicine

MDPI

Article

Hematological Composite Scores in Patients with Inflammatory Bowel Disease

Marta Carrillo-Palau [1], Belén Vera-Santana [1], Andrea Morant-Domínguez [1], Alejandro Hernández-Camba [2], Laura Ramos [1], Inmaculada Alonso-Abreu [1], Noemi Hernández Álvarez-Buylla [1], Laura Arranz [2], Milagros Vela [2], Manuel Hernández-Guerra [1], Cristina Gómez-Moreno [3], Miguel Á. González-Gay [4,5,*] and Iván Ferraz-Amaro [6,7,*]

1 Division of Gastroenterology, Hospital Universitario de Canarias, 38320 Tenerife, Spain; mcarpal@gobiernodecanarias.org (M.C.-P.); bversanq@gobiernodecanarias.org (B.V.-S.); amordom@gobiernodecanarias.org (A.M.-D.); lrlopez@gobiernodecanarias.org (L.R.); ialoabr@gobiernodecanarias.org (I.A.-A.); nheralv@gobiernodecanarias.org (N.H.Á.-B.); mhernand@ull.edu.es (M.H.-G.)
2 Division of Gastroenterology, Hospital Universitario de Nuestra Señora de la Candelaria, 38010 Tenerife, Spain; ahercamxl@gobiernodecanarias.org (A.H.-C.); larrher@gobiernodecanarias.org (L.A.); mvelgon@gobiernodecanarias.org (M.V.)
3 Fundación Jiménez Díaz School of Nursing of Madrid, Autonomous University of Madrid, 28040 Madrid, Spain; cgomezm@fdj.es
4 Division of Rheumatology, Instituto de Investigación Sanitaria Fundación Jiménez Díaz, 28040 Madrid, Spain
5 Department of Medicine, University of Cantabria, 39005 Santander, Spain
6 Division of Rheumatology, Hospital Universitario de Canarias, 38320 Tenerife, Spain
7 Department of Internal Medicine, Universidad de La Laguna (ULL), 38200 Tenerife, Spain
* Correspondence: miguel.ggay@quironsalud.es (M.Á.G.-G.); iferraza@ull.edu.es (I.F.-A.)

Abstract: The neutrophil-to-lymphocyte ratio (NLR), platelet-to-lymphocyte ratio (PLR), monocyte-to-lymphocyte ratio (MLR), and the systemic immune-inflammatory index (SIRI, neutrophils × monocytes/lymphocytes) have been identified as potential inflammatory biomarkers. In this work we aimed to analyze whether the hematological composite scores differ between inflammatory bowel disease (IBD) patients and healthy controls, and if they are related to disease activity. A total of 197 IBD patients—130 Crohn's (CD) disease and 67 ulcerative colitis (UC)—and 208 age- and sex-matched healthy controls were enrolled. C-reactive protein and fecal calprotectin were assessed. Multivariable linear regression analysis was executed. After adjustment, NLR and PLR, but not SIRI and MLR, were significantly higher in IBD patients compared to controls. C-reactive protein and SIRI and NLR were correlated in IBD patients. However, fecal calprotectin was not related to any of these blood scores. Furthermore, disease activity parameters were not associated with any of the blood composite scores in both CD and UC patients. In conclusion, NLR and PLR, but not SIRI and MLR, are independently higher in IBD patients compared to controls. However, the four hematological scores are not related to disease activity in either CD or UC patients. Based on these results, blood-based inflammatory scores may not serve as subrogated biomarkers of disease activity in IBD.

Keywords: inflammatory bowel disease; systemic immune-inflammatory index; hematological inflammatory scores

1. Introduction

The Systemic Inflammation Response Index (SIRI) is a novel prognostic marker that relies on the relative proportions of peripheral neutrophils, monocytes, and lymphocytes, calculated by multiplying the neutrophil count by the monocyte count and then dividing by the lymphocyte count [1]. This score is part of the group of other hematological scores previously described, such as the neutrophil-lymphocyte ratio (NLR) [2], the platelet-lymphocyte ratio (PLR) [3], and the lymphocyte-monocyte ratio (LMR) [4]. These are regarded as markers of inflammation because white blood cells and platelets are typically present in acute and chronic inflammatory settings, where they release cytokines, proteases, angiogenic factors, and chemokines [5]. In recent years, these scores have generated interest and have gained relevance because they have been described as relating to or predicting certain outcomes in chronic inflammatory, autoimmune [6–8], and cardiovascular diseases [9], as well as in cancer [10] or infections [11].

Inflammatory bowel disease (IBD) comprises two main disorders: ulcerative colitis (UC) and Crohn's disease (CD). While UC affects the colon, CD can affect any component of the gastrointestinal tract from the mouth to the perianal area. Both are considered inflammatory conditions characterized by relapsing and remitting episodes. Inflammation in UC is limited to the mucosal layer of the colon whereas CD is characterized by transmural inflammation and by skip areas of involvement. Recent findings indicate that subjective assessments of disease activity in IBD may be misleading [12]. Moreover, while objective inflammation markers are closely linked to significant long-term results, they frequently necessitate invasive and costly procedures like ileocolonoscopy and cross-sectional imaging techniques involving computed tomography or magnetic. For this reason, in practice, serum or fecal markers such as C-reactive protein (CRP) and fecal calprotectin are used as measures of intestinal inflammation. However, they are not specific for IBD [13,14], cut-off points have not been defined for both that determine activity [15,16], and their diagnostic or predictive capacity for relapse is doubtful [17–19]. For this reason, the challenge persists for locating inflammation markers that are more precise, sensitive, and adaptive, with the aim of enhancing IBD management.

In the present work we sought to determine if blood composite scores differ between IBD patients and controls. In a second step, we aimed to analyze whether these scores are related to acute phase reactants, fecal calprotectin or specific disease activity scores in patients with IBD, including UC and CD. If these scores were related to the activity of the disease, they could be proposed as surrogate biomarkers of the disease and, perhaps, be used as such in clinical practice.

2. Materials and Methods

2.1. Study Participants

A cross-sectional study was conducted, involving 197 consecutive patients diagnosed with IBD and 208 age-matched controls, all of whom were 18 years of age or older. IBD individuals were under the care of gastroenterologists and received periodic follow-ups at gastroenterology outpatient clinics. Inclusion criteria were a diagnosis of IBD based on clinical, endoscopic, and histological criteria with a disease duration of $\geq$1 year. Exclusion criteria for both groups included a history of cancer, any other inflammatory or autoimmune chronic disease, or evidence of active infection (because this could lead to upregulation of different blood cell types). The control group consisted of individuals from the community recruited by general practitioners in primary health centers. The study protocol was approved by the Institutional Review Committees at Hospital Universitario de Canarias and Hospital Universitario Nuestra Señora de La Candelaria, both located in Spain, and all participants provided written informed consent (approval no. CHUC_2019_103). Research involving human subjects adhered to the principles of the Helsinki Declaration.

2.2. Data Collection

Questionnaires regarding clinical history were conducted in both IBD patients and control groups to evaluate cardiovascular risk factors and medication usage. Hypertension was characterized as having a systolic blood pressure exceeding 140 mmHg or a diastolic blood pressure exceeding 90 mmHg. Disease activity in patients with CD was determined using two measures: the Crohn's Disease Activity Index (CDAI) and the Harvey-Bradshaw Index (HBI) [20]. Disease activity in UC was calculated through the partial Mayo Clinic score [21]. Dyslipidemia was determined based on meeting one or more of the following criteria: total cholesterol exceeding 200 mg/dL, triglyceride levels exceeding 150 mg/dL, HDL-cholesterol lower than 40 mg/dL in men or less than 50 mg/dL in women, or LDL-cholesterol surpassing 130 mg/dL. Hematological composite scores were computed as follows: neutrophil-to-lymphocyte ratio (NLR) = neutrophils/lymphocytes; monocyte-to-lymphocyte ratio (MLR) = monocytes/lymphocytes; platelet-to-lymphocyte ratio (PLR) = platelets/lymphocytes; systemic inflammation response index (SIRI) = neutrophils multiplied by monocytes, divided by lymphocytes. Neutrophils, monocytes, lymphocytes, and platelets were measured per 1000 cells/μL, except for platelets, which were measured per 100,000 cells/μL. Information regarding the therapies used in the disease was collected including the use of mesalazine, prednisone (as binary or mg/day), azathioprine and methotrexate, and biological therapies.

2.3. Statistical Analysis

In a previous work by our group, 430 patients with rheumatoid arthritis had a SIRI value of 1.22 ± 0.81 [8]. We have estimated that we would expect to find a difference in patients with IBD of 0.1. Thus, assuming an alpha error of 0.05 for a power of 80% and for an allocation between groups of 1:1, 194 subjects per group would have to be recruited. Demographic and clinical characteristics were presented as frequencies for binary variables. Continuous variable data were expressed as either mean ± standard deviation (SD) or as a median and interquartile range (IQR) for variables that did not follow a normal distribution. To assess univariate differences between patients and the control group, various statistical tests were employed, including Student's *t*-test, the Mann–Whitney U-test, the chi-squared test, or Fisher's exact test, depending on factors like distribution normality or sample size. Differences between IBD patients and controls in terms of hematological scores were examined using multivariable linear regression analysis, with the control group as the reference category. Confounding variables were selected from demographic factors and traditional cardiovascular risk factors if their p-values were less than 0.20 in the univariate analysis comparing patients and controls. All statistical analyses were carried out utilizing Stata software, version 17/SE (StataCorp, College Station, TX, USA), and a significance level of 5% was adopted for two-sided tests. A p value of less than 0.05 was considered indicative of statistical significance.

3. Results

3.1. Demographics and Disease-Related Data

A total of 197 IBD patients and 208 sex-matched controls with a mean ± SD age of 49 ± 10 and 50 ± 15 years, respectively, were included in this study. Demographic and disease-related characteristics of the participants are detailed in Table 1. The body mass index was higher in controls than in IBD patients (27 ± 5 vs. 29 ± 4 kg/m^2, $p \leq 0.001$). No significant differences were observed in smoking prevalence or dyslipidemia, but a higher proportion of controls had diabetes and hypertension. Among the patients, 66% had CD, and 32% had UC. The median disease duration for IBD was 12 years (IQR 8–19). In patients with CD, the predominant phenotypes were ileal and non-stricturing, non-penetrating. The median CDAI score was 39 (IQR 7–80), and 89% of the patients were classified as being in asymptomatic remission. Similarly, the Harvey–Bradshaw Index had a median score of 2 (IQR 0–4), with 82% of patients in the remission category based on this index. For UC, 52% had experienced pancolitis, and 78% had a partial Mayo score of less than 2 points. Further details concerning disease-related data can be found in Table 1.

Table 1. Characteristics of patients with inflammatory bowel disease and controls.

	Controls	IBD Patients	
	(n = 208)	(n = 197)	p
Age, years	50 ± 15	49 ± 10	0.25
Female, n (%)	124 (59)	107 (54)	0.28
Body mass index, kg/m^2	**29 ± 4**	**27 ± 5**	**<0.001**
Abdominal circumference, cm	93 ± 8	94 ± 12	0.49
Cardiovascular co-morbidity			
Smoking, n (%)	45 (22)	39 (20)	0.65
Diabetes, n (%)	**29 (14)**	**11 (6)**	**0.004**
Hypertension, n (%)	**63 (30)**	**35 (18)**	**0.003**
Dyslipidemia, n (%)	190 (77)	157 (80)	0.53
Obesity, n (%)	57 (27)	55 (28)	0.91
Statins, n (%)	**47 (23)**	**21 (11)**	**0.001**
IBD related data			
Ulcerative colitis, n (%)		67 (34)	
Crohn's disease, n (%)		130 (66)	
Disease duration since diagnosis, years		12 (8-19)	
CRP, mg/L	2.0 (1.0–4.8)	1.8 (0.9–3.8)	0.30
Ulcerative Colitis related data, n (%)			
Partial Mayo score		1 (0-1)	
<2		52 (78)	
≥2		15 (21)	
Pancolitis		34 (52)	
Left-sided colitis		23 (35)	
Proctosigmoiditis		7 (10)	
Crohn's Disease related data, n (%)			
A1 below 16 years		19 (15)	
A2 between 17 and 40 years		81 (62)	
A3 above 40 years		27 (21)	
B1 non-stricturing, non-penetrating		73 (56)	
B2 stricturing		46 (35)	
B3 penetrating		14 (11)	
L1 ileal		56 (43)	
L2 colonic		23 (18)	
L3 ileocolonic		51 (39)	
L4 isolated upper disease		11 (8)	
Harvey-Bradshaw Index		2 (0–4)	
Clinical remission		106 (82)	
Mildly active disease		14 (11)	
Moderately active disease		8 (6)	
Severely active disease		1 (1)	
CDAI score		39 (7–80)	
Asymptomatic remission		116 (89)	
Mildly to moderately active Crohn disease		10 (8)	
Moderately to severely active Crohn disease		3 (2)	
Severely active to fulminant disease		0 (0)	
Fecal calprotectin, mcg/g		113 (30–251)	
>150		96 (49)	
≥150		71 (36)	
Perianal disease, n (%)		23 (12)	
Previous surgery, n (%)		55 (28)	
Oral mesalazine, n (%)		175 (89)	
Prednisone, mg/day		8 (5–20)	
Current prednisone, n (%)		6 (2)	
Methotrexate, n (%)		22 (11)	
Azathioprine, n (%)		61 (31)	
Anti-TNF therapy, n (%)		58 (29)	
Ustekinumab, n (%)		8 (4)	
Vedolizumab, n (%)		5 (3)	
Tofacitinib, n (%)		4 (2)	

Data represent mean ± SD or median (interquartile range) when data were not normally distributed. BMI: body mass index; CRP: C reactive protein; TNF: tumor necrosis factor. CDAI was categorized as 0 to 149: asymptomatic remission; 150 to 220 points: mildly to moderately active; 221 to 450 points: moderately to severely active; 451 to 1100 points: severely active to fulminant disease. The Harvey-Bradshaw Index was categorized as 0 to 4 points: clinical remission; 5 to 7 points: mildly active disease, 8 to 16 points: moderately active disease; 17 to 100 points: severely active disease. Dyslipidemia was characterized by meeting any of the following criteria: total cholesterol exceeding 200 mg/dL, triglyceride levels surpassing 150 mg/dL, HDL-cholesterol below 40 mg/dL in men or under 50 mg/dL in women, or LDL-cholesterol exceeding 130 mg/dL. Significant p values are depicted in bold.

3.2. Differences between Patients and Controls in Hematological Count Cells and Scores

Red cell, leucocyte and platelet count differences between patients with IBD and controls are shown in Table 2. Regarding red blood cells, although hemoglobin and hematocrit values did not differ between both groups, the mean corpuscular volume and the mean corpuscular hemoglobin were higher, and the mean corpuscular hemoglobin concentration was lower in IBD patients compared to controls after multivariable analysis. Furthermore, lymphocytes, eosinophils, and basophils were significantly lower in IBD patients compared to healthy controls after adjustment for covariates. However, platelets and the mean platelet volume did not show differences between patients and controls (Table 2). Regarding composite hematological scores, after multivariable analysis, NLR and PLR were higher in patients with IBD than in controls. This difference was not observed for SIRI and MLR. Similar results were found when this analysis was performed separately in patients with CD and UC (Supplementary Table S1). In this regard, NLR and PLR, but not SIRI or MLR, differed between patients with CD and healthy controls. Additionally, only PLR, but not SIRI, NLR or MLR, disclosed significant differences between patients with UC and healthy subjects (Supplementary Table S1).

Table 2. Multivariable analysis of the differences between patients and controls in hematological count cells and scores.

	Controls (n = 208)	IBD Patients (n = 197)	p	Beta Coef. (95%CI)	p
	Univariable			Multivariable	
Red blood cells, $\times 10^6/\text{mm}^3$	4.76 ± 0.49	4.67 ± 0.47	0.056	−0.09 (−0.19–0.01)	0.076
Hemoglobin, g/dL	14.0 ± 1.5	14.0 ± 1.5	0.77		
Hematocrit, %	42.9 ± 4.1	42.7 ± 3.9	0.63		
Mean corpuscular volume, fL	**90.3 ± 5.8**	**91.7 ± 5.6**	**0.011**	**1.6 (0.5–2.8)**	**0.006**
Mean corpuscular hemoglobin, pg	**29.6 ± 2.5**	**30.3 ± 2.6**	**0.003**	**0.8 (0.3–1.3)**	**0.003**
Mean corpuscular hemoglobin concentration, g/dL	**32.7 ± 1.2**	**30.9 ± 5.8**	**<0.001**	**−1.6 (−2.5–(−0.8))**	**<0.001**
Leucocytes/mm^3	**7480 ± 1941**	**7003 ± 2079**	**0.019**	−292 (−701–118)	0.16
Neutrophils/mm^3	4154 ± 1504	4139 ± 1615	0.92		
Lymphocytes/mm^3	**2427 ± 827**	**2037 ± 835**	**<0.001**	**−339 (−509–(−169))**	**<0.001**
Monocytes/mm^3	600 ± 171	584 ± 249	0.48		
Eosinophils/mm^3	**245 ± 176**	**196 ± 169**	**0.005**	**−44 (−80–(−8))**	**0.016**
Basophils/mm^3	**50 ± 26**	**43 ± 25**	**0.006**	**−6 (−11–(−1))**	**0.027**
Platelets $\times 10^3/\text{mm}^3$	263 ± 59	270 ± 69	0.27		
Mean platelet volume, fL	10.2 ± 0.9	10.2 ± 1.0	0.69		
Composite hematological scores					
Systemic inflammation response index (SIRI) $\times 10^{-3}$	1. 23 ± 1.20	1.36 ± 0.94	0.26		
Neutrophil-to-lymphocyte ratio	**1.99 ± 1.57**	**2.32 ± 1.24**	**0.022**	**0.3 (0.03–0.6)**	**0.033**
Monocyte-to-lymphocyte ratio	0.29 ± 0.23	0.34 ± 0.38	0.085	0.05 (−0.01–0.1)	0.13
Platelet-to-lymphocyte ratio	**125 ± 79**	**156 ± 80**	**<0.001**	**27 (11–44)**	**0.001**

In the multivariable analysis controls is considered the reference category. IBD: Inflammatory bowel disease. Multivariable analysis is adjusted for body mass index, diabetes, hypertension, and statins intake. Significant p values are depicted in bold.

3.3. Relationship of C-Reactive Protein, Fecal Calprotectin and Disease Activity Scores to Composite Hematological Scores

The relationship between CRP, fecal calprotectin and disease activity scores with composite blood-based scores is shown in Table 3. While CRP and SIRI and NLR were significantly and positively correlated, no relationship was found between CRP and MLR and PLR. Remarkably, fecal calprotectin did not disclose association with any of the hematological scores. In addition, concerning disease activity scores, CDAI score and Harvey-Bradshaw index, that correspond to CD, were not related to any composite blood scores. Similarly, partial Mayo score, that represents UC disease activity, was not significantly associated with the hematological scores (Table 3).

Table 3. Relationship of C-reactive protein, fecal calprotectin and disease activity scores to composite hematological scores.

	Beta Coef. (95%CI), *p*							
	SIRI		NLR		MLR		PLR	
CRP, mg/L	**55 (25–84)**	**<0.001**	**0.06 (0.02–0.1)**	**0.003**	0.007 (−0.01–0.01)	0.91	1 (−1–4)	0.28
Fecal calprotectin, mcg/g	0.1 (−0.2–0.4)	0.44	0.00005 (−0.0004–0.0005)	0.82	3×10^{-6} (−0.0001–0.0001)	0.97	0.009 (−0.02–0.03)	0.50
Crohn's disease								
CDAI score	0.6 (−2–3)	0.65	0.001 (−0.002–0.004)	0.50	−0.0004 (−0.001–0.0008)	0.52	0.06 (−0.1–0.3)	0.54
Asymptomatic remission	ref.		ref.		ref.		ref.	
Mildly to moderately active	309 (−372–991)	0.37	0.4 (−0.5–1.3)	0.35	0.02 (−0.3–0.3)	0.89	17 (−40–73)	0.56
Moderately to severely active	−97 (−1246–1054)	0.87	−0.6 (−2.1–0.9)	0.40	−0.1 (−0.6–0.4)	0.66	−23 (−118–71)	0.63
Harvey-Bradshaw Index	6 (−53–65)	0.84	0.009 (−0.07–0.08)	0.83	−0.02 (−0.04–0.01)	0.21	−3 (−8–1)	0.16
Clinical remission	ref.		ref.		ref.		ref.	
Mildly active disease	−32 (−595–531)	0.91	−0.3 (−1.1–0.4)	0.38	−0.08 (−0.3–0.2)	0.52	−44 (−89–1)	0.056
Moderately to severity active	−72 (−797–652)	0.34	−0.1 (−1.0–0.9)	0.90	−0.1 (−0.5–0.2)	0.44	−46 (−104–12)	0.12
Ulcerative Colitis related data								
Partial Mayo score	−3 (−138–133)	0.97	0.03 (−0.2–0.2)	0.73	−0.008 (−0.3–0.01)	0.50	−2 (−15–11)	0.79
<2	ref.		ref.		ref.		ref.	
≥2	−48 (−535–438)	0.84	0.2 (−0.4–0.9)	0.52	−0.01 (−0.09–0.07)	0.73	3 (−43–49)	0.91

Hematological scores are the dependent variables in this analysis. CDAI was categorized as 0 to 149: asymptomatic remission; 150 to 220 points: mildly to moderately active; 221 to 450 points: moderately to severely active; 451 to 1100 points: severely active to fulminant disease. The Harvey-Bradshaw Index was categorized as 0 to 4 points: clinical remission; 5 to 7 points: mildly active disease; 8 to 16 points: moderately active disease; 17 to 100 points: severely active disease. Significant *p* values are depicted in bold.

4. Discussion

In the present study we have analyzed four hematological scores, which have shown a relationship with certain outcomes in cancer, autoimmune, cardiovascular and inflammatory diseases, in a large series of patients with IBD. Based on our findings, NLR and PLR were significantly higher in IBD patients but this was not the case for SIRI and MLR. However, none of them showed a relationship with markers of systemic inflammation, fecal calprotectin or activity scores of both UC and CD.

In a previous work that evaluated SIRI in 87 patients with UC, patients were divided into active and non-active disease groups based on the Mayo score. In that study, SIRI was discovered to be superior in patients with active disease compared with UC in remission, and correlated with CRP [22]. Similarly, in a report of 187 patients with UC and 185 age- and sex-matched controls, higher SIRI levels were observed in moderate and severe UC subgroups compared to mild or remission subgroups [23]. Moreover, correlation analysis displayed that the SIRI levels were positively related with the Mayo score. This correlation maintained its significance after multivariable analysis. Similar findings were found in a work in 167 patients with UC and 106 controls [24]. SIRI significantly augmented in patients with UC and was closely correlated with the Mayo clinical score, Mayo endoscopic score, and Nancy histological index.

Regarding other blood-based scores, NLR and PLR have been found to be significantly elevated in UC subjects compared to controls in a report of 187 consecutive patients with UC and 185 age- and sex-matched healthy controls [23]. Similarly, in a work of UC patients in which 151 were active, and 36 in remission, NLR and PLR were significantly higher in the active group [25].

Few studies have assessed composite hematological scores in CD. In this regard, in a report of 44 patients with active CD, 66 patients with inactive CD, and 55 healthy blood donors, NLR values were found to be elevated in active CD compared to inactive CD patients plus controls, but no statistical differences were found between the active and inactive CD groups [26]. In contrast, in a report of 24 active and 25 inactive CD patients, the NLR was found to be higher in the active group [27].

Regarding MLR, a recent systematic review and meta-analysis that included nine studies found that MLR values were significantly higher in active IBD patients as compared to those under remission being these results consistent in both UC and CD patients with active disease [28]. However, our study does not support these previous findings. It should be noted that our sample size allowed us to perform multivariable analysis. Furthermore, the characterization of our series of patients has been broader than in previous works. On the other hand, in the studies discussed above, disease activity was generally dichotomized. In this regard, in our work we evaluated the scores in a continuous and binary manner. Moreover, it is important to take into account that the majority of patients from our series, both in UC and CD, had low disease activity. This would support the fact that these scores are not valid to measure disease activity in patients when the disease is under control.

In our study we found that patients with IBD had a BMI in the overweight range but significantly lower than controls. This is in line with previous studies in which it has been described that patients with IBD have lower BMI values compared to controls [29]. This is believed to be due to the inflammatory activity of the disease. However, we believe this fact may have not affected our results since the differences in hematological scores between patients and controls were adjusted for this BMI.

We acknowledge the limitation that for UC subjects, partial Mayo score and not complete Mayo score was available for these patients. Furthermore, the cross-sectional design of our work prevents concluding causality. Additionally, patients with IBD may present hematological disruptions caused by certain therapies used in the disease such as methotrexate or azathioprine.

5. Conclusions

In conclusion, the SIRI, NLR, MLR and PLR hematological-based scores are not appropriate for the monitoring of disease activity in patients with IBD that are in the range of low or moderate activity.

Supplementary Materials: The following supporting information can be downloaded at: https://www.mdpi.com/article/10.3390/jcm12237248/s1, Table S1: Univariable analysis of the differences between patients with Crohn's disease and ulcerative colitis and controls in hematological count cells and scores.

Author Contributions: I.F.-A. and M.Á.G.-G.: Conception, design, and interpretation of the data; M.C.-P., B.V.-S., A.M.-D., A.H.-C., L.R., I.A.-A., N.H.Á.-B., M.H.-G., L.A., M.V. and C.G.-M.: Acquisition of the data. All authors have read and agreed to the published version of the manuscript.

Funding: This work was supported by a grant to I. Ferraz-Amaro from the Spanish Ministry of Health, Instituto de Salud Carlos III (ISCIII), co-funded by European Union (grant number: PI20/00084).

Institutional Review Board Statement: The study protocol received approval from the Institutional Review Committee at both Hospital Universitario de Canarias and Hospital Universitario Nuestra Señora de La Candelaria, both in Spain. All participating individuals provided written informed consent (approval number CHUC_2019_103). The research was conducted in strict adherence to applicable guidelines and regulations, as well as in accordance with the principles outlined in the Declaration of Helsinki.

Informed Consent Statement: Informed consent was obtained from all subjects involved in the study.

Data Availability Statement: The data sets used and/or analyzed in the present study are available from the corresponding author upon request.

Conflicts of Interest: The authors report no conflict of interest. However, it is worth noting that Iván Ferraz-Amaro has received research grants and support from Abbott, MSD, Janssen, and Roche, and has also received consulting fees from speaker bureaus associated with Abbott, Pfizer, Roche, Sanofi, Celgene. Additionally, M.A. González-Gay has received consulting fees and participated in company-sponsored speaker bureaus with Sanofi, Lilly, and Amgen.

References

1. Qi, Q.; Zhuang, L.; Shen, Y.; Geng, Y.; Yu, S.; Chen, H.; Liu, L.; Meng, Z.; Wang, P.; Chen, Z. A Novel Systemic Inflammation Response Index (SIRI) for Predicting the Survival of Patients with Pancreatic Cancer after Chemotherapy. *Cancer* **2016**, *122*, 2158–2167. [CrossRef]
2. Buonacera, A.; Stancanelli, B.; Colaci, M.; Malatino, L. Neutrophil to Lymphocyte Ratio: An Emerging Marker of the Relationships between the Immune System and Diseases. *Int. J. Mol. Sci.* **2022**, *23*, 3636. [CrossRef]
3. Balta, S.; Ozturk, C. The Platelet-Lymphocyte Ratio: A Simple, Inexpensive and Rapid Prognostic Marker for Cardiovascular Events. *Platelets* **2015**, *26*, 680–681. [CrossRef] [PubMed]
4. Balta, S.; Demirer, Z.; Aparci, M.; Yildirim, A.O.; Ozturk, C. The Lymphocyte-Monocyte Ratio in Clinical Practice. *J. Clin. Pathol.* **2016**, *69*, 88–89. [CrossRef] [PubMed]
5. Kany, S.; Vollrath, J.T.; Relja, B. Cytokines in Inflammatory Disease. *Int. J. Mol. Sci.* **2019**, *20*, 6008. [CrossRef] [PubMed]
6. Xu, Y.; He, H.; Zang, Y.; Yu, Z.; Hu, H.; Cui, J.; Wang, W.; Gao, Y.; Wei, H.; Wang, Z. Systemic Inflammation Response Index (SIRI) as a Novel Biomarker in Patients with Rheumatoid Arthritis: A Multi-Center Retrospective Study. *Clin. Rheumatol.* **2022**, *41*, 1989–2000. [CrossRef] [PubMed]
7. Liu, B.; Wang, J.; Li, Y.Y.; Li, K.P.; Zhang, Q. The Association between Systemic Immune-Inflammation Index and Rheumatoid Arthritis: Evidence from NHANES 1999–2018. *Arthritis Res. Ther.* **2023**, *25*, 34. [CrossRef] [PubMed]
8. González-Sierra, M.; Quevedo-Rodríguez, A.; Romo-Cordero, A.; González-Chretien, G.; Quevedo-Abeledo, J.C.; de Vera-González, A.; González-Delgado, A.; Martín-González, C.; González-Gay, M.Á.; Ferraz-Amaro, I. Relationship of Blood Inflammatory Composite Markers with Cardiovascular Risk Factors and Subclinical Atherosclerosis in Patients with Rheumatoid Arthritis. *Life* **2023**, *13*, 1469. [CrossRef]
9. Dziedzic, E.A.; Gąsior, J.S.; Tuzimek, A.; Paleczny, J.; Junka, A.; Dąbrowski, M.; Jankowski, P. Investigation of the Associations of Novel Inflammatory Biomarkers-Systemic Inflammatory Index (SII) and Systemic Inflammatory Response Index (SIRI)-With the Severity of Coronary Artery Disease and Acute Coronary Syndrome Occurrence. *Int. J. Mol. Sci.* **2022**, *23*, 9553. [CrossRef]
10. Zhou, Q.; Su, S.; You, W.; Wang, T.; Ren, T.; Zhu, L. Systemic Inflammation Response Index as a Prognostic Marker in Cancer Patients: A Systematic Review and Meta-Analysis of 38 Cohorts. *Dose-Response* **2021**, *19*, 15593258211064744. [CrossRef]

11. Muhammad, S.; Fischer, I.; Naderi, S.; Jouibari, M.F.; Abdolreza, S.; Karimialavijeh, E.; Aslzadeh, S.; Mashayekhi, M.; Zojaji, M.; Kahlert, U.D.; et al. Systemic Inflammatory Index Is a Novel Predictor of Intubation Requirement and Mortality after SARS-CoV-2 Infection. *Pathogens* **2021**, *10*, 58. [CrossRef] [PubMed]
12. Sands, B.E. Biomarkers of Inflammation in Inflammatory Bowel Disease. *Gastroenterology* **2015**, *149*, 1275–1285.e2. [CrossRef] [PubMed]
13. Van Rheenen, P.F.; Van De Vijver, E.; Fidler, V. Faecal Calprotectin for Screening of Patients with Suspected Inflammatory Bowel Disease: Diagnostic Meta-Analysis. *BMJ* **2010**, *341*, 188. [CrossRef]
14. Menees, S.B.; Powell, C.; Kurlander, J.; Goel, A.; Chey, W.D. A Meta-Analysis of the Utility of C-Reactive Protein, Erythrocyte Sedimentation Rate, Fecal Calprotectin, and Fecal Lactoferrin to Exclude Inflammatory Bowel Disease in Adults with IBS. *Am. J. Gastroenterol.* **2015**, *110*, 444–454. [CrossRef]
15. Kristensen, V.; Moum, B. Correspondence: Fecal Calprotectin and Cut-off Levels in Inflammatory Bowel Disease. *Scand. J. Gastroenterol.* **2015**, *50*, 1183–1184. [CrossRef] [PubMed]
16. Guardiola, J.; Lobatón, T.; Rodríguez-Alonso, L.; Ruiz-Cerulla, A.; Arajol, C.; Loayza, C.; Sanjuan, X.; Sánchez, E.; Rodríguez-Moranta, F. Fecal Level of Calprotectin Identifies Histologic Inflammation in Patients with Ulcerative Colitis in Clinical and Endoscopic Remission. *Clin. Gastroenterol. Hepatol.* **2014**, *12*, 1865–1870. [CrossRef] [PubMed]
17. Osterman, M.T.; Aberra, F.N.; Cross, R.; Liakos, S.; McCabe, R.; Shafran, I.; Wolf, D.; Hardi, R.; Nessel, L.; Brensinger, C.; et al. Mesalamine Dose Escalation Reduces Fecal Calprotectin in Patients with Quiescent Ulcerative Colitis. *Clin. Gastroenterol. Hepatol.* **2014**, *12*, 1887–1893.e3. [CrossRef]
18. Kallel, L.; Ayadi, I.; Matri, S.; Fekih, M.; Mahmoud, N.B.; Feki, M.; Karoui, S.; Zouari, B.; Boubaker, J.; Kaabachi, N.; et al. Fecal Calprotectin Is a Predictive Marker of Relapse in Crohn's Disease Involving the Colon: A Prospective Study. *Eur. J. Gastroenterol. Hepatol.* **2010**, *22*, 340–345. [CrossRef]
19. Laharie, D.; Mesli, S.; El Hajbi, F.; Chabrun, E.; Chanteloup, E.; Capdepont, M.; Razaire, S.; De Lédinghen, V.; Zerbib, F. Prediction of Crohn's Disease Relapse with Faecal Calprotectin in Infliximab Responders: A Prospective Study. *Aliment. Pharmacol. Ther.* **2011**, *34*, 462–469. [CrossRef]
20. Harvey, R.F.; Bradshaw, J.M. A Simple Index of Crohn's-Disease Activity. *Lancet* **1980**, *315*, 514. [CrossRef]
21. Schroeder, K.W.; Tremaine, W.J.; Ilstrup, D.M. Coated Oral 5-Aminosalicylic Acid Therapy for Mildly to Moderately Active Ulcerative Colitis. *N. Engl. J. Med.* **1987**, *317*, 1625–1629. [CrossRef]
22. Pakoz, Z.B.; Ustaoglu, M.; Vatansever, S.; Yuksel, E.S.; Topal, F. Serum Immune-Inflammation Index Assessment in the Patients with Ulcerative Colitis. *Gastroenterol. Res. Pract.* **2022**, *2022*, 1–5. [CrossRef] [PubMed]
23. Xie, Y.; Zhuang, T.; Ping, Y.; Zhang, Y.; Wang, X.; Yu, P.; Duan, X. Elevated Systemic Immune Inflammation Index Level Is Associated with Disease Activity in Ulcerative Colitis Patients. *Clin. Chim. Acta* **2021**, *517*, 122–126. [CrossRef]
24. Yan, J.; Deng, F.; Tan, Y.; Zhou, B.; Liu, D. Systemic Immune-Inflammation Index as a Potential Biomarker to Monitor Ulcerative Colitis. *Curr. Med. Res. Opin.* **2023**, *39*, 1321–1328. [CrossRef] [PubMed]
25. Lin, H.; Bai, Z.; Wu, Q.; Chu, G.; Zhang, Y.; Guo, X.; Qi, X. Inflammatory Indexes for Assessing the Severity and Disease Progression of Ulcerative Colitis: A Single-Center Retrospective Study. *Front. Public Health* **2022**, *10*, 851295. [CrossRef]
26. Gao, S.Q.; Huang, L.D.; Dai, R.J.; Chen, D.D.; Hu, W.J.; Shan, Y.F. Neutrophil-Lymphocyte Ratio: A Controversial Marker in Predicting Crohn's Disease Severity. *Int. J. Clin. Exp. Pathol.* **2015**, *8*, 14779.
27. Eraldemir, F.C.; Musul, M.; Duman, A.E.; Oztas, B.; Baydemir, C.; Hulagu, S. The Relationship between Neutrophil/Lymphocyte and Platelet/Lymphocyte Ratios with Oxidative Stress in Active Crohn's Disease Patients. *Hippokratia* **2016**, *20*, 368. [PubMed]
28. Gao, L.; Zhan, Y.; Hu, X.; Liao, S. Platelet-Lymphocyte Ratio and Lymphocyte-Monocyte Ratio in Inflammatory Bowel Disease and Disease Activity: A Systematic Review and Meta-Analysis. *Scott. Med. J.* **2023**, *68*, 101–109. [CrossRef]
29. Dong, J.; Chen, Y.; Tang, Y.; Xu, F.; Yu, C.; Li, Y.; Pankaj, P.; Dai, N. Body Mass Index Is Associated with Inflammatory Bowel Disease: A Systematic Review and Meta-Analysis. *PLoS ONE* **2015**, *10*, e0144872. [CrossRef]

Journal of
Clinical Medicine

MDPI

Article

Intensification with Intravenous Ustekinumab in Refractory Crohn's Disease

Cristina Suárez Ferrer [1,2,*], José Arroyo Argüelles [1], Jose Luis Rueda García [1,2], Laura García Ramírez [1,2], Eduardo Martin Arranz [1,2], María Sánchez Azofra [1,2], Joaquín Poza Cordón [1,2], Jesús Noci Belda [1] and Maria Dolores Martin-Arranz [1,2,3]

1 Inflammatory Bowel Disease Unit, Digestive Medicine Service, Hospital Universitario La Paz, 28046 Madrid, Spain; jmarroyo94@gmail.com (J.A.A.); eiiclapaz@gmail.com (L.G.R.); emarranz@salud.madrid.org (E.M.A.); maryazofra@gmail.com (M.S.A.); mmartinarranz@gmail.com (M.D.M.-A.)

2 IdiPAZ Study Group for Immune-Mediated Gastrointestinal Diseases, 28049 Madrid, Spain

3 Faculty de Medicina, Universidad Autónoma de Madrid, 28049 Madrid, Spain

* Correspondence: cristinajsuarezferrer@gmail.com

Abstract: Background: The rates of clinical and biochemical responses in Crohn's disease (CD) patients treated with intravenous (IV) ustekinumab (UST) intensification are scarcely described. Methods: Patients with diagnosis of CD who were under intensified IV ustekinumab treatment (130 mg every 4 weeks) were retrospectively included, evaluating the clinical and biochemical response 12 weeks after the change in treatment regimen (switch from SC to IV), as well as the serum levels of the drug. Results: Twenty-seven patients, all of whom had transitioned to intensified intravenous ustekinumab treatment due to a secondary loss of response to the drug, were included in the retrospective analysis. At the baseline visit, prior to changing IV UST, differences in levels were observed between intensified and non-intensified patients (7216 vs. 2842 ng/mL, $p = 0.00005$). However, no significant differences were found between these two groups 12 weeks after IV intensification (7949 vs. 7937 ng/mL; $p = 0.99$). In patients with previous intensified UST SC, a decrease in fecal calprotectin was observed 12 weeks after starting IV intensification, going from a mean of 1463 ug/g to 751 ug/g, although the differences were not significant ($p = 0.14$). Conclusion: In our experience, intensifying treatment with IV UST leads to clinical and biochemical improvements in CD patients with a secondary loss of response to SC maintenance with this drug, and an increase in drug levels was observed 12 weeks after IV UST intensification.

Keywords: Crohn's disease; ustekinumab

1. Introduction

In recent years, we have witnessed a rapid development in the therapeutic arsenal for the management and treatment of inflammatory bowel disease (IBD).

The first anti-TNF drugs were introduced in 2002 and remain a fundamental pillar for the treatment of our patients, being the most commonly used biological drugs. More recently, other biologicals with different therapeutic targets have been approved for use, such as Vedolizumab (an anti-integrin drug) or ustekinumab (anti-IL-12 and IL-23) [1].

Undoubtedly, this variety of treatments has expanded our treatment options, achieving better control of the disease with higher response rates and achieving deep remission in most of our patients.

However, the options to optimize biological treatments when there is a loss of response to the medication, that is, the intensification guidelines, are not clearly established, especially when we refer to more recent drugs such as ustekinumab or vedolizumab [2].

Ustekinumab is recommended in Crohn's disease for patients who have had an inadequate response, a had loss of response, or are intolerant (mainly due to the occurrence of adverse effects) to conventional treatment or anti-TNF, or where there are medical contraindications. It has shown the ability to induce and maintain remission in some patients, reducing the symptoms and intestinal inflammation associated with the disease.

In other words, ustekinumab is proposed as a second-line biological treatment after anti-TNF failure (or first-line treatment if there is a contraindication to the immunomodulatory or anti-TNF treatment) [3]. However, in real-life studies [4], most of the patients treated with ustekinumab have previously failed an anti-TNF or even two or three biologicals. Despite that, the clinical response to Ustekinumab stands at around 50% by week 52, with clinical remission rates reaching up to 39%.

This means that patients receiving ustekinumab are often refractory to treatment [4] and in a scenario where therapeutic alternatives are more limited. This probably translates into a greater need for treatment intensification.

In a recent review that included a network meta-analysis [5], drugs targeting IL-23 (ustekinumab and risankizumab) were identified as a potentially more effective strategy in patients with previous exposure to TNF antagonists.

The need to intensify ustekinumab for Crohn's disease arises primarily due to the loss of response to the drug. Over time, some patients might experience reduced effectiveness or diminished response to the standard dosage of ustekinumab. In such cases, intensifying the treatment involves increasing the dose or frequency of ustekinumab administration to regain a better therapeutic response and effectively manage the symptoms of Crohn's disease.

Evidence on the usefulness of treatment intensification comes from some real-life studies, in which benefits have been reported by shortening the regimen every 4 weeks and, even in some cases, every 3 weeks or even with an individualized regimen according to experience [6].

In previous studies in real life [7], it has been observed that after intensifying the subcutaneous ustekinumab regimen to 90 mg every 4 weeks, remission rates of up to 31% and clinical response rates of 61% are achieved.

Likewise, previous studies have explored the effectiveness of reinduction with intravenous ustekinumab (to subsequently continue with the subcutaneous regimen). A significant decrease in the Harvey Bradshaw index has been identified (reduction by 2.4 points ($p = 0.0034$)) [8]. Similarly, with the intensified regimen performed subcutaneously every 4 weeks, not only an improvement in the clinical indices has been observed, but also a biochemical response, especially in those patients with greater underlying inflammatory activity.

However, not all patients achieve a response after shortening the administration interval [9], so it is necessary in the management of our patients to explore other alternatives for drug intensification, such as intravenous drug transfer.

The proactive determination of biological drug levels in IBD, although yielding controversial results in previous studies, seems to be associated with better disease control and improved long-term outcomes. However, this correlation between drug levels and efficacy has been established with antiTNF drugs, not with other biological medications.

However, monitoring ustekinumab levels in the blood in the treatment of CD [10] can help to determine the appropriate amount of medication needed to control disease symptoms and maintain long-term remission. Therefore, the interpretation of these levels may vary depending on the patients, and, currently, the therapeutic range has not been established.

The objective of our study is to analyze the clinical response, biochemical response, and endoscopic/ultrasound improvements after intensifying treatment with an intravenous regimen every 4 weeks. Likewise, the goal is to determine the change in drug levels in the blood after switching from ustekinumab to intravenous maintenance treatment and ultimately establish if there is a relationship between drug levels and drug efficacy.

2. Material and Methods

A study was conducted where patients with a previously established diagnosis of Crohn's disease, undergoing treatment with intensified intravenous ustekinumab every 4 weeks, were retrospectively included. At our center, the cost of intravenous ustekinumab is lower than the subcutaneous form. Therefore, for those patients undergoing drug intensification every 4 weeks in clinical practice, there was a switch to the intravenous form of the medication.

Only those with stable follow-up in the IBD unit of Hospital La Paz were chosen, so it was possible to retrospectively assess the evolution and response to treatment.

Data related to patients' baseline characteristics were collected. Likewise, data related to the patients' previous pharmacological and surgical treatment for their IBD, as well as the previous ustekinumab regimen (start date, dose, and regimen), were included.

Clinical activity was assessed before switching to intravenous treatment, 12 weeks after the switch, and at the end of follow-up. The follow-up time was calculated from the date of the switch to intravenous treatment with ustekinumab every 4 weeks until the date of the last appointment. Clinical response was considered as a decrease in the Harvey Bradshaw score (HBI) [11] of $\geq$3.

Biochemical response was also assessed, as well as fecal calprotectin and C-reactive protein in blood, prior to the change to intravenous ustekinumab (considering the baseline level) and 12 weeks after the change to intravenous.

Finally, in those patients in whom it was available, endoscopic and radiological activities were investigated using intestinal ultrasound prior to the change to intravenous (baseline) and 12 weeks after it. Given the retrospective nature of the study, with the possible difficulty of having a baseline endoscopic and/or radiological study, examinations performed in the 6 months prior to the intravenous intensification of ustekinumab were included, provided that there were no clinical or treatment changes in this period. To assess the endoscopic response, the SES-CD index was used [11], considering remission $\leq$3 points.

As per usual clinical practice, in our center, trough levels of the drug (ustekinumab) are requested prior to each administration. Levels were assessed prior to switching to intravenous treatment (considering this as baseline levels) as well as after 12 weeks of the intensified regimen.

A descriptive analysis of the baseline characteristics and those related to their IBD was performed. For continuous variables, the mean and standard deviation were calculated; for the categorical, the percentages and 95% confidence intervals were calculated. Provided that the variables have a normal distribution (verified using the Shapiro–Wilk test), the categorical variables were compared using the c2 test, and the quantitative variables using the Student's T test. Otherwise, the corresponding non-parametric test was applied. A value of $p < 0.05$ was considered statistically significant. The analysis was carried out using Stata version 16 for Mac.

3. Results

A total of 27 patients with Crohn's disease receiving intensified treatment with ustekinumab, 130 mg intravenously every 4 weeks, were retrospectively included. All of them had undergone previous treatment with UST SC. Among them, five patients (18.5%) were receiving concomitant treatment with azathioprine.

Baseline and IBD-related characteristics of the included patients are summarized in Table 1.

Regarding previous treatment received by the patients, 4/27 (14.8%) were under treatment with UST on the first line, 10/27 (37%) on the second line, and 9/27 (33.4%) on the third line; 4/27 (14.8%) had failed three biologicals. The median number of previous biologicals was 2, IQR: 1–2.

The reason for intensification with IV UST was the secondary loss of response in all included patients, seven of whom (25.93%) were found in the context of post-surgical recurrence.

Table 1. Patient baseline characteristics.

Variables	Number of Patients, %			
Sex	Women		Men	
	(12) 44.4%		(15) 55.5%	
Tobacco	No	Yes	Former smoker	
	(16) 59.3%	(6) 22.2%	(5) 18.5%	
Extraintestinal manifestations	No		Yes	
	(22) 81.5%		(5) 18.5%	
Location (Montreal)	L1	L2	L3	L4
	(18) 66.6%	(0), 0%	(6), 22.2%	(3), 11.1%
Phenotype (Montreal)	B1	B2	B3	
	(6) 22.2%	(15) 55.5%	(6) 22.2%	
Perianal involvement	No		Yes	
	(18) 66.7%		(9) 33.3%	
Previous surgeries	No	1	2	3
	(18), 66.6%	(4), 14.8%	(4), 14.8%	(1), 3.7%
Concomitant immunosuppression	No		Yes	
	(22), 81.4%		(5), 18.5%	

It should be noted regarding the subcutaneous regimen prior to switching to intravenous that 10 patients (37.03%) were already under treatment with intensified SC UST (9 patients every 4 weeks and 1 patient every 6 weeks), while the remaining 17 patients (62.96%) were under treatment with a standard schedule of SC UST every 8 weeks.

No adverse effects related to the use of intravenous ustekinumab were observed during the study.

When assessing the clinical activity of the included patients, 70% (19 patients) had baseline activity (HBI $\geq$ 5), with no clinically or statistically significant changes at 12 weeks of treatment and at the last follow-up visit (70%, 67%, respectively). However, if we consider the severity of the clinical activity, it is noteworthy that 10 patients (37%) had severe baseline activity (HBI $\geq$ 9), decreasing to 14.8% (4 patients) 12 weeks after switching to intravenous and 11% (3 patients) at the end of follow-up Figure 1.

Among the 17 patients without prior intensified treatment before the switch to intravenous, baseline activity was mild in 26.7%, moderate in 26.7%, and severe in 6.6%. In this group, at 12 weeks after the intravenous intensification, mild activity was observed in 60%, 13.3% had moderate activity, and no patient exhibited severe activity. However, these differences did not reach statistical significance.

Overall, taking into account all the patients, a reduction in fecal calprotectin levels was observed at 12 weeks (463 vs. 272.5 ug/g), $p = 0.08$ Figure 2.

In patients with intensified sc UST, fecal calprotectin decreased 12 weeks after starting IV intensification, from a mean of 1463 to 751 ug/g, although the differences were not statistically significant ($p = 0.14$).

Likewise, a reduction in CRP was detected after 12 weeks of IV treatment (6.6 vs. 4.1 mg/L), although statistical significance was not reached ($p = 0.3$).

A significant increase in ustekinumab levels was observed 12 weeks after intensifying intravenous treatment and shortening the regimen (in those patients who initiated treatment with ustekinumab every 8 weeks sc), 7216 vs. 2842 ng/mL ($p = 0.0005$) Figure 3.

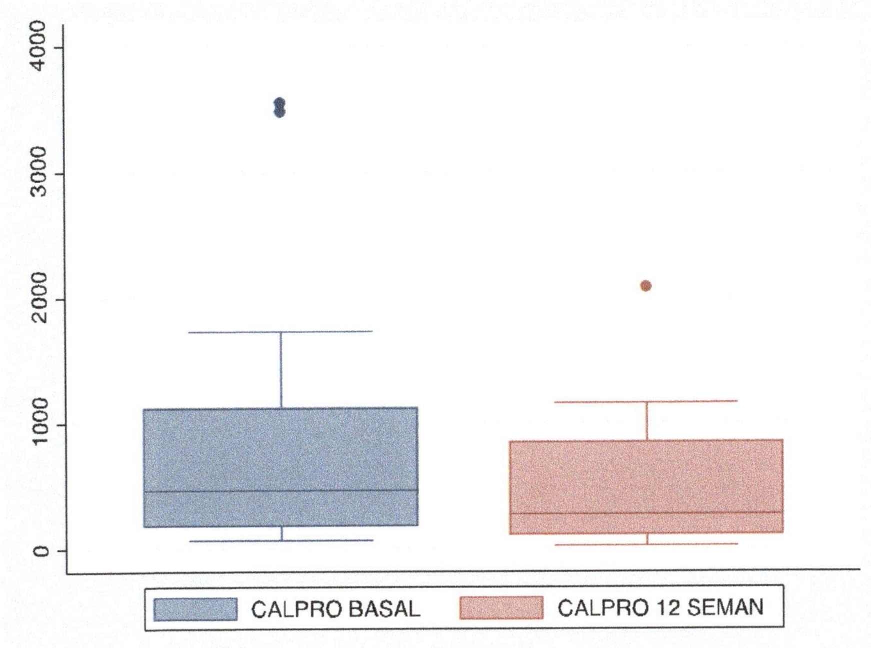

Figure 1. Improvement in fecal calprotectin levels 12 weeks after intravenous drug intensification.

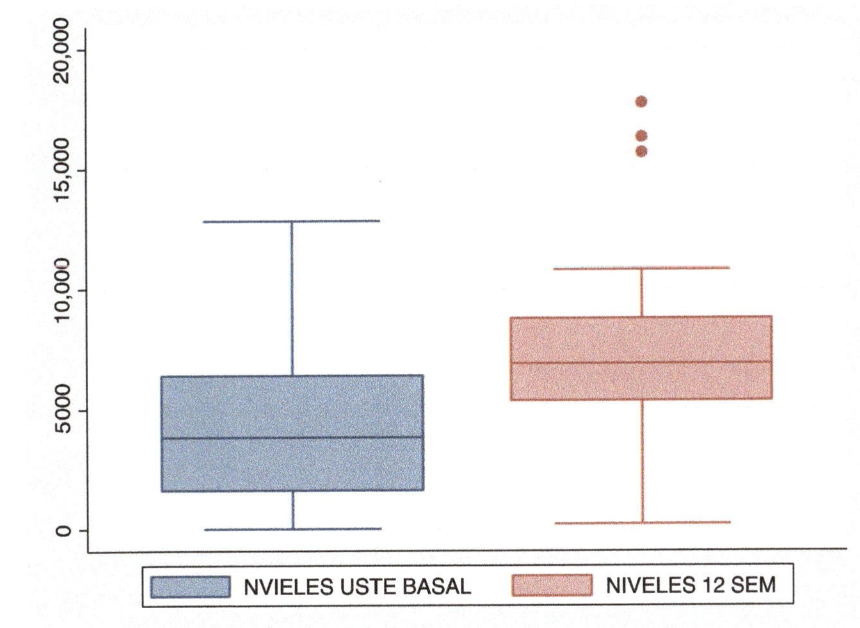

Figure 2. Improvement in ustekinumab levels 12 weeks after intravenous drug intensification.

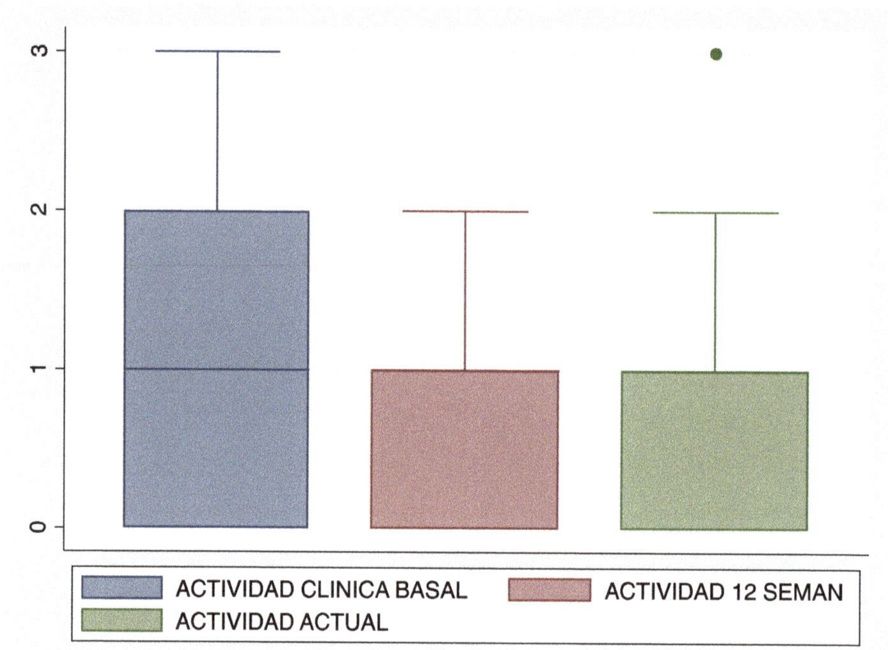

Figure 3. Clinical activity at baseline, 12 weeks after switching to ustekinumab iv, and at the end of follow-up.

The previous results are summarized in Table 2.

Table 2. Analysis of clinical activity, CRP, fecal calprotectin, and UST levels before and after (at 12 weeks) starting UST IV.

Variables	Basal				12 Weeks			
Clinical activity (n, %)	No	Mild	Moderate	Serious	No	Mild	Moderate	Serious
	8 29.6%	9 33.3%	8 29.6%	2 7.4%	9 33.3%	13 48.1%	5 18.5%	0 0%
PCR	Median		I.Q.R.		Median		I.Q.R.	
	6.6		10.7		4.1		6.7	
Calprotectin	Median		I.Q.R.		Median		I.Q.R.	
	463		946.5		272.5		749.5	
UST levels	Median		I.Q.R.		Median		I.Q.R.	
	3810		4840		6870		3510	

Despite these differences in drug levels after 12 weeks of IV treatment, no differences were observed among those patients who started with the intensified drug at the baseline visit (7949 vs. 7937 ng/mL; $p = 0.99$).

No correlation was found between higher drug levels at week 12 and the absence of clinical activity when analyzing the subgroup of patients without prior intensified drug regimens (8413.56 vs. 6672.5; $p = 0.5$).

Finally, the endoscopic study at baseline and at week 12 was available in only three patients. Two of them were in a situation of post-surgical recurrence and one with luminal activity. Endoscopic improvement was identified in two of the three patients, with a reduction in endoscopic activity indices (i3 at baseline vs. i1 at week 12, and SES-CD 26 vs. SES-CD 7).

As for ultrasound activity, it was available in 10 patients (at baseline and at 12 weeks), with significant improvements (no significant ultrasound activity) in 3 of them.

4. Discussion

Ustekinumab has been proven to be a safe and effective drug in patients with Crohn's disease both in clinical trials [12] and in real-life cohorts [13–16], also demonstrating excellent treatment survival in patients responding to the drug [17].

However, there is little evidence on what to do if there is an inadequate response or the disease relapses during maintenance. A recent meta-analysis [18] showed that reinduction with UST or interval shortening may be effective therapeutic alternatives in this setting, especially in patients coming from a standard maintenance regimen of sc ustekinumab every 8 weeks.

It should be noted that our study not only investigated the possibility of intensifying the maintenance treatment period (every 4 weeks), but also of administering the medication intravenously. In addition, 37% of the included patients had already started an intensified ustekinumab regimen before switching to intravenous (subcutaneous every 4 or 6 weeks).

In our experience, we observed a clinical and biochemical improvement (reduction in fecal calprotectin and CRP levels) 12 weeks after switching to the intravenous regimen, even in those patients who switched from the intensified subcutaneous regimen. It should be noted that most of the studies on the subject assessed the effectiveness of treatment intensification solely with clinical criteria and not biochemical criteria as in our study [19].

We have previous evidence [20–22] on the possible relationship between blood drug levels and therapeutic efficacy. However, in the case of ustekinumab, this is an underexplored field. In our study, an overall increase in ustekinumab blood levels was observed after intravenous intensification, although these differences did not reach statistical significance in those patients who switched from the intensified subcutaneous regimen.

Ustekinumab has shown, in previous studies, not only clinical, but also endoscopic [23,24], ultrasonographic [25,26], and even histological [27] improvements. Despite this, studies addressing the efficacy of intensification strategies in the face of loss of response during maintenance often measure targets only with clinical or biochemical response. In the present study, we do not have power to draw conclusions in this regard. However, it should be noted that in a cohort of highly refractory patients, endoscopic improvement was quite common.

One of the main limitations of our study is the limited sample size. In fact, we cannot rule out, given the good results obtained, the absence of statistical significance being related to the sample size (type II error). More studies on a wider population are needed.

However, since this is a study in real clinical practice, increasing the sample size is complex, and the inclusion rate is unpredictable.

On the other hand, one of the main strengths to highlight is that, to our knowledge, this is the first study that addresses the possibility of intensifying the treatment, not only by reducing the regimen, but also by switching to intravenous administration as maintenance treatment, also obtaining good results and broadening the therapeutic possibilities in these patients.

5. Conclusions

In our experience, intensifying ustekinumab treatment, not only by reducing the interval (to 4 weeks) but also by transitioning to intravenous administration, is a safe and effective option for a significant proportion of patients.

When assessing the clinical activity of these patients, around 70% exhibited baseline activity, with no significant changes observed after 12 weeks of treatment. However, among those with severe baseline activity, a notable reduction was seen to 14.8% after 12 weeks of intravenous treatment. Although overall fecal calprotectin levels reduced at 12 weeks, statistical significance was not reached. Similarly, C-reactive protein (CRP) levels showed a decrease after 12 weeks of intravenous treatment, although this is not statistically significant.

Moreover, there was a substantial increase in ustekinumab levels after 12 weeks of intensified intravenous treatment in patients who initially received the drug every 8 weeks subcutaneously. Nevertheless, no differences in drug levels were observed among those who started with intensified drug treatment from the beginning. Endoscopic improvement was detected in a small subset of patients, while ultrasound activity showed significant improvement in three out of ten patients evaluated at both the baseline and 12 weeks.

Notably, no adverse effects were noted with the intravenous administration of ustekinumab during the study.

Author Contributions: Methodology, C.S.F. and L.G.R.; Formal analysis, C.S.F.; Investigation, J.A.A.; Data curation, J.A.A.; Writing—original draft, C.S.F.; Writing—review & editing, J.L.R.G., L.G.R., E.M.A., M.S.A., J.P.C., J.N.B. and M.D.M.-A. All authors have read and agreed to the published version of the manuscript.

Funding: We have not received any funding for the execution of this article.

Institutional Review Board Statement: The inclusion of patients in the database was carried out after approval from the ethics committee of La Paz University Hospital.

Informed Consent Statement: All patients signed the corresponding informed consent.

Data Availability Statement: The data is available in a locally anonymized file in case further studies are required in the future, and it will be preserved for a minimum of 4 years.

Conflicts of Interest: The authors declare that they have no conflicts of interest that could affect the execution of the present manuscript.

References

1. Mao, R.; Hu, P.J. The Future of IBD Therapy: Where Are We and Where Should We Go Next? *Dig. Dis.* **2016**, *34*, 175–179. [CrossRef] [PubMed]
2. Torres, J.; Bonovas, S.; Doherty, G.; Kucharzik, T.; Gisbert, J.P.; Raine, T.; Adamina, M.; Armuzzi, A.; Bachmann, O.; Bager, P.; et al. ECCO Guidelines on Therapeutics in Crohn's Disease: Medical Treatment. J Crohns Colitis. *J. Crohn's Colitis* **2020**, *14*, 4–22. [CrossRef] [PubMed]
3. Feagan, B.G.; Sandborn, W.J.; Gasink, C.; Jacobstein, D.; Lang, Y.; Friedman, J.R.; Blank, M.A.; Johanns, J.; Gao, L.-L.; Miao, Y.; et al. Ustekinumab as Induction and Maintenance Therapy for Crohn's Disease. *N. Engl. J. Med.* **2016**, *375*, 1946–1960. [CrossRef] [PubMed]
4. Miranda, A.; Gravina, A.G.; Cuomo, A.; Mucherino, C.; Sgambato, D.; Facchiano, A.; Granata, L.; Priadko, K.; Pellegrino, R.; de Filippo, F.R.; et al. Efficacy of ustekinumab in the treatment of patients with Crohn's disease with failure to previous conventional or biologic therapy: A prospective observational real-life study. *J. Physiol. Pharmacol.* **2021**, *72*, 537–543. [CrossRef]
5. Singh, S.; Murad, M.H.; Fumery, M.; Sedano, R.; Jairath, V.; Panaccione, R.; Sandborn, W.J.; Ma, C. Comparative efficacy and safety of biologic therapies for moderate-to-severe Crohn's disease: A systematic review and network meta-analysis. *Lancet Gastroenterol. Hepatol.* **2021**, *6*, 1002–1014. [CrossRef] [PubMed]
6. Barré, A.; Colombel, J.F.; Ungaro, R. Review article: Predictors of response to vedolizumab and ustekinumab in inflammatory bowel disease. *Aliment. Pharmacol. Ther.* **2018**, *47*, 896–905. [CrossRef] [PubMed]
7. Chateau, T.; Peyrin-Biroulet, L. Two cases of inflammatory bowel disease patients treated with ustekinumab 90 mg every 3 weeks. *Inflamm. Bowel Dis* **2020**, *26*, e7. [CrossRef]
8. Fumery, M.; Peyrin-Biroulet, L.; Nancey, S.; Altwegg, R.; Gilletta, C.; Veyrard, P.; Bouguen, G.; Viennot, S.; Poullenot, F.; Filippi, J.; et al. Effectiveness and Safety of Ustekinumab Intensification At 90 Mg Every Four Weeks In Crohn's Disease: A Multicenter Study. *J. Crohn's Colitis* **2020**, *15*, 222–227. [CrossRef]
9. Sedano, R.; Guizzetti, L.; McDonald, C.; Jairath, V. Intravenous Ustekinumab Reinduction Is Effective in Prior Biologic Failure Crohn's Disease Patients Already on Every-4-Week Dosing. *Clin. Gastroenterol. Hepatol.* **2021**, *19*, 1497–1498.e1. [CrossRef]
10. Ollech, J.E.; Normatov, I.; Peleg, N.; Wang, J.; Patel, S.A.; Rai, V.; Yi, Y.; Singer, J.; Dalal, S.R.; Sakuraba, A.; et al. Effectiveness of ustekinumab dose escalation in patients with Crohn's disease. *Clin. Gastroenterol. Hepatol.* **2020**, *19*, 104–110. [CrossRef]
11. Harvey, R.F.; Bradshaw, J.M. A simple index of Crohn's-disease activity. *Lancet* **1980**, *1*, 514. [CrossRef] [PubMed]
12. Daperno, M.; D'Haens, G.; Van Assche, G.; Baert, F.; Bulois, P.; Maunoury, V.; Sostegni, R.; Rocca, R.; Pera, A.; Gevers, A.; et al. Development and validation of a new, simplified endoscopic activity score for Crohn's disease: The SES-CD. *Gastrointest. Endosc.* **2004**, *60*, 505–512. [CrossRef] [PubMed]

13. Papamichael, K.; Afif, W.; Drobne, D.; Dubinsky, M.C.; Ferrante, M.; Irving, P.M.; Kamperidis, N.; Kobayashi, T.; Kotze, P.G.; Lambert, J.; et al. Therapeutic drug monitoring of biologics in inflammatory bowel disease: Unmet needs and future perspectives. *Lancet Gastroenterol. Hepatol.* **2022**, *7*, 171–185. [CrossRef] [PubMed]
14. Siegmund, B.; Nitschmann, S. Ustekinumab als Therapeutikum bei Morbus Crohn: UNITI-IM-UNITI [Ustekinumab for the treatment of Crohn's disease: UNITI-IM-UNITI]. *Internist* **2017**, *58*, 424–426; Erratum in *Internist* **2017**, *58*, 426. (In Germany) [CrossRef] [PubMed]
15. Engel, T.; Yung, D.E.; Ma, C.; Pariente, B.; Wils, P.; Eliakim, R.; Ungar, B.; Ben-Horin, S.; Kopylov, U. Effectiveness and safety of Ustekinumab for Crohn's disease; systematic review and pooled analysis of real-world evidence. *Dig Liver Dis.* **2019**, *51*, 1232–1240. [CrossRef] [PubMed]
16. Khorrami, S.; Ginard, D.; Marín-Jiménez, I.; Chaparro, M.; Sierra, M.; Aguas, M.; Sicilia, B.; García-Sánchez, V.; Suarez, C.; Villoria, A.; et al. Ustekinumab for the Treatment of Refractory Crohn's Disease: The Spanish Experience in a Large Multicentre Open-label Cohort. *Inflamm. Bowel Dis.* **2016**, *22*, 1662–1669. [CrossRef]
17. Eberl, A.; Hallinen, T.; Björkesten, C.-G.A.; Heikkinen, M.; Hirsi, E.; Kellokumpu, M.; Koskinen, I.; Moilanen, V.; Nielsen, C.; Nuutinen, H.; et al. Ustekinumab for Crohn's disease: A nationwide real-life cohort study from Finland (FINUSTE). *Scand. J. Gastroenterol.* **2019**, *54*, 718–725. [CrossRef]
18. Wils, P.; Bouhnik, Y.; Michetti, P.; Flourie, B.; Brixi, H.; Bourrier, A.; Allez, M.; Duclos, B.; Serrero, M.; Buisson, A.; et al. Long-term efficacy and safety of ustekinumab in 122 refractory Crohn's disease patients: A multicentre experience. *Aliment. Pharmacol. Ther.* **2018**, *47*, 588–595. [CrossRef]
19. Sandborn, W.J.; Rutgeerts, P.; Gasink, C.; Jacobstein, D.; Zou, B.; Johanns, J.; Sands, B.E.; Hanauer, S.B.; Targan, S.; Ghosh, S.; et al. Long-term efficacy and safety of ustekinumab for Crohn's disease through the second year of therapy. *Aliment. Pharmacol. Ther.* **2018**, *48*, 65–77. [CrossRef]
20. Meserve, J.; Ma, C.; Dulai, P.S.; Jairath, V.; Singh, S. Effectiveness of Reinduction and/or Dose Escalation of Ustekinumab in Crohn's Disease: A Systematic Review and Meta-analysis. *Clin. Gastroenterol. Hepatol.* **2022**, *20*, 2728–2740.e1. [CrossRef]
21. Vermeire, S.; Gils, A. Value of drug level testing and antibody assays in optimising biological therapy. *Frontline Gastroenterol.* **2013**, *4*, 41–43. [CrossRef] [PubMed]
22. Hirayama, H.; Morita, Y.; Imai, T.; Takahashi, K.; Yoshida, A.; Bamba, S.; Inatomi, O.; Andoh, A. Ustekinumab trough levels predicting laboratory and endoscopic remission in patients with Crohn's disease. *BMC Gastroenterol.* **2022**, *22*, 195. [CrossRef] [PubMed]
23. Adedokun, O.J.; Xu, Z.; Gasink, C.; Jacobstein, D.; Szapary, P.; Johanns, J.; Gao, L.L.; Davis, H.M.; Hanauer, S.B.; Feagan, B.G.; et al. Pharmacokinetics and Exposure Response Relationships of Ustekinumab in Patients with Crohn's Disease. *Gastroenterology* **2018**, *154*, 1660–1671. [CrossRef] [PubMed]
24. Proietti, E.; Pauwels, R.W.M.; van der Woude, C.J.; Doukas, M.; Oudijk, L.; Peppelenbosch, M.P.; Grohmann, U.; Crombag, M.B.S.; de Vries, A.C.; Fuhler, G.M. Ustekinumab Tissue and Serum Levels in Patients with Crohn's Disease Are Closely Correlated Though Not Consistently Associated with Objective Response After Induction. *Inflamm. Bowel Dis.* **2022**, *29*, 1038–1046. [CrossRef]
25. Danese, S.; Vermeire, S.; D'Haens, G.; Panés, J.; Dignass, A.; Magro, F.; Nazar, M.; Le Bars, M.; Lahaye, M.; Ni, L.; et al. Treat to target versus standard of care for patients with Crohn's disease treated with ustekinumab (STARDUST): An open-label, multicentre, randomised phase 3b trial. *Lancet Gastroenterol. Hepatol.* **2022**, *7*, 294–306; Erratum in *Lancet Gastroenterol. Hepatol.* **2022**, *7*, e8. [CrossRef]
26. Rutgeerts, P.; Gasink, C.; Chan, D.; Lang, Y.; Pollack, P.; Colombel, J.-F.; Wolf, D.C.; Jacobstein, D.; Johanns, J.; Szapary, P.; et al. Efficacy of Ustekinumab for Inducing Endoscopic Healing in Patients with Crohn's Disease. *Gastroenterology* **2018**, *155*, 1045–1058. [CrossRef]
27. Kucharzik, T.; Wilkens, R.; Maconi, G.; A D'agostino, M.; Le Bars, M.; Nazar, M.; Sloan, S.; Lahaye, M.; Ni, L.; Ercole, E.; et al. DOP10 Intestinal ultrasound response and transmural healing after ustekinumab induction in Crohn's disease: Week 16 interim analysis of the STARDUST trial substudy. *J. Crohn's Colitis* **2020**, *14*, S046–S048. [CrossRef]

Journal of
Clinical Medicine

MDPI

Article

Longitudinal Measurements of Blood Biomarkers in Patients with Crohn's Disease or Ulcerative Colitis Treated with Infliximab: Only the Latest Values in the Induction Period Predict Treatment Failure

Kim Oren Gradel [1,2,*], Bente Mertz Nørgård [1,2], Sonia Friedman [1,3], Jens Kjeldsen [4,5] and Michael Due Larsen [1,2,6]

1 Center for Clinical Epidemiology, Odense University Hospital, 5000 Odense, Denmark; bente.noergaard@rsyd.dk (B.M.N.); sfriedman1@tuftsmedicalcenter.org (S.F.); michael.d.larsen@ntnu.no (M.D.L.)
2 Research Unit of Clinical Epidemiology, Department of Clinical Research, University of Southern Denmark, 5230 Odense, Denmark
3 Gastroenterology Division, Tufts Medical School, Tufts Medical Center, Boston, MA 02111, USA
4 Department of Medical Gastroenterology S, Odense University Hospital, 5000 Odense, Denmark; jens.kjeldsen@rsyd.dk
5 Research Unit of Medical Gastroenterology, Department of Clinical Research, University of Southern Denmark, 5230 Odense, Denmark
6 Department of Clinical and Molecular Medicine, Norwegian University of Science and Technology, 7034 Trondheim, Norway
* Correspondence: kim.gradel@rsyd.dk

Abstract: Background: Few studies have incorporated longitudinal assessments or used combinations of blood biomarkers as predictors of loss of response to biologic therapy for patients with Crohn's disease (CD) or ulcerative colitis (UC). **Methods:** This is a population-based cohort study comprising Danish patients with CD or UC from 2008 to 2018. We used logistic regression to analyze whether levels and changes in levels of C-reactive protein (CRP), serum albumin, and hemoglobin, routinely measured during a 14-week infliximab induction period, predicted a change to another biologic medication or cessation of biologic therapy. **Results:** During the induction period, 2883 (1626 CD, 1257 UC) patients had 12,730, 12,040, and 13,538 specimens with CRP, serum albumin, and hemoglobin, respectively. In all, 284 patients (9.9%) switched to another biologic medication, and 139 (4.8%) ceased biologic therapy in the follow-up period. Only the most recent CRP and hemoglobin levels predicted the efficacy of infliximab treatment at approximately 14 weeks, a time point when the clinician often determines whether to continue treatment. **Conclusion:** Measurement of blood biomarkers prior to the clinical assessment does not predict the effectiveness of infliximab.

Keywords: blood biomarkers; longitudinal measurements; infliximab; prediction; Crohn's disease; ulcerative colitis

1. Introduction

Prediction of response to medical treatment is one of the main challenges in caring for patients with Crohn's disease (CD) and ulcerative colitis (UC). This is particularly important for biologic medications because of their high cost and potentially serious side effects. Current guidelines recommend an individualized empiric strategy for handling the loss of response to biological treatment. This includes intensifying biologic therapy, changing within the class of biologic therapy, changing to another class of biologic therapy, optimizing concomitant treatment with conventional immunosuppressives, and finally, surgery [1,2]. This strategy assumes that it is preferable to completely exhaust one treatment option before discontinuing or changing the biologic therapy. Although tumor necrosis factor (TNF)-blocking therapy has resulted in long-term remission for CD and UC, up to 35% of the patients may have primary failure to this therapy [3]. Induction therapy for infliximab consists of three infusions: at day 0 and after 2 and 6 weeks, followed by maintenance therapy every 8 weeks. The effectiveness of the therapy is typically evaluated at the fourth treatment—that is, around 14 weeks after its initiation. If this induction therapy is not beneficial, whatever the reason, the clinician will change to an alternative therapy. An early prediction of treatment failure will facilitate the supervision of vulnerable patients and the decisions to change or supplement treatments earlier in the disease course. Whether an early prediction is possible can be assessed in longitudinal biomarker studies, preferably by combinations of biomarkers.

The blood biomarkers C-reactive protein (CRP), serum albumin, and hemoglobin are often used as standard biomarkers when starting and continuing biologic therapy. Among these, the inflammatory marker CRP has gained the most attention [3]. Serum albumin is a negative inflammatory biomarker [4] and a strong prognostic predictor in many diseases [5,6]. Anemia has a high prevalence in patients with inflammatory bowel disease (IBD) [7]. The hemoglobin level is included in prognostic indices for acute severe UC [8] and CD [9], and it has been evaluated as a prognostic predictor in a few studies [10].

There is no ideal blood biomarker, and the combination of two or more biomarkers has been recommended for prognostic studies [11]. Moreover, the vast majority of prognostic studies have only assessed one-time values of the biomarker, with a few exceptions for studies of CRP [12–14]. Studies with changes in CRP levels, rather than single measurements, have been recommended for patients with IBD [14], and the same may apply to serum albumin and hemoglobin.

CRP, serum albumin, and hemoglobin are routinely measured in patients with IBD. The little knowledge on whether their values, separately or in combination, could be used longitudinally for the prognosis thus prompted us to conduct this study.

In this population-based study, we examined whether levels of and changes in CRP, serum albumin, and/or hemoglobin during the 14-week induction period with infliximab treatment could predict a treatment failure, defined as a shift to another biologic therapy or cessation of biological treatment altogether.

2. Materials and Methods

2.1. Setting

This unselected study cohort is based on data from national Danish health registries. In Denmark (population approximately 5.8 million), all citizens have access to free public healthcare, and this enables us to develop a population-based study design based on an unselected nationwide study population [15]. The Danish healthcare system is tax-financed and thus free for the individual patient [16]. All patients with IBD are diagnosed and treated in public hospitals, with high completeness and validity of recorded IBD diagnoses and procedure codes [17,18]. Data from administrative registries can be linked by the unique personal identifier given to all Danish residents [15].

2.2. Study Population

We refer to Figure 1 for further details.

In brief, the study population initially comprised patients in the Danish National Patient Registry [18] from which we retrieved patients treated with infliximab. In Denmark, anti-TNFs, interleukin inhibitors, and anti-integrin drugs are administered only in public hospitals or hospital-based out-patient settings, and procedure codes for each treatment and dates of administration are recorded in the Danish National Patient Registry [18]. The system holds a complete record of individuals receiving biological therapy and its associated consequences.

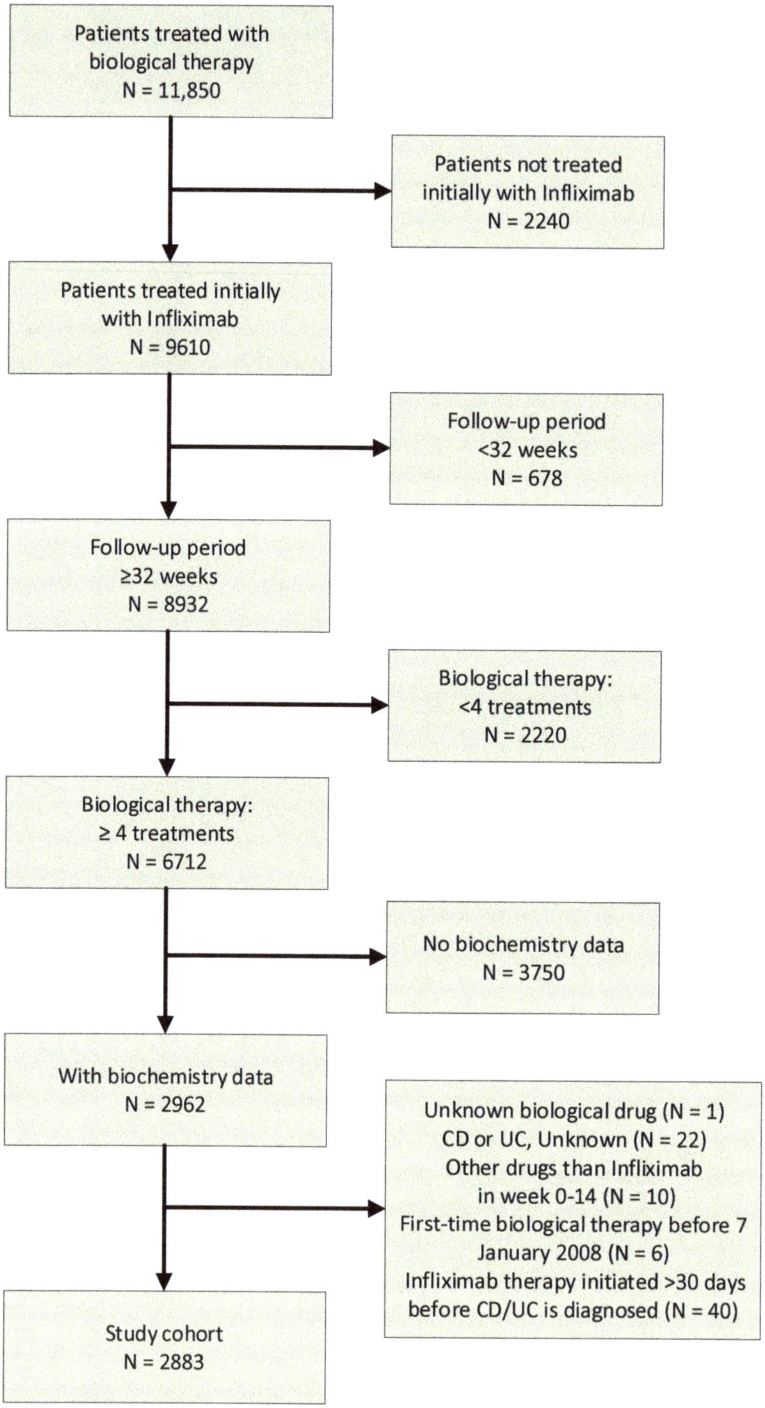

Figure 1. Derivation of the study population.

We restricted the inclusion of patients to those who fulfilled induction therapy (≥4 infliximab treatments) and ≥32 weeks of follow-up after the induction therapy period. We retrieved data for CRP, serum albumin, and hemoglobin in blood specimens from a laboratory database hosted by the Danish Health Data Authority, which covers all of Denmark as of 2008, except the Central Denmark Region (21% of Denmark's population) [19]. The final study population included patients treated with infliximab, initiated between 7 January 2008 and 30 June 2018, and with blood specimen levels for CRP, serum albumin, or hemoglobin. From the Danish Civil Registration System [15], we retrieved data on the vital status up to 21 September 2020, including the date of death or emigration, if relevant.

2.3. Outcome

The outcome of this study was treatment failure, which we defined as either a shift to a biologic other than infliximab or cessation of biologic treatment altogether in the follow-up period. The follow-up spanned from 98 days (14 weeks) through 224 days (32 weeks) after the first-time infliximab treatment.

2.4. Statistical Analyses

We computed a contingency table with the patients' baseline characteristics for all patients and stratified them into patients with CD or UC. Figure 2 gives the timeline for the study.

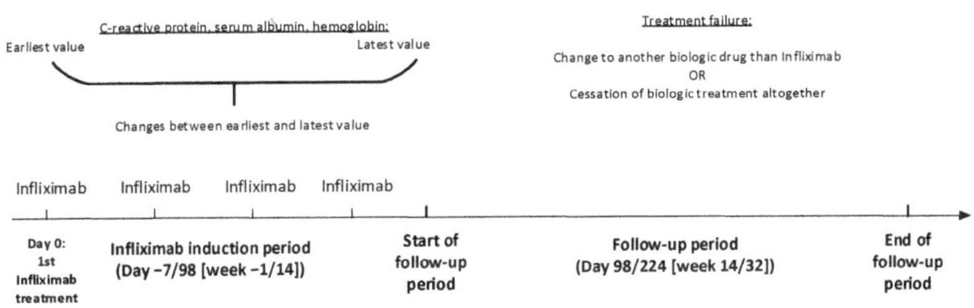

Figure 2. Timeline for the study.

We included blood specimens for CRP, serum albumin, and hemoglobin, from 7 days (1 week) before through 98 days (14 weeks) after the first-time infliximab treatment. Because CRP was not normally distributed, we used its base-10 logarithm (CRP10), whereas serum albumin and hemoglobin values were not changed due to their normal distribution. Within this −7 to 98-day induction period, we focused on the earliest and the latest specimens and computed the days and changes in levels between these.

For each of the three biomarkers, we graphically depicted trajectories of daily mean levels in the −7 to 98-day period, separately for patients with and without treatment failure.

For the outcome, we computed logistic regression analyses with odds ratios (ORs) and 95% confidence intervals (CIs). These analyses were undertaken separately for CRP10, serum albumin, and hemoglobin and within each of these for the earliest and the latest levels, as well as for changes between these, divided them into percentiles (0–25%, 25–75%, and 75–100%). As the earliest levels contributed little to the outcome, these were omitted from the multivariate analyses in which we applied the following models:

Model A: the latest level of CRP10, serum albumin, and hemoglobin
Model B: Model A + changes in CRP10, serum albumin, and hemoglobin levels
Model C: Model A + changes in hemoglobin levels
Model D: the latest levels of CRP10 and hemoglobin + changes in hemoglobin levels
Model E: Model D + gender, age groups (0–16, 17–39, 40–59, ≥60 years), body mass index (BMI) (<18.5, ≥18.5 and <25, ≥25 and <30, ≥30 and <35, ≥35, missing), and quartiles of time from diagnosis of IBD to first-time treatment with infliximab (0–187, 188–808, 809–3053, 3054–14,652 days).

We computed areas under the receiver operating characteristic curves (AUROCs) for all the logistic regression analyses. For Models A–E, we compared these mutually by C-statistics [20].

Because of the retrospective nature of our data, in which values were not missing at random, we could not perform genuine longitudinal analyses [21]. Consequently, we reiterated all analyses in the following subgroups to assess the robustness of the data: (i) patients with CD; (ii) patients with UC; (iii) patients with 2 or more biomarker specimens in the −7 to 98 day period (the earliest and latest specimen comprised CRP10, serum albumin, and hemoglobin, and there were 1–83 days between the earliest and the latest specimen); (iv) as iii, but with 84–105 days between the earliest and latest specimen; (v) for patients with 3 or more biomarker specimens in the −7/98 day induction period, we replaced the latest level in the induction period by the level from the induction period's 3rd biomarker specimen; (vi) where a change to another biologic drug was the only outcome, i.e., we skipped patients for whom biologic therapy was stopped altogether; (vii) for patients with UC, we divided the follow-up period into analyses before and from 1 April 2012 (date of approval of adalimumab); (viii) for all patients, we divided the follow-up period into analyses before and from 1 May 2014 (date of approval of vedolizumab).

In all analyses, a two-sided p-value of <0.05 was considered significant. The program Stata®, vs. 17, (StataCorp., College Station, TX, USA) was used for all analyses.

3. Results

A total of 2883 patients were included in the final study cohort (Figure 1), of whom 1626 (56.4%) had CD and 1257 (43.6%) had UC (Table 1).

Table 1. Descriptive characteristics of patients with Crohn's disease or ulcerative colitis introduced to infliximab therapy from 2008 through 2018.

Characteristic	All Patients (n = 2883)	Crohn's Disease (n = 1626)	Ulcerative Colitis (n = 1257)
Gender			
Females	1487 (51.6)	853 (52.5)	634 (50.4)
Males	1396 (48.4)	773 (47.5)	623 (49.6)
Age, years [1]			
Range	1.1–89.3	1.1–82.3	3.7–89.3
Median (IQR)	34.0 (23.0–47.6)	30.9 (21.6–46.2)	36.9 (25.5–50.0)
Body mass index [1]			
<18.5	52 (1.8)	38 (2.3)	14 (1.1)
≥18.5, <25	544 (18.9)	310 (19.1)	234 (18.6)
≥25, <30	329 (11.4)	177 (10.9)	152 (12.1)
≥30, <35	142 (4.9)	84 (5.2)	58 (4.6)
≥35	62 (2.2)	30 (1.9)	32 (2.6)
Missing	1754 (60.8)	987 (60.7)	767 (61.0)
C-reactive protein, measured [2]			
Patients	2817 (97.7)	1594 (98.0)	1223 (97.3)
Number of values			
All	12,730	6208	6522
Per patient			
Range	1–51	1–51	1–45
Median (IQR)	3 (2–5)	3 (2–4)	4 (3–6)
Serum albumin, measured [2]			
Patients	2709 (94.0)	1543 (94.9)	1166 (92.8)
Number of values			
All	12,040	5876	6164
Per patient			
Range	1–52	1–52	1–37
Median (IQR)	3 (2–5)	3 (2–4)	4 (3–6)

Table 1. *Cont.*

Characteristic	All Patients (n = 2883)	Crohn's Disease (n = 1626)	Ulcerative Colitis (n = 1257)
Hemoglobin, measured [2]			
Patients	2880 (99.9)	1624 (99.9)	1256 (99.9)
Number of values			
All	13,538	6594	6944
Per patient			
Range	1–49	1–49	1–46
Median (IQR)	4 (3–5)	2 (3–5)	4 (3–7)
Gastrointestinal surgery [3]	18 (0.6)	8 (0.5)	10 (0.8)
Shift to another biological drug [4]	284 (9.9)	140 (8.6)	144 (11.5)
Ceasing biological treatment [4]	139 (4.8)	56 (3.4)	83 (6.6)

[1] On the date of initiating biological therapy. [2] From 7 days (1 week) before through 98 days (14 weeks) after initiating biological therapy. [3] Nordic Classification of Surgical Procedures, codes KJFH* (total colectomy) or KJFB* (intestinal resection), from 7 days (1 week) before through 98 days (14 weeks) after initiating biological therapy. [4] From 98 days (14 weeks) through 224 days (32 weeks) after initiating biological therapy.

There were no material differences between patients with CD and UC for any baseline characteristics in Table 1. Most of the patients had CRP, serum albumin, and hemoglobin measured, ranging from 92.8% for serum albumin for patients with UC to 99.9% for hemoglobin for the whole study population. In the period from 7 days before through 98 days after starting the infliximab treatment, each patient had a median (IQR) of 3 (2–5) specimens for CRP and serum albumin and 4 (3–5) for hemoglobin.

3.1. *Trajectories of Mean Daily Levels*

During the day −7 to day 98 induction period, daily mean levels of CRP10 were generally higher and levels of serum albumin and hemoglobin were generally lower among patients with treatment failure in comparison to patients without treatment failure (Figure 3).

The fitted lines deviated more from each other with the progression from day −7 to-ward day 98, most notably for hemoglobin, less for serum albumin, and least for CRP10.

3.2. *Logistic Regression Analyses Separately for the Three Biomarkers*

In the six models, in which either the earliest or the latest biomarker level was the only covariate, only models with the latest level were significant (Table 2).

Hence, only the latest levels were combined with changes in the equivalent biomarker levels. In these models, the ORs (95% CIs) for the latest levels changed immaterially in comparison to the models without the changes. Changes were non-significant for CRP10 or serum albumin, although they were close to significant for serum albumin. For hemoglobin, changes were significant, with a trend of lower ORs with higher percentile changes. AUROCs ranged from 0.523 (for the earliest CRP10 level) to 0.594 (for the model with the latest hemoglobin level and hemoglobin changes). The results differed insignificantly between patients with CD and UC.

3.3. *Multivariate Logistic Regression Analyses*

When the latest levels of each biomarker were combined (Model A), CRP10 and hemoglobin were significantly associated with the outcome (Table 3).

With the amendment of changes in levels (Model B), only changes for hemoglobin were significant. We, therefore, excluded changes in levels for CRP10 and serum albumin (Model C) and further excluded the latest serum albumin level in Model D. ORs or 95% CIs did not change materially for the same covariates when these were compared between Models A, B, C, and D. The AUROC was 0.595 for Model A and very similar in Models B D (ranging from 0.610 to 0.616). In the final Model E, the amendment of other possible confounders (gender, age, BMI, and time from diagnosis to first-time treatment with infliximab) did not change ORs or 95% CIs for the biomarker covariates in comparison to Model D (Table 3). Moreover, none of the amended confounders were significant.

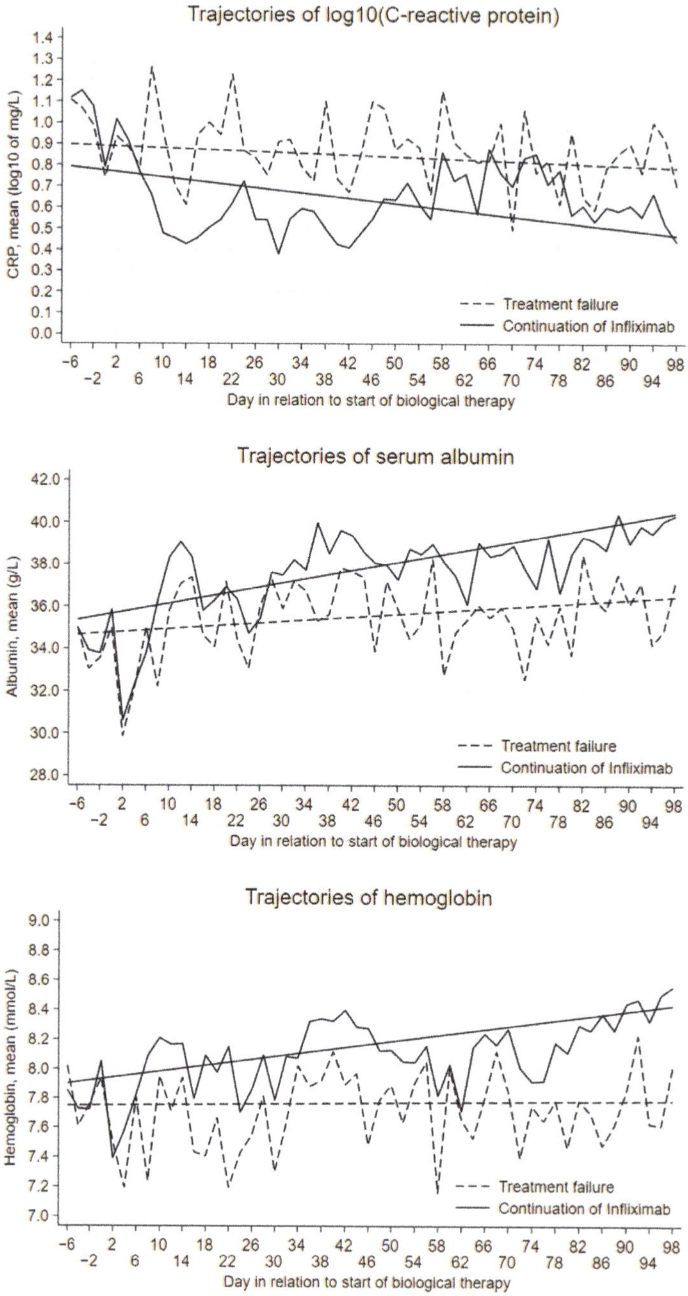

Figure 3. Daily mean levels of biomarkers, with fitted lines, days −7/98 in relation to starting biological therapy.

Table 2. Odds ratio (OR) and area under the receiver operating characteristic curve (AUROC) for the biomarker levels and their changes as predictors for treatment failure.

Model	OR (95% CI)	AUROC [1]
log10 of CRP [1], earliest	1.12 (0.94–1.34)	0.523
log10 of CRP, latest	1.72 (1.39–2.13)	0.568
Serum albumin, earliest	0.98 (0.96–1.00)	0.529
Serum albumin, latest	0.95 (0.93–0.97)	0.570
Hemoglobin, earliest	0.90 (0.81–1.00)	0.528
Hemoglobin, latest	0.74 (0.67–0.83)	0.575
log10 of CRP, 0–25 percentile change log10 of CRP, 25–75 percentile change log10 of CRP, 75–100 percentile change log10 of CRP, latest	1 (ref.) 0.92 (0.68–1.26) 0.90 (0.68–1.21) 1.76 (1.41–2.20)	0.572
Serum albumin, 0–25 percentile change Serum albumin, 25–75 percentile change Serum albumin, 75–100 percentile change Serum albumin, latest	1 (ref.) 0.76 (0.57–1.02) 0.73 (0.52–1.02) 0.95 (0.93–0.98)	0.576
Hemoglobin, 0–25 percentile change Hemoglobin, 25–75 percentile change Hemoglobin, 75–100 percentile change Hemoglobin, latest	1 (ref.) 0.74 (0.57–0.96) 0.60 (0.44–0.82) 0.78 (0.70–0.88)	0.594

[1] The base-10 logarithm of C-reactive protein.

3.4. AUROCs for Models A–E

In pairwise comparisons of AUROCs between the models, only Model A differed from Model E ($p = 0.03$), whereas the other comparisons were non-significant.

3.5. Subgroup Analyses

A total of 1800 patients had 2 or more biomarker specimens where both the earliest and latest specimens comprised CRP, serum albumin, and hemoglobin. The median time between the earliest and the latest specimen was 84 days, which we chose as a cut-off for dividing into patients with 1–83 (n = 867) and 84–105 days (n = 933). The results did not differ materially between these two groups or in comparison to the whole study population.

A number of 1565 patients had 3 or more biomarker specimens, and 1440 of these (92.0%) could be used for the logistic regression analyses due to non-missing data for all the models' variables. The results were very similar to those for the whole study population.

In the analyses where the outcome was restricted to change to another biologic drug than infliximab, all results were essentially the same as for the results in which stopping biologic treatment was included in the outcome definition.

The results of the analyses in the divided follow-up periods (before vs. after 1 April 2012 for patients with UC and before vs. after 1 May 2014 for all patients) did not deviate materially from the overall results either.

Table 3. Logistic regression analyses, combined for the three biomarkers, in addition to adjustment for gender, age, body mass index, and time between diagnosis and start of infliximab treatment.

Cofactor	Model A (0.595) [1]	Model B (0.616)	Model C (0.614)	Model D (0.610)	Model E (0.623)
log10 of CRP, latest	1.43 (1.12–1.82)	1.41 (1.09–1.82)	1.39 (1.09–1.77)	1.48 (1.19–1.85)	1.49 (1.18–1.87)
Serum albumin, latest	0.98 (0.95–1.01)	0.98 (0.95–1.01)	0.98 (0.95–1.01)		
Hemoglobin, latest	0.80 (0.70–0.91)	0.85 (0.74–0.98)	0.84 (0.73–0.96)	0.83 (0.73–0.94)	0.81 (0.71–0.93)

Table 3. *Cont.*

Cofactor	Model A (0.595) [1]	Model B (0.616)	Model C (0.614)	Model D (0.610)	Model E (0.623)
log10 of CRP, 0–25 percentile difference		1 (reference)			
log10 of CRP, 25–75 percentile difference		0.95 (0.67–1.35)			
log10 of 75–100 percentile difference		0.93 (0.65–1.32)			
Serum albumin, 0–25 percentile difference		1 (reference)			
Serum albumin, 25–75 percentile difference		0.85 (0.62–1.19)			
Serum albumin, 75–100 percentile difference		0.98 (0.65–1.47)			
Hemoglobin, 0–25 percentile difference		1 (reference)	1 (reference)	1 (reference)	1 (reference)
Hemoglobin, 25–75 percentile difference		0.74 (0.55–0.99)	0.73 (0.55–0.97)	0.71 (0.54–0.93)	0.70 (0.53–0.93)
Hemoglobin, 75–100 percentile difference		0.54 (0.37–0.80)	0.56 (0.39–0.80)	0.56 (0.40–0.78)	0.57 (0.41–0.80)
Males					0.96 (0.75–1.23)
Age, 0–16 years					1 (reference)
Age, 17–39 years					1.00 (0.57–1.76)
Age, 40–59 years					1.48 (0.82–2.68)
Age, ≥60 years					1.33 (0.69–2.55)
Body mass index, <18.5					0.55 (0.19–1.62)
Body mass index, ≥18.5 and <25					1 (reference)
Body mass index, ≥25 and <30					0.82 (0.54–1.25)
Body mass index, ≥30 and <35					0.98 (0.57–1.67)
Body mass index, ≥35					0.59 (0.25–1.38)
Body mass index, missing					0.78 (0.58–1.05)
Time, diag-biol [2], 0–187 days					1 (reference)
Time, diag-biol, 188–808 days					1.15 (0.83–1.59)
Time, diag-biol, 809–3053 days					1.07 (0.76–1.50)
Time, diag-biol, 3054–14,652 days					1.00 (0.70–1.42)

[1] Brackets: area under the receiver operating characteristic curve for the model, based on the 2103 patients in Models A–C (in order to enable comparisons between the models). [2] Time from diagnosis of inflammatory bowel disease to start of infliximab treatment.

4. Discussion

We hypothesized that levels of and changes in the routinely retrieved biomarkers CRP, serum albumin, and hemoglobin could predict whether treatment with infliximab would be clinically valuable after its 14-week induction period. Ultimately, we hoped that the earliest measured levels could predict treatment failure sooner. However, statistical significance was seen only for the latest measured CRP and hemoglobin levels in the induction period and for changes in the hemoglobin levels. These latest measurements occurred at a time point when the clinician will likely assess the patient's condition anyway, including decisions on whether treatment with infliximab needs to continue or change to another drug, which we defined as treatment failure. Moreover, AUROCs below 0.7, regardless of the model, reflected non-acceptable discrimination [22].

Approximately one-third of patients will be non-responders to infliximab (and other biologics) and will require alternative treatment. It would be ideal if biomarkers collected at the beginning of the biologic therapy period could predict a clinical response. Patients would be able to avoid a prolonged flare and further clinical decline by choosing a medication other than infliximab. This large study finds, rather, that patients must undergo a full infliximab induction, and only biomarker measurements around 14 weeks will be reflective of clinical response. CRP and hemoglobin are helpful insofar as they are reflective of the clinical response to infliximab induction and can help differentiate common concurrent diagnoses such as irritable bowel syndrome or chronic pain syndrome, which may obscure clinical response.

The fecal calprotectin level is the gold standard for assessing the severity of IBD [3,14]. Our real-life data were too sparse to incorporate this specimen type in the prognostic assessment, as only 993 patients (34.4%) had fecal calprotectin specimens, and among these, 578 (58.2%) had one specimen only, which hampered longitudinal analyses. Consequently, the study was based on CRP, serum albumin, and hemoglobin from blood specimens, which are normally retrieved concomitantly with the infliximab treatment. Still, half of the patients received their fourth treatment after the 14-week induction period, some up to 32 weeks thereafter. This was also reflected in varying numbers of biomarker specimens in the day −7 to day 98 period, to which we restricted our analyses to minimize heterogeneity.

We were inspired by a previous study, in which CRP levels ≥10 mg/L or a clinical score ≥5 (the Harvey–Bradshaw index for CD and the Simple Clinical Colitis Activity Index for UC) predicted a nearly fourfold increased risk of steroid therapy or surgery after the 14-week induction therapy period [23]. In the present study, we focused on the utility of longitudinal aspects of CRP, serum albumin, and hemoglobin, as well as of their combinations. This was also the reason for not incorporating clinical scores, which were recorded for the end of the induction therapy period and, therefore, did not contribute to an earlier prognostic assessment.

Most biomarker studies in patients with IBD are either cross-sectional, in which biomarkers were compared with clinical scores [24], or one-time levels that predicted future adverse outcomes, such as complications after surgery [25], increased risk of surgery or medication [26], prolonged hospitalizations [27], or steroid non-response [28]. Newer studies have incorporated one-time levels of CRP and serum albumin, often as the CRP/serum albumin ratio (CAR) [24]. To assess the separate impact of CRP, serum albumin, and hemoglobin, we did not use CAR in our study, and because serum albumin had little impact in models with hemoglobin, it was skipped in the final analyses. Fewer studies have evaluated changes in biomarker levels as predictors of an adverse outcome. Studies from European countries have incorporated CRP levels at baseline, after 4/10/14 weeks, and the difference or ratio between these, for patients with UC [29] or CD [12,13,30–32], all treated with infliximab. Comparison to our results is difficult due to the various follow-up periods and outcomes or the rates only computed for patients with high first-time CRP levels. A Belgian study of 614 patients with CD found that the baseline CRP level did not predict a sustained clinical benefit of infliximab during a 5-year follow-up period, whereas a drop of >50% from the baseline level or normalization to <3 mg/L did [32]. This is in accordance with our results and supports the recommendation of longitudinal assessments of biomarker levels [14]; however, no AUROCs were reported in the Belgian study. A Japanese study of 72 UC patients used the ratio between the week 0 and 2 levels of both CRP and serum albumin to predict the response to infliximab at week 14 [33]. The ratio of CRP, but not of serum albumin, was a predictor with a good discriminatory ability (AUROC = 0.799). A few older studies from the UK have reported longitudinal data for serum albumin and hemoglobin, but the low number of patients (50 or fewer) precludes firm conclusions [34–38]. In our study, there were no differences between patients with UC and CD. For CRP, this is not in accordance with several studies, which state that a high CRP response is mainly seen in patients with CD but not with UC [3]. For hemoglobin, the reverse has been reported, i.e., it is prognostic in patients with UC but not with CD [10]. Comparison between our results and other studies is difficult due to different settings and outcomes and the few studies that have assessed longitudinal aspects.

Our study is population-based and includes a high number of patients, both with UC and CD. Among the studies with longitudinal analyses, the highest number of patients was 718 [31], and we have not encountered other studies that combined CRP, serum albumin, and hemoglobin. Both the diagnoses of IBD and the procedure recordings of infliximab treatment have high completeness and validity [17,18]. The outcome is relevantly based on the physicians' assessments after the 14-week induction therapy period.

Our study also has limitations that deserve further consideration. First, real-life data with varying numbers of specimens and time intervals between these hamper genuine longitudinal analyses [21]. However, stratifying the analyses into 1–83 and 84–105 days between the earliest and latest specimens did not change our results materially. Moreover, ORs changed little between various models or when the last specimen was replaced by the third. Thus, our results seemed robust despite the heterogeneous data. Second, we do not know to what degree the outcome (i.e., the physicians' decisions) was based on the biomarker results. Hence, possible predictors may be part of the outcome, although the magnitude of this is difficult to quantify for a holistic clinical assessment. However, this pitfall would have been a bigger problem if the results had shown that the biomarkers were strong predictors. Third, the inclusion of fecal calprotectin in the analyses would be beneficial, but the number of specimens did not allow this. Fourth, as in other retrospectively derived data, there are unknown confounders such as intake of other drugs, smoking, or alcohol intake. The intake of other drugs may, however, be related to exacerbations of IBD symptoms, which are also correlated to levels of CRP, serum albumin, and hemoglobin, so confounding by indication is a pitfall if other drugs than infliximab are included in the analyses. Moreover, the amendment of possible confounders in Model E did not change the ORs for the biomarkers or the AUROCs materially, and it is unlikely that this would differ for other possible confounders. Finally, 18 patients underwent gastrointestinal surgery in the induction treatment period, which is an undesirable outcome regardless of the decision regarding infliximab continuation. These patients had more biomarker specimens (median 19.5, IQR 7–32), and 16 (88.9%) experienced the outcome, but their exclusion did not change the analyses materially.

5. Conclusions

Results from specimens of CRP, serum albumin, and hemoglobin retrieved before the end of the 14-week induction treatment period with infliximab were weak predictors of whether infliximab treatment should be continued thereafter. Additional studies, including genetics, serology, and correlation with specific IBD subtypes, need to be performed in order to find more clinically predictive biomarkers.

Author Contributions: Conceptualization, all authors; methodology, all authors; software, K.O.G. and M.D.L.; validation, M.D.L.; formal analysis, K.O.G. and M.D.L.; investigation, K.O.G. and M.D.L.; data curation, K.O.G. and M.D.L.; writing—original draft preparation, K.O.G.; writing—review and editing, all authors; visualization, K.O.G.; supervision, B.M.N., S.F. and J.K.; project administration, K.O.G., B.M.N. and M.D.L.; funding acquisition, irrelevant. All authors have read and agreed to the published version of the manuscript.

Funding: This research received no external funding.

Institutional Review Board Statement: This study abides by all applicable Danish laws regarding scientific research. This study was approved by the Danish Patient Safety Authority (ref. MITW, rec. no. 3-3013-3126/1, 9 August 2019) and notified at the Danish Data Protection Agency under the current joint notification of the Region of Southern Denmark (rec. no. 18/43305, 9 August 2019).

Informed Consent Statement: This study was not interventional and did not require direct patient contact or influence on the patient's treatment.

Data Availability Statement: This register-based non-interventional study follows the STROBE guideline [39]. The authors of this paper have no special access privileges to the data used in this study, and other researchers may apply for access to the data through an application to the Research Service at the Danish Health Data Authority.

Conflicts of Interest: The authors declare no conflicts of interest.

References

1. Harbord, M.; Eliakim, R.; Bettenworth, D.; Karmiris, K.; Katsanos, K.; Kopylov, U.; Kucharzik, T.; Molnar, T.; Raine, T.; Sebastian, S.; et al. Third European Evidence-based Consensus on Diagnosis and Management of Ulcerative Colitis. Part 2: Current Management. *J. Crohn's Colitis* **2017**, *11*, 769–784. [CrossRef]
2. Torres, J.; Bonovas, S.; Doherty, G.; Kucharzik, T.; Gisbert, J.P.; Raine, T.; Adamina, M.; Armuzzi, A.; Bachmann, O.; Bager, P.; et al. ECCO Guidelines on Therapeutics in Crohn's Disease: Medical Treatment. *J. Crohn's Colitis* **2020**, *14*, 4–22. [CrossRef] [PubMed]
3. Tarapatzi, G.; Filidou, E.; Kandilogiannakis, L.; Vradelis, S.; Kolios, G. Biomarkers in Inflammatory Bowel Diseases: Predicting the Indication and the Effect of Biologics. *J. Gastrointest. Liver Dis.* **2022**, *31*, 229–243. [CrossRef] [PubMed]
4. Wiedermann, C.J. Hypoalbuminemia as Surrogate and Culprit of Infections. *Int. J. Mol. Sci.* **2021**, *22*, 4496. [CrossRef] [PubMed]
5. Levitt, D.G.; Levitt, M.D. Human serum albumin homeostasis: A new look at the roles of synthesis, catabolism, renal and gastrointestinal excretion, and the clinical value of serum albumin measurements. *Int. J. Gen. Med.* **2016**, *9*, 229–255. [CrossRef] [PubMed]
6. Vincent, J.L.; Dubois, M.J.; Navickis, R.J.; Wilkes, M.M. Hypoalbuminemia in acute illness: Is there a rationale for intervention? A meta-analysis of cohort studies and controlled trials. *Ann. Surg.* **2003**, *237*, 319–334. [CrossRef] [PubMed]
7. Koutroubakis, I.E.; Ramos-Rivers, C.; Regueiro, M.; Koutroumpakis, E.; Click, B.; Schoen, R.E.; Hashash, J.G.; Schwartz, M.; Swoger, J.; Baidoo, L.; et al. Persistent or Recurrent Anemia Is Associated with Severe and Disabling Inflammatory Bowel Disease. *Clin. Gastroenterol. Hepatol.* **2015**, *13*, 1760–1766. [CrossRef]
8. Truelove, S.C.; Witts, L.J. Cortisone in ulcerative colitis; final report on a therapeutic trial. *Br. Med. J.* **1955**, *2*, 1041–1048. [CrossRef]
9. Best, W.R.; Becktel, J.M.; Singleton, J.W.; Kern, F., Jr. Development of a Crohn's disease activity index. National Cooperative Crohn's Disease Study. *Gastroenterology* **1976**, *70*, 439–444. [CrossRef]
10. Gisbert, J.P.; Chaparro, M. Predictors of Primary Response to Biologic Treatment [Anti-TNF, Vedolizumab, and Ustekinumab] in Patients with Inflammatory Bowel Disease: From Basic Science to Clinical Practice. *J. Crohn's Colitis* **2020**, *14*, 694–709. [CrossRef]
11. Dragoni, G.; Innocenti, T.; Galli, A. Biomarkers of Inflammation in Inflammatory Bowel Disease: How Long before Abandoning Single-Marker Approaches? *Dig. Dis.* **2021**, *39*, 190–203. [CrossRef]
12. Reinisch, W.; Wang, Y.; Oddens, B.J.; Link, R. C-reactive protein, an indicator for maintained response or remission to infliximab in patients with Crohn's disease: A post-hoc analysis from ACCENT I. *Aliment. Pharmacol. Ther.* **2012**, *35*, 568–576. [CrossRef]
13. Cornillie, F.; Hanauer, S.B.; Diamond, R.H.; Wang, J.; Tang, K.L.; Xu, Z.; Rutgeerts, P.; Vermeire, S. Postinduction serum infliximab trough level and decrease of C-reactive protein level are associated with durable sustained response to infliximab: A retrospective analysis of the ACCENT I trial. *Gut* **2014**, *63*, 1721–1727. [CrossRef]
14. Ma, C.; Battat, R.; Khanna, R.; Parker, C.E.; Feagan, B.G.; Jairath, V. What is the role of C-reactive protein and fecal calprotectin in evaluating Crohn's disease activity? *Best Pract. Res. Clin. Gastroenterol.* **2019**, *38–39*, 101602. [CrossRef]
15. Schmidt, M.; Schmidt, S.A.J.; Adelborg, K.; Sundboll, J.; Laugesen, K.; Ehrenstein, V.; Sorensen, H.T. The Danish health care system and epidemiological research: From health care contacts to database records. *Clin. Epidemiol.* **2019**, *11*, 563–591. [CrossRef]
16. Christiansen, T. Organization and financing of the Danish health care system. *Health Policy* **2002**, *59*, 107–118. [CrossRef] [PubMed]
17. Fonager, K.; Sørensen, H.T.; Rasmussen, S.N.; Moller-Petersen, J.; Vyberg, M. Assessment of the diagnoses of Crohn's disease and ulcerative colitis in a Danish hospital information system. *Scand. J. Gastroenterol.* **1996**, *31*, 154–159. [CrossRef]
18. Schmidt, M.; Schmidt, S.A.; Sandegaard, J.L.; Ehrenstein, V.; Pedersen, L.; Sørensen, H.T. The Danish National Patient Registry: A review of content, data quality, and research potential. *Clin. Epidemiol.* **2015**, *7*, 449–490. [CrossRef] [PubMed]
19. Arendt, J.F.H.; Hansen, A.T.; Ladefoged, S.A.; Sorensen, H.T.; Pedersen, L.; Adelborg, K. Existing Data Sources in Clinical Epidemiology: Laboratory Information System Databases in Denmark. *Clin. Epidemiol.* **2020**, *12*, 469–475. [CrossRef] [PubMed]
20. Hanley, J.A.; McNeil, B.J. A method of comparing the areas under receiver operating characteristic curves derived from the same cases. *Radiology* **1983**, *148*, 839–843. [CrossRef]
21. Singer, J.D.; Willett, J.B. *Applied Longitudinal Data Analysis—Modeling Change and Event Occurrence*, 1st ed.; Oxford University Press: New York, NY, USA, 2003.
22. Hosmer, D.W.; Lemeshow, S. Assessing the fit of the model. In *Applied Logistic Regression*, 2nd ed.; Hosmer, D.W., Lemeshow, S., Eds.; John Wiley & Sons, Inc.: New York, NY, USA, 2000; Volume 1, pp. 143–202.
23. Larsen, M.D.; Nørgård, B.M.; Kjeldsen, J. Does Disease Activity After Induction Treatment with Biologics Predict Short-Term Outcome in Crohn's Disease and Ulcerative Colitis? *Inflamm. Bowel Dis.* **2022**, *28*, 1658–1666. [CrossRef]
24. Feng, W.; Zhu, L.; Liu, Y.; Xu, L.; Shen, H. C-reactive protein/albumin ratio and IL-6 are associated with disease activity in patients with ulcerative colitis. *J. Clin. Lab. Anal.* **2023**, *37*, e24843. [CrossRef]
25. Ghoneima, A.S.; Flashman, K.; Dawe, V.; Baldwin, E.; Celentano, V. High risk of septic complications following surgery for Crohn's disease in patients with preoperative anaemia, hypoalbuminemia and high CRP. *Int. J. Color. Dis.* **2019**, *34*, 2185–2188. [CrossRef] [PubMed]
26. Ziade, F.; Rungoe, C.; Kallemose, T.; Paerregaard, A.; Wewer, A.V.; Jakobsen, C. Biochemical Markers, Genotype, and Inflammation in Pediatric Inflammatory Bowel Disease: A Danish Population-Based Study. *Dig. Dis.* **2019**, *37*, 140–146. [CrossRef] [PubMed]
27. Yerushalmy-Feler, A.; Singer, D.; Berkovitch, G., Lubetzky, R.; Dotan, I.; Ziv-Baran, T.; Cohen, S. Predictors for poor outcome of hospitalized children with inflammatory bowel disease. *Eur. J. Pediatr.* **2019**, *179*, 157–164. [CrossRef] [PubMed]

28. Gibson, D.J.; Hartery, K.; Doherty, J.; Nolan, J.; Keegan, D.; Byrne, K.; Martin, S.T.; Buckley, M.; Sheridan, J.; Horgan, G.; et al. CRP/Albumin Ratio: An Early Predictor of Steroid Responsiveness in Acute Severe Ulcerative Colitis. *J. Clin. Gastroenterol.* **2018**, *52*, e48–e52. [CrossRef] [PubMed]
29. Arias, M.T.; Vande Casteele, N.; Vermeire, S.; de Buck van Overstraeten, A.; Billiet, T.; Baert, F.; Wolthuis, A.; Van Assche, G.; Noman, M.; Hoffman, I.; et al. A panel to predict long-term outcome of infliximab therapy for patients with ulcerative colitis. *Clin. Gastroenterol. Hepatol.* **2015**, *13*, 531–538. [CrossRef] [PubMed]
30. Magro, F.; Rodrigues-Pinto, E.; Santos-Antunes, J.; Vilas-Boas, F.; Lopes, S.; Nunes, A.; Camila-Dias, C.; Macedo, G. High C-reactive protein in Crohn's disease patients predicts nonresponse to infliximab treatment. *J. Crohn's Colitis* **2014**, *8*, 129–136. [CrossRef]
31. Jürgens, M.; Mahachie John, J.M.; Cleynen, I.; Schnitzler, F.; Fidder, H.; van Moerkercke, W.; Ballet, V.; Noman, M.; Hoffman, I.; van Assche, G.; et al. Levels of C-reactive protein are associated with response to infliximab therapy in patients with Crohn's disease. *Clin. Gastroenterol. Hepatol.* **2011**, *9*, 421–427.e1. [CrossRef]
32. Schnitzler, F.; Fidder, H.; Ferrante, M.; Noman, M.; Arijs, I.; Van Assche, G.; Hoffman, I.; Van Steen, K.; Vermeire, S.; Rutgeerts, P. Long-term outcome of treatment with infliximab in 614 patients with Crohn's disease: Results from a single-centre cohort. *Gut* **2009**, *58*, 492–500. [CrossRef]
33. Iwasa, R.; Yamada, A.; Sono, K.; Furukawa, R.; Takeuchi, K.; Suzuki, Y. C-reactive protein level at 2 weeks following initiation of infliximab induction therapy predicts outcomes in patients with ulcerative colitis: A 3 year follow-up study. *BMC Gastroenterol.* **2015**, *15*, 103. [CrossRef] [PubMed]
34. Lees, C.W.; Heys, D.; Ho, G.T.; Noble, C.L.; Shand, A.G.; Mowat, C.; Boulton-Jones, R.; Williams, A.; Church, N.; Satsangi, J.; et al. A retrospective analysis of the efficacy and safety of infliximab as rescue therapy in acute severe ulcerative colitis. *Aliment. Pharmacol. Ther.* **2007**, *26*, 411–419. [CrossRef] [PubMed]
35. Wells, C.W.; Lewis, S.; Barton, J.R.; Corbett, S. Effects of changes in hemoglobin level on quality of life and cognitive function in inflammatory bowel disease patients. *Inflamm. Bowel Dis.* **2006**, *12*, 123–130. [CrossRef] [PubMed]
36. Travis, S.P.; Farrant, J.M.; Ricketts, C.; Nolan, D.J.; Mortensen, N.M.; Kettlewell, M.G.; Jewell, D.P. Predicting outcome in severe ulcerative colitis. *Gut* **1996**, *38*, 905–910. [CrossRef]
37. Buckell, N.A.; Lennard-Jones, J.E.; Hernandez, M.A.; Kohn, J.; Riches, P.G.; Wadsworth, J. Measurement of serum proteins during attacks of ulcerative colitis as a guide to patient management. *Gut* **1979**, *20*, 22–27. [CrossRef]
38. De Dombal, F.T. Prognostic value of the serum proteins during severe attacks of ulcerative colitis. *Gut* **1968**, *9*, 144–149. [CrossRef]
39. von Elm, E.; Altman, D.G.; Egger, M.; Pocock, S.J.; Gøtzsche, P.C.; Vandenbroucke, J.P. The Strengthening the Reporting of Observational Studies in Epidemiology (STROBE) statement: Guidelines for reporting observational studies. *J. Clin. Epidemiol.* **2008**, *61*, 344–349. [CrossRef]

Journal of
Clinical Medicine

MDPI

Article

Low ALT Is Associated with IBD and Disease Activity: Results from a Nationwide Study

Asher Shafrir [1,2,3,*], Lior H. Katz [2,3], Michal Shauly-Aharonov [4,5], Adar Zinger [2,3], Rifaat Safadi [3,6], Joshua Stokar [3,7] and Itay Kalisky [2,3]

1 Meuhedet Health Medical Organization, Jerusalem District, Tel Aviv 6203854, Israel
2 Institute of Gastroenterology and Hepatology, Hadassah Medical Center, Jerusalem 1200, Israel; klior@hadassah.org.il (L.H.K.); adar@hadassah.org.il (A.Z.); itayk@hadassah.org.il (I.K.)
3 Faculty of Medicine, Hebrew University of Jerusalem, Jerusalem 9190500, Israel; safadi@hadassah.org.il (R.S.); ystokar@hadassah.org.il (J.S.)
4 Braun School of Public Health and Community Medicine, Hebrew University of Jerusalem, Jerusalem 9190500, Israel; michal.shauly@mail.huji.ac.il
5 The Jerusalem College of Technology, Jerusalem 9190401, Israel
6 The Liver Institute, Hadassah Medical Organization, Jerusalem 91120, Israel
7 Department of Endocrinology, Hadassah Medical Center, Faculty of Medicine, Hebrew University of Jerusalem, Jerusalem 9190500, Israel
* Correspondence: ashershaf@gmail.com

Abstract: Background: Sarcopenia is underdiagnosed in patients with inflammatory bowel disease (IBD). Low alanine transaminase (ALT) is associated with sarcopenia. We evaluated the association between low ALT and the presence of IBD and disease activity. **Methods**: Data were collected from a national Israeli health insurer cohort comprising 976,615 patients. Patients with a diagnosis of IBD were compared to healthy controls. After exclusion of patients with liver disease, ALT > 40 IU/L and age < 18, a total of 233,451 patients were included in the analysis. Low ALT was defined as <10 IU/L. **Results**: Low ALT was more common amongst patients with IBD than in healthy controls (7.76% vs. 5.7% $p < 0.001$). Low ALT was found in 148 (7.9%) of the patients with CD and 69 (6.9%) of the patients with UC. For CD, low ALT was associated with increased fecal calprotectin (FC) and CRP (223.00 μg/mg [63.45–631.50] vs. 98.50 [31.98–324.00], $p < 0.001$, 9.10 mg/L [3.22–19.32] vs. 3.20 [1.30–8.30], $p < 0.001$) and decreased albumin and hemoglobin (3.90 g/dL [3.60–4.20] vs. 4.30 [4.00–4.50], $p < 0.001$,12.20 g/dL [11.47–13.00] vs. 13.60 [12.60–14.70], $p < 0.001$). For UC, low ALT was associated with higher FC and CRP (226.50 μg/mg [143.00–537.00] vs. 107.00 [40.85–499.50], $p = 0.057$, 4.50 mg/L [1.90–11.62] vs. 2.30 [1.00–6.20], $p < 0.001$) and with lower albumin and hemoglobin (4.00 g/dL [3.62–4.18] vs. 4.30 [4.10–4.40], $p < 0.001$, 12.40 g/dL [11.60–13.20] vs. 13.60 [12.60–14.60], $p < 0.001$). These findings remained consistent following multivariate regression and in a propensity score-matched cohort. **Conclusions**: Low ALT is more common in patients with IBD and is associated with biochemical disease activity indices.

Keywords: inflammatory bowel disease; alanine transaminase; sarcopenia; calprotectin

1. Introduction

Inflammatory bowel disease (IBD), including ulcerative colitis (UC) and Crohn's disease (CD), is characterized by chronic intestinal inflammation due to a complex interaction between genetic factors, disturbed epithelial barriers, uncontrolled inflammatory signals, loss of tolerance, and environmental triggers [1]. IBD is frequently complicated by malnutrition, defined as "a state resulting from lack of intake or uptake of nutrition that leads to altered body composition (decreased fat-free mass) and body cell mass leading to diminished physical and mental function and impaired clinical outcome from disease" [2]. Malnutrition is a crucial factor in the state of muscle loss known as sarcopenia [2]. Patients with quiescent disease have higher muscle mass than those with active bowel disease who are more likely to be malnourished and sarcopenic [3]. Even amongst patients with IBD who have a normal body mass index (BMI, calculated as kg/m^2) and serum albumin level, body cell mass and handgrip strength are lower than in healthy controls. [4,5]. Sarcopenia is also associated with a higher risk of surgical complications [3,6,7]. Patients with IBD and sarcopenia are also more likely to suffer from osteopenia and osteoporosis [5]. A normal BMI cannot rule out the presence of sarcopenia, since a high percentage of patients with IBD are obese; thus, sarcopenia can be frequently underdiagnosed [8]. The clinical importance of sarcopenia warrants incorporating muscle strength when evaluating and tailoring management of IBD [9]. However, as many of these tests are time-consuming and are not available in many IBD centers, surrogate markers that could show patients at risk for malnutrition and sarcopenia are warranted.

Alanine aminotransferase [ALT, also known as serum glutamic-pyruvic transaminase (SGPT)] is a critical enzyme in the alanine cycle that is responsible for the transfer of the α-amino group from an α-amino acid to an α-keto acid, transforming pyruvate to alanine in skeletal muscle and catalyzing alanine to pyruvate in the liver [10]. Elevated ALT is a marker of liver damage as it is released to the blood by damaged hepatocytes [11]. Conversely, multiple studies have shown that low ALT is associated with increased mortality [12–17]. Low ALT is also associated with frailty, sarcopenia, and disability, which may all explain the increase in mortality [18–20]. Patients with lower skeletal muscle mass index have lower ALT than patients with a normal skeletal mass index [21]. Low ALT is also more prevalent in the geriatric population [18,22].

The association of IBD with elevated liver enzymes, including ALT, is well established [23] and in some studies has predicted complications and a worse prognosis [24,25]. Conversely, a higher prevalence of low ALT was reported in two small retrospective studies among pediatric and adult IBD patients [26,27]. However, data concerning the association of low liver enzymes, specifically ALT, with IBD are still scarce.

This study aims to explore the prevalence of low ALT amongst patients with IBD and the possible associations of low ALT with serum markers of disease activity in a nationwide health organization.

2. Methods

The Meuhedet health maintenance organization (HMO) is one of Israel's four state-mandated HMOs. It serves over 1,300,000 individuals and is the third largest HMO in Israel. Meuhedet's EMR (electronic medical record) includes real-time input from all physician visits, medical diagnoses, laboratory results, hospitalizations, and dispensing data on prescription and over-the-counter medications. Data of 976,615 patients were collected as part of a prospective study following all HMO patients who underwent SARS-CoV-2 testing from March 2020 to 31 December 2021. Data gathered included diagnoses documented in the EMR and blood tests in the year prior. As all data were from before any possible COVID-19 infection, there were no concerns regarding a confounding effect of COVID-19 on laboratory results. Based on ICD-9 coding, patients diagnosed with IBD were compared to a healthy controls. ALT levels were divided into three groups, low (ALT < 10 IU/L), normal (10–40 IU/L), and high (ALT > 40 IU/L). As high ALT levels point to liver disease, patients with ALT > 40 were excluded from the study [28].

Within the IBD cohort, various inflammatory and metabolic markers correlated with disease activity were compared between patients with low ALT with those with normal ALT. Patients with ICD-9 diagnoses of chronic liver disease, cirrhosis, a diagnosis of both CD and UC (indeterminate IBD), ALT > 40 IU/L, those who did not have an ALT level from the year prior to the study cohort, and those of age < 18 were excluded.

The study was conducted in accordance with the Declaration of Helsinki and approved by the research ethics committee and internal review board of Meuhedet HMO (02-24-08-20). Helsinki approval was granted on 2 September 2020.

Statistical Analysis

For descriptive analyses, counts and percentages were used for categorical variables. Continuous normally distributed variables were summarized as means ± standard deviations (SD). Variables not normally distributed were summarized as medians with an interquartile rang. The Chi-squared test was used to compare categorical variables; Student's *t*-test was used to compare means of normally distributed continuous variables; and the Wilcoxon rank test was used for variables not normally distributed. Multivariate logistic regression was performed to assess the association of IBD with low ALT while controlling for age, gender, smoking status, socioeconomic status (SES), and sector. The SES index is an integral part of the Meuhedet HMO electronic database and is provided by Points Location Intelligence (https://points.co.il/ (accessed on 4 March 2024)), being rated on a scale of 1–10. The index uses data that include average family size, income, educational level, unemployment rate, number of cars per family, and median age in the specific area in which the patient lives. Sector was categorized into Arab, ultra-orthodox Jewish, and orthodox/secular Jewish and is loosely identified based on the clinic's location. For the analysis within the IBD cohort, multivariate linear and logistic regression models were constructed to evaluate the association between low ALT and different laboratory outcomes such as serum albumin, fecal calprotectin (FC), vitamin B12, ferritin, C reactive protein (CRP), and low vitamin D (>20 ng/mL). Additionally, 1:2 propensity score-matching (PSM) was used to compare patients based on age, sex, disease type, BMI, smoking, SES, and sector. Inflammatory and metabolic biomarkers were compared using a paired t-test or chi-square tests according to the compared variable. A *p*-value of less than 0.05 was considered statistically significant in all analyses. Statistical analysis was performed using R software version 3.6 (R Development Core Team, 2018).

3. Results

Starting from a total of 976,615 patients in the database, 233,451 patients remained after application of the exclusion criteria. Compared with patients with normal ALT, those with low ALT were younger (45.72 ± 22.84 vs. 46.90 ± 18.47, *p*-value < 0.001), more likely to be female (11,222 (83.8%) vs. 134,462 (61.1%), *p*-value < 0.001), and had a lowerBMI (25.62 ± 5.66 vs. 26.78 ± 5.41 *p*-value < 0.001). Additional comparisons are described in Table 1.

Low ALT was more common amongst patients with IBD (7.76% vs. 5.7% *p*-value < 0.001), which also remained statistically significant after application of multivariate logistic regression including age, gender, smoking, BMI, socioeconomic status, and sector (OR 1.51, 95% CI 1.29–1.76, *p*-value < 0.001).

Amongst patients with established IBD, 1869 (66.58%) had CD and 938 (33.44%) had UC. Amongst those with CD, 148 (7.9%) had ALT < 10, and 1721(92.1%) had normal ALT. The proportion of females was higher in the low-ALT group (111 (75.0%) vs. 898 (52.2%) *p*-value < 0.001), and BMI was lower (23.35 ± 4.81 vs. 25 ± 5.25, *p*-value < 0.001). Age and smoking were not significantly different between the two groups. Amongst patients with UC, 69 (6.9%) had low ALT and 930 (93.1%) had normal ALT. Amongst patients with UC, compared to those with normal ALT, patients with low ALT were younger (42.43 ± 19.53 vs. 48.98 ± 17.51, *p*-value = 0.003), more likely female (82.6% vs. 48.98%, *p*-value < 0.001), and had a lower BMI (24.19 ± 5.27 vs. 25.72 ± 4.77, *p*-value = 0.029). See Table 2 for additional comparisons.

Table 1. Comparison of demographic and medical history of the study population with low and normal ALT levels.

	ALT < 10	10 ≤ ALT < 40	*p*-Value
N	13,391	220,060	
Age (mean ± SD)	45.72 ± 22.84	46.90 ± 8.47	<0.001

Table 1. *Cont.*

	ALT < 10	10 ≤ ALT < 40	*p*-Value
Female	11,222 (83.8%)	134,462 (61.1%)	<0.001
BMI (mean ± SD)	25.62 ± 5.66	26.78 ± 5.41	<0.001
Smoking	1360 (10.2%)	29,371 (13.3%)	<0.001
Sector (%)			<0.001
Arab	2669 (19.9%)	38,413 (17.5%)	
Non Arab, Non Ultra-Orthodox	7632 (57.0%)	135,592 (61.6%)	
Ultra-Orthodox	3088 (23.1%)	45,990 (20.9%)	
Socioeconomic Status (mean ± SD)	5.03 (2.03)	5.29 (2.05)	<0.001
IBD (%)	217 (1.6%)	2580 (1.2%)	<0.001
Hypertension (%)	1432 (10.7%)	20,393 (9.3%)	<0.001
Diabetes Mellitus (%)	1715 (12.8%)	23,413 (10.6%)	<0.001
Ischemic Heart Disease (%)	837 (6.3%)	11,072 (5.0%)	<0.001

BMI—Body mass index, IBD—Inflammatory bowel disease.

Table 2. Comparison of demographic and laboratory parameters in IBD patients with low and normal ALT levels.

	Crohn's Disease				Ulcerative Colitis			
	ALT < 10	10 ≤ ALT < 40	*p*-Value	*p* -Value in Multivariate Regression	ALT < 10	10 ≤ ALT < 40	*p*-Value	*p*-Value in Multivariate Regression
n	148	1721			69	859		
Age (mean ± SD)	39.99 ± 17.21	41.33 ± 16.20	0.337		42.43 ± 19.53	49.27 ± 17.60	0.002	
Female (%)	111 (75.0%)	898 (52.2%)	<0.001		57 (82.6%)	473 (55.1%)	<0.001	
BMI (mean ± SD)	23.35 ± 4.81	25.02 ± 5.25	0.001		24.19 ± 5.27	25.60 ± 4.70	0.041	
Smoking (%)	16 (10.8%)	250 (14.5%)	0.263		9 (13.0%)	66 (7.7%)	0.18	
Sector (%)			0.08				0.526	
Arab	8 (5.4%)	141 (8.2%)			6 (8.7%)	64 (7.5%)		
Non Arab/non Ultra-Orthodox	92 (62.2%)	1155 (67.1%)			45 (65.2%)	615 (71.6%)		
Ultra-Orthodox	48 (32.4%)	425 (24.7%)			18 (26.1%)	180 (21.0%)		
FC (median [IQR])	223.00 [63.45, 631.50]	98.50 [31.98, 324.00]	<0.001	0.009	226.50 [143.00, 537.00]	107.00 [40.85, 499.50]	0.057	0.69
FC > 150 (%)	41 (57.7)	301 (39.2)	0.004	0.016	19 (73.1)	105 (46.1)	0.016	0.015
CRP (median [IQR])	9.10 [3.22, 19.32]	3.20 [1.30, 8.30]	<0.001	<0.001	4.50 [1.90, 11.62]	2.30 [1.00, 6.20]	0.001	<0.001
Albumin (median [IQR])	3.90 [3.60, 4.20]	4.30 [4.00, 4.50]	<0.001	<0.001	4.00 [3.62, 4.18]	4.30 [4.10, 4.40]	<0.001	<0.001
Platelet (median [IQR])	295.00 [215.75, 356.00]	260.00 [216.00, 311.00]	0.003	0.001	286.00 [234.00, 342.00]	253.00 [209.00, 302.00]	0.002	0.054
Hemoglobin (median [IQR])	12.20 [11.47, 13.00]	13.60 [12.60, 14.70]	<0.001	<0.001	12.40 [11.60, 13.20]	13.60 [12.60, 14.60]	<0.001	<0.001
Vitamin D < 20 ng/mL (%)	38 (49.4)	324 (34.6)	0.014	0.012	17 (53.1)	157 (33.5)	0.04	0.22
Vitamin B12 < 280 (%)	39 (37.5)	290 (28.8)	0.082	0.016	12 (30.0)	101 (20.0)	0.192	0.29

FC—fecal calprotectin, SD—standard deviation., IQR—interquartile range.

3.1. Association with Inflammatory Biomarkers

Amongst patients with CD and low ALT, median fecal calprotectin was higher at 223.00 μg/mg [63.45–631.50] vs. 98.50 [31.98–324.00], *p*-value < 0.001, Figure 1A), as were CRP (9.10 mg/L [3.22–19.32] vs. 3.20 [1.30–8.30], *p*-value < 0.001, Figure 1B) and platelet levels (295,000 U/mL [215,750–350,000] vs. 260,000 U/mL [216,000–311,000], *p*-value = 0.003,

Figure 2) compared to those with normal ALT. Additionally, the proportion of patients with elevated FC (>150 µg/mg) was higher in the low-ALT group (27.7% vs. 17.48%, p-value = 0.004). These findings were consistent when using a multivariate linear regression model controlling for age, gender, smoking status, BMI, socioeconomic status, sector, and IBD disease (Table 2).

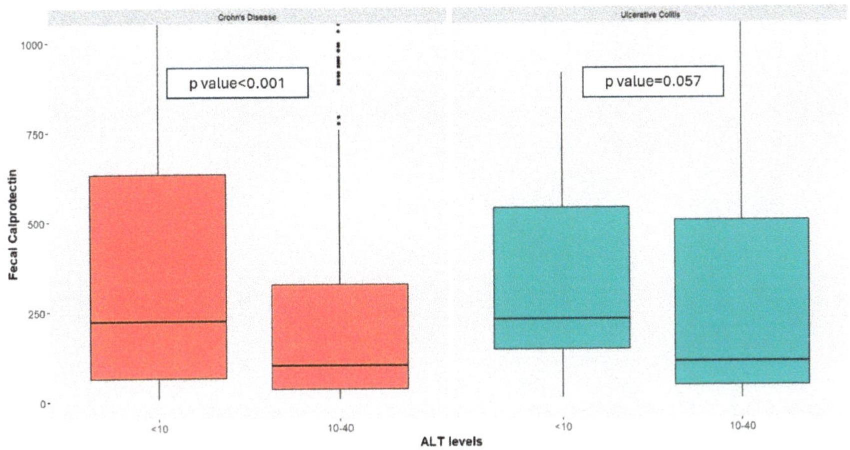

(A)

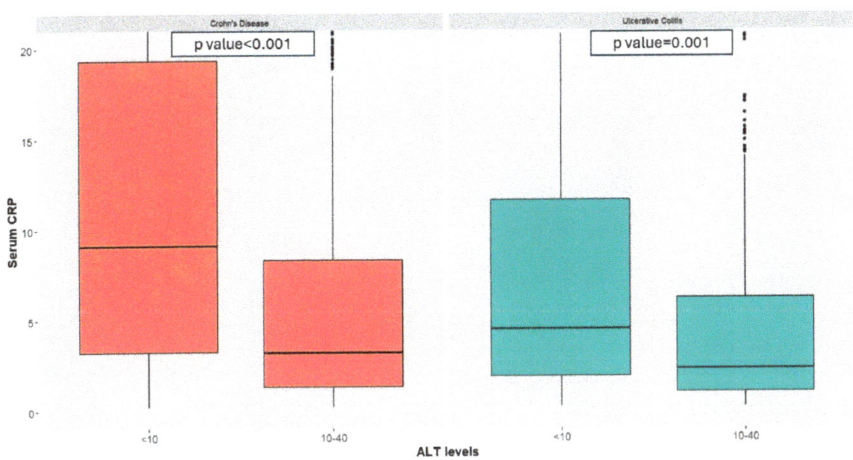

(B)

Figure 1. Fecal calprotectin (**A**) and CRP levels (**B**) amongst patients with UC and CD with low and normal ALT.

In patients with UC, low ALT was associated with higher FC (226.50 µg/mg vs. 107.00 [40.85–499.50], p-value = 0.057, Figure 1A), higher CRP (4.50 mg/L [1.90–11.62] vs. 2.30 [1.00–6.20], p-value < 0.001, Figure 1B), and a higher platelet count (286,000 U/mL [234,000–342,000] vs. 253,000 [209,000–302,000], p-value = 0.002, Figure 2). The proportion of patients with elevated FC (>150 µg/mg) was also higher (27.56% vs. 13.38%, p-value = 0.015) in patients with low ALT. These findings were consistent when using a multivariate linear regression model controlling for age, gender, smoking status, BMI, socioeconomic status, sector, and IBD disease (Table 2).

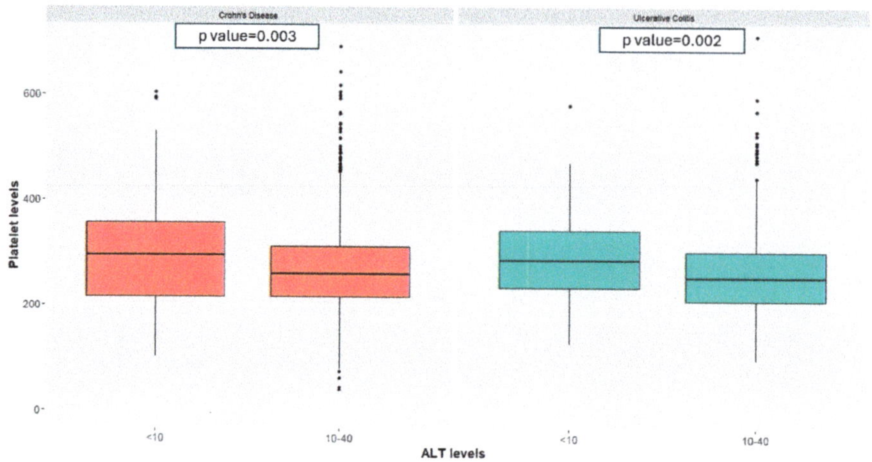

Figure 2. Platelet levels amongst patients with UC and CD with low and normal ALT.

3.2. Association with Metabolic Markers

Amongst patients with CD and low ALT, serum albumin (3.90 g/dL [3.60–4.20] vs. 4.30 [4.00–4.50], *p*-value < 0.001, Figure 3A) and hemoglobin levels (12.20 g/dL [11.47–13.00] vs. 13.60 [12.60–14.70], *p*-value < 0.001, Figure 3B) were lower when compared to those in the normal group. A low vitamin D level (<20 ng/mL) was more common in the low ALT group (49.4% vs. 34.6%, *p*-value < 0.001, Figure 4). These findings remained statistically significant after application of a linear regression model controlling for age, sex, smoking status, type of IBD disease, BMI, SES, and sector (Table 2).

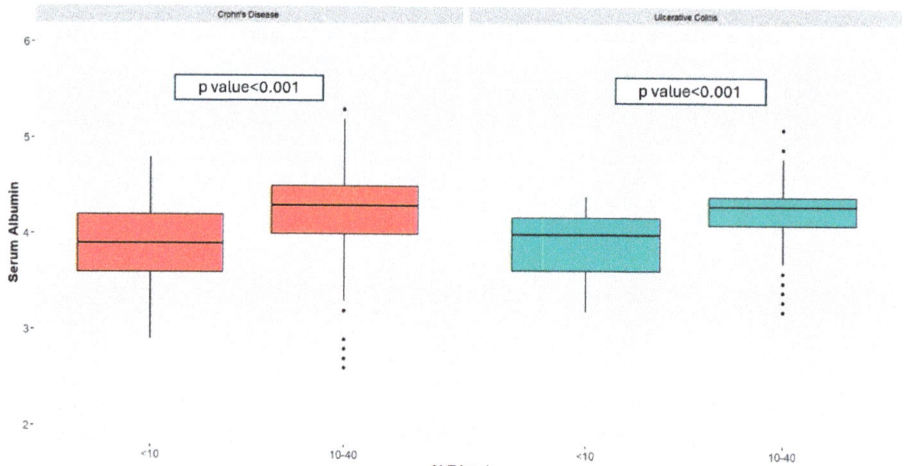

(**A**)

Figure 3. *Cont.*

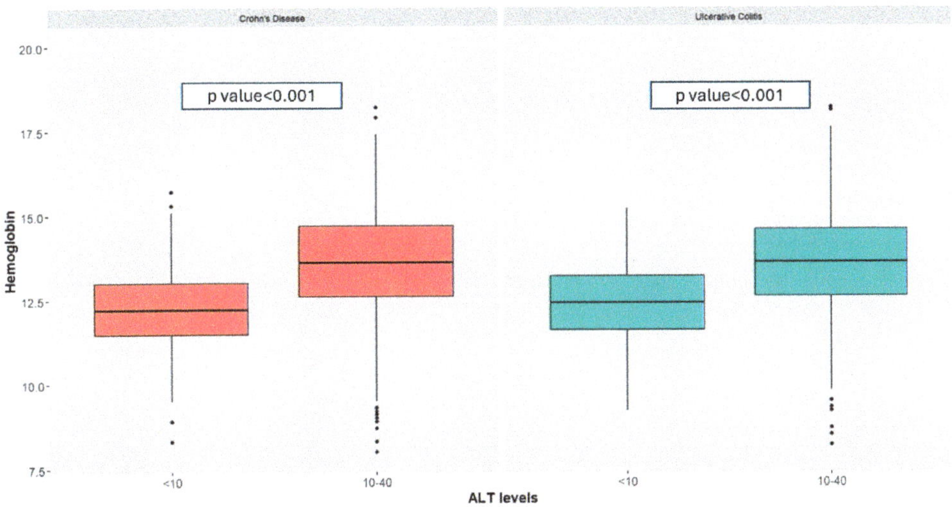

(**B**)

Figure 3. Serum albumin (**A**) and hemoglobin (**B**) amongst patients with UC and CD with low and normal ALT.

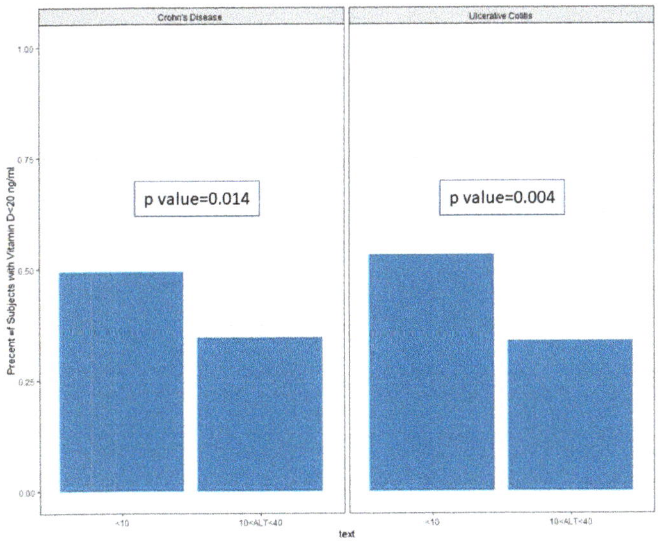

Figure 4. Proportion of patients with serum vitamin D levels < 20 ng/mL amongst low- and normal-ALT groups.

Amongst patients with UC, low ALT was associated with lower albumin (4.00 g/dL [3.62–4.18] vs. 4.30 [4.10–4.40], *p*-value < 0.001, Figure 3A) and lower hemoglobin (12.40 g/dL [11.60–13.20] vs. 13.60 [12.60–14.60], *p*-value < 0.001, Figure 3B). A low level of vitamin D (<20 ng/mL) was more common amongst patients in the low-ALT group (53.1% vs. 33.5%, *p*-value = 0.04), see Figure 4.

3.3. Propensity Score-Matching

Using a propensity score-matched algorithm, 134 subjects with IBD and low ALT were compared to 268 patients with normal ALT. In this cohort, there was no significant difference in age, gender, BMI, sector, socioeconomic status, and smoking status. In the low ALT group, fecal calprotectin, serum CRP, and platelet count were higher (205.50 g/mg [71.90–793.00] vs. 115.00 [40.70–389.00], *p*-value = 0.005, 6.90 mg/L [2.10–15.70] vs. 3.10 mg/L [1.17–8.10], *p*-value < 0.001, 306,500 U/mL [244,000–364,000] vs. 269,500 U/mL [225,000–319,250], *p*-value = 0.001, respectively). Regarding metabolic biomarkers, patients with low ALT had lower albumin (4.00 [3.69–4.20] vs. 4.20 [4.00–4.40], *p*-value < 0.001.), see Table 3. Table 4 describes the same cohort with patients only compared to those with the same disease. Despite the smaller sample size in this comparison, the results were overall still statistically significant.

Table 3. Propensity score-matched cohort.

	ALT < 10	**10 ≤ ALT < 40**	***p*-Value**
N	134	268	
Age (mean ± SD)	38.66 (16.75)	39.38 (16.36)	0.615
Female (%)	212 (79.1%)	216 (80.6%)	0.747
BMI (mean ± SD)	23.44 (4.90)	23.65 (4.77)	0.627
Ulcerative Colitis (%)	84 (31.3%)	84 (31.3%)	1
Smoking (%)	34 (12.7%)	29 (10.8%)	0.592
Sector (%)			0.905
Arab	22 (8.2%)	23 (8.6%)	
Non Arab/non Ultra-Orthodox	170 (63.4%)	165 (61.6%)	
Ultra-Orthodox	76 (28.4%)	80 (29.9%)	
SES (mean ± SD)	5.51 (2.10)	5.45 (2.10)	0.743
CRP (median [IQR])	6.90 [2.10, 15.70]	3.00 [1.00, 8.10]	<0.001
Fecal Calprotectin (median [IQR])	205.50 [71.90, 793.00]	111.00 [40.70, 461.00]	0.006
FC > 150 (%)	86 (61.4%)	55 (44.0%)	0.007
Albumin (median [IQR])	4.00 [3.69, 4.20]	4.20 [4.00, 4.40]	<0.001
Platelets (median [IQR])	306.50 [244.00, 364.00]	265.00 [223.00, 319.00]	<0.001
Vitamin B12 (median [IQR])	327.00 [238.00, 438.75]	384.00 [282.25, 514.75]	0.003
Vitamin D < 20 ng/mL (%)	78 (52.7%)	57 (36.3%)	0.006

SES—socioeconomic status, CRP—C reactive protein. IQR—interquartile range.

Table 4. Propensity score-matched cohort according to specific disease.

	Ulcerative Colitis			**Crohn's Disease**		
	ALT < 10	**10 ≤ ALT < 40**	***p*-Value**	**ALT < 10**	**10 ≤ ALT <40**	***p*-Value**
n	42	84		92	184	
Age (mean ± SD)	38.90 (19.38)	43.49 (18.55)	0.119	38.54 (15.46)	37.50 (14.94)	0.511
Female (%)	70 (83.3%)	75 (89.3%)	0.369	142 (77.2%)	141 (76.6%)	1
BMI (mean ± SD)	24.18 (5.30)	23.74 (4.22)	0.551	23.11 (4.69)	23.61 (5.02)	0.326

Table 4. *Cont.*

	Ulcerative Colitis			Crohn's Disease		
	ALT < 10	**10 ≤ ALT < 40**	***p*-Value**	**ALT < 10**	**10 ≤ ALT <40**	***p*-Value**
Smoking (%)	12 (14.3%)	3 (3.6%)	0.03	22 (12.0%)	26 (14.1)	0.642
Sector (%)			0.604			0.53
Arab	8 (9.5%)	5 (6.0%)		14 (7.6%)	18 (9.8%)	
Non Arab/non Ultra-Orthodox	52 (61.9%)	57 (67.9%)		118 (64.1%)	108 (58.7%)	
Ultra-Orthodox	24 (28.6%)	22 (26.2%)		52 (28.3%)	58 (31.5%)	
SES (mean ± SD)	5.33 (2.04)	5.83 (2.11)	0.121	5.59 (2.13)	5.27 (2.08)	0.152
CRP (median [IQR])	3.75 [1.90, 12.30]	2.65 [0.90, 6.50]	0.007	8.15 [2.82, 16.92]	3.10 [1.17, 8.72]	<0.001
Fecal Calprotectin (median [IQR])	224.00 [159.75, 734.75]	74.60 [40.70, 490.50]	0.026	193.00 [59.75, 911.50]	141.00 [41.18, 442.50]	0.074
FC > 150 (%)	30 (78.9%)	10 (32.3%)	<0.001	56 (54.9)	45 (47.9)	0.4
Albumin (median [IQR])	4.00 [3.70, 4.11]	4.20 [4.00, 4.40]	0.001	4.00 [3.67, 4.23]	4.20 [4.00, 4.40]	<0.001
Platelets (median [IQR])	302.00 [244.00, 354.00]	270.00 [218.00, 315.25]	0.024	306.50 [243.50, 365.00]	264.00 [228.00, 321.25]	<0.001
Vitamin B12 (median [IQR])	310.00 [262.00, 488.00]	413.00 [358.75, 527.50]	0.06	327.50 [224.75, 430.50]	364.50 [272.75, 501.50]	0.026
Vitamin D < 20 ng/mL (%)	22 (55.0%)	18 (39.1%)	0.209	56 (51.9%)	39 (35.1%)	0.018

4. Discussion

Alanine aminotransferase (ALT) is a pyridoxal enzyme that catalyzes the reversible interconversion of L-alanine and 2-oxoglutarate to pyruvate and L-glutamate. Serum ALT is generally used to assess liver health. The reported prevalence of IBD-associated hepatobiliary diseases and resulting elevated liver enzymes ranges from 3% to greater than 50% depending on the exact definition used [29]. Elevated liver enzymes can be attributed to multiple etiologies including fatty liver disease [30], drug-related liver injury [31–34], use of total parenteral nutrition (TPN) [35], systemic inflammatory processes [36], cholelithiasis [23], and primary sclerosing cholangitis [37]. Liver enzyme abnormalities were observed in adults and children with IBD [36]. In a retrospective study of 383 newly diagnosed adult patients with CD, elevated liver enzymes at diagnosis predicted a more complicated course including hospitalizations, surgeries, and mortality [24]. In a recent study by Yanai et al., serum ALT > 25 IU/L was incorporated as part of a predictive model for complicated disease in treatment naïve IBD patients [38].

Multiple studies have shown that low ALT is associated with frailty, sarcopenia, and increased mortality [13,14]. However, the prevalence and effect of low ALT in patients with IBD have not been adequately investigated. In a small study amongst pediatric patients with patients, almost half were reported to have ALT < 5 IU/L (29% at initial admission, 18% during follow-up) [26]. A Danish study performed on 127 adults with IBD found that almost all the patients with CD had subnormal ALT on at least one occasion across a 10-year follow-up. Only one patient with UC had a subnormal ALT. It should be noted that patients older than 50 years were excluded from the study, a population where low ALT is more common [27].

In this current population-based study, we showed that low ALT levels are more common in patients with IBD than in the general population. This finding remained statistically significant after controlling for multiple covariates such as age, gender, socioeconomic status, and sector. In our cohort, the overall prevalence of low ALT amongst patients with

IBD was much lower than previous reports. Possible explanations for this disparity may be the shorter duration of follow-up, the more restricted definition of low ALT, and the larger cohort included in our study.

It should be noted that while other liver enzymes exist, such as aspartate aminotransferase (AST), only two patients in our IBD cohort had AST levels < 10 IU/L. This may point to ALT being a more sensitive biomarker than IBD-related inflammatory and metabolic markers.

Our study shows that amongst patients with IBD, low ALT levels was associated with increased inflammatory markers such as FC, CRP, and platelet count, and with decreased metabolic markers such as hemoglobin, albumin, and vitamin D.

Low ALT was found to be associated with a significant risk of relapse, steroid dependency, and a low level of albumin, hemoglobin, folic acid, and penetrating phenotype in a small cohort of pediatric patients with IBD [21]. Low ALT has been proposed as a surrogate marker for low muscle mass and sarcopenia [39], and patients with low ALT have a lower L3 muscle mass index [40]. In patients with IBD, multiple studies have demonstrated an increased incidence of sarcopenia amongst patients with active disease [6,41]. Thus, we can hypothesize that IBD patients' low ALT levels in our cohort may be related to IBD activity and attributable to sarcopenia.

The most common nutrient deficiencies in IBD are of iron, vitamin B12, vitamin D, vitamin K, folic acid, selenium, zinc, vitamin B6, and vitamin B1 [34]. The ALT enzyme requires active vitamin B6 to function; thus, vitamin B6 deficiency may decrease ALT levels in inflammatory diseases, as well as in elderly patients and individuals suffering with alcohol addiction [42,43]. Nutritional deficiencies are more common in CD than in UC [44], as well as in active disease vs. remission. Thus, the higher prevalence of low ALT in CD patients in our study is consistent with this pattern. Although smoking likely lowers ALT in healthy patients and increases it in people with liver disease [45], the multivariate logistic regression model used in the current study controlled for smoking as an effecting factor.

The strength of this study is its large and heterogenous population, with data extracted from a national health insurance provider covering a diverse range of populations. Multivariate analysis and propensity score-matching methods were employed to reduce the influence of potential confounders. The results showed a consistent correlation between low ALT and inflammatory and metabolic markers.

This work has several limitations. Its retrospective nature and the absence of endoscopic evidence of IBD activity may lead to misguided conclusions. Additional research is needed to investigate whether low ALT can predict treatment failure and the frequency of flare ups. We also did not introduce any direct evidence linking low ALT with sarcopenia, for example, from imaging or muscle strength tests. Hence, this link remains a hypothesis warranting further studies.

5. Conclusions

In conclusion, in this large population-based cohort, low ALT, defined as ALT < 10 IU/L, is more prevalent in patients with IBD and associated with low BMI, increased inflammatory markers, and low metabolic indices. Low ALT can be used as a surrogate for disease activity and metabolic deficiencies in patients with IBD.

Author Contributions: Methodology, A.S. and I.K.; Formal analysis, A.S.; Investigation, M.S.-A.; Writing—original draft, A.S. and I.K.; Writing—review & editing, L.H.K., A.Z., R.S. and J.S. All authors have read and agreed to the published version of the manuscript.

Funding: This research received no funding.

Institutional Review Board Statement: This study was conducted in accordance with the Declaration of Helsinki and approved by the research ethics committee and internal review board of Meuhedet HMO (02-24-08-20). Helsinki approval was granted on 2 September 2020.

Informed Consent Statement: Patient consent was waived as the data were anonymized, and no intervention took place.

Data Availability Statement: The datasets presented in this article are not readily available because there are ethical restrictions on sharing our data set because data contains potentially identifying patient information. These restrictions were imposed by the Ethics Committee of Meuhedet HMO who owns the data. Requests to access the datasets should be directed to Liron Yitzchaki, coordinator of Meuhedet Research Center, liron.y3@meuhedet.co.il.

Conflicts of Interest: The authors declare no conflicts of interest.

References

1. Ashton, J.J.; Harden, A.; Beattie, R.M. Paediatric inflammatory bowel disease: Improving early diagnosis. *Arch. Dis. Child.* **2018**, *103*, 307–308. [CrossRef] [PubMed]
2. Cederholm, T.; Barazzoni, R.; Austin, P.; Ballmer, P.; Biolo, G.; Bischoff, S.C.; Compher, C.; Correia, I.; Higashiguchi, T.; Holst, M.; et al. ESPEN guidelines on definitions and terminology of clinical nutrition. *Clin. Nutr.* **2017**, *36*, 49–64. [CrossRef] [PubMed]
3. Zhang, T.; Ding, C.; Xie, T.; Yang, J.; Dai, X.; Lv, T.; Li, Y.; Gu, L.; Wei, Y.; Gong, J.; et al. Skeletal muscle depletion correlates with disease activity in ulcerative colitis and is reversed after colectomy. *Clin. Nutr.* **2017**, *36*, 1586–1592. [CrossRef] [PubMed]
4. Valentini, L.; Schaper, L.; Buning, C.; Hengstermann, S.; Koernicke, T.; Tillinger, W.; Guglielmi, F.W.; Norman, K.; Buhner, S.; Ockenga, J.; et al. Malnutrition and impaired muscle strength in patients with Crohn's disease and ulcerative colitis in remission. *Nutrition* **2008**, *24*, 694–702. [CrossRef]
5. Bryant, R.V.; Ooi, S.; Schultz, C.G.; Goess, C.; Grafton, R.; Hughes, J.; Lim, A.; Bartholomeusz, F.D.; Andrews, J.M. Low muscle mass and sarcopenia: Common and predictive of osteopenia in inflammatory bowel disease. *Aliment. Pharmacol. Ther.* **2015**, *41*, 895–906. [CrossRef]
6. Ryan, E.; McNicholas, D.; Creavin, B.; Kelly, M.E.; Walsh, T.; Beddy, D. Sarcopenia and Inflammatory Bowel Disease: A Systematic Review. *Inflamm. Bowel Dis.* **2018**, *25*, 67–73. [CrossRef]
7. Zhang, T.; Cao, L.; Cao, T.; Yang, J.; Gong, J.; Zhu, W.; Li, N.; Li, J. Prevalence of Sarcopenia and Its Impact on Postoperative Outcome in Patients With Crohn's Disease Undergoing Bowel Resection. *J. Parenter. Enter. Nutr.* **2017**, *41*, 592–600. [CrossRef]
8. Adams, D.W.; Gurwara, S.; Silver, H.J.; Horst, S.N.; Beaulieu, D.B.; Schwartz, D.A.; Seidner, D.L. Sarcopenia Is Common in Overweight Patients with Inflammatory Bowel Disease and May Predict Need for Surgery. *Inflamm. Bowel Dis.* **2017**, *23*, 1182–1186. [CrossRef]
9. Dhaliwal, A.; Quinlan, J.I.; Overthrow, K.; Greig, C.; Lord, J.M.; Armstrong, M.J.; Cooper, S.C. Sarcopenia in Inflammatory Bowel Disease: A Narrative Overview. *Nutrients* **2021**, *13*, 656. [CrossRef] [PubMed]
10. Sherman, K.E. Alanine Aminotransferase in Clinical Practice: A Review. *Arch. Intern. Med.* **1991**, *151*, 260–265. [CrossRef] [PubMed]
11. van Beek, J.H.; de Moor, M.H.; de Geus, E.J.; Lubke, G.H.; Vink, J.M.; Willemsen, G.; Boomsma, D.I. The genetic architecture of liver enzyme levels: GGT, ALT and AST. *Behav. Genet.* **2013**, *43*, 329–339. [CrossRef]
12. Ramaty, E.; Maor, E.; Peltz-Sinvani, N.; Brom, A.; Grinfeld, A.; Kivity, S.; Segev, S.; Sidi, Y.; Kessler, T.; Sela, B. Low ALT blood levels predict long-term all-cause mortality among adults. A historical prospective cohort study. *Eur. J. Intern. Med.* **2014**, *25*, 919–921. [CrossRef]
13. Ruhl, C.E.; Everhart, J.E. The association of low serum alanine aminotransferase activity with mortality in the US population. *Am. J. Epidemiol.* **2013**, *178*, 1702–1711. [CrossRef]
14. Le Couteur, D.G.; Blyth, F.M.; Creasey, H.M.; Handelsman, D.J.; Naganathan, V.; Sambrook, P.N.; Seibel, M.J.; Waite, L.M.; Cumming, R.G. The association of alanine transaminase with aging, frailty, and mortality. *J. Gerontol. Ser. A Biomed. Sci. Med. Sci.* **2010**, *65*, 712–717. [CrossRef] [PubMed]
15. Koehler, E.M.; Sanna, D.; Hansen, B.E.; van Rooij, F.J.; Heeringa, J.; Hofman, A.; Tiemeier, H.; Stricker, B.H.; Schouten, J.N.L.; Janssen, H.L.A. Serum liver enzymes are associated with all-cause mortality in an elderly population. *Liver Int.* **2014**, *34*, 296–304. [CrossRef] [PubMed]
16. Elinav, E.; Ackerman, Z.; Maaravi, Y.; Ben-Dov, I.Z.; Ein-Mor, E.; Stessman, J. Low Alanine Aminotransferase Activity in Older People Is Associated with Greater Long-Term Mortality. *J. Am. Geriatr. Soc.* **2006**, *54*, 1719–1724. [CrossRef]
17. Genzel, D.; Katz, L.H.; Safadi, R.; Rozenberg, A.; Milgrom, Y.; Jacobs, J.M.; Shafrir, A. Patients with low ALT levels are at increased risk for severe COVID-19. *Front. Med.* **2023**, *10*, 1231440. [CrossRef] [PubMed]
18. Vespasiani-Gentilucci, U.; De Vincentis, A.; Ferrucci, L.; Bandinelli, S.; Antonelli Incalzi, R.; Picardi, A. Low Alanine Aminotransferase Levels in the Elderly Population: Frailty, Disability, Sarcopenia, and Reduced Survival. *J.Gerontol. Ser. A* **2017**, *73*, 925–930. [CrossRef] [PubMed]
19. Anani, S.; Goldhaber, G.; Brom, A.; Lasman, N.; Turpashvili, N.; Shenhav-saltzman, G.; Avaky, C.; Negru, L.; Agbaria, M.; Ariam, S.; et al. Frailty and Sarcopenia Assessment upon Hospital Admission to Internal Medicine Predicts Length of Hospital Stay and Re-Admission: A Prospective Study of 980 Patients. *J. Clin. Med.* **2020**, *9*, 2659. [CrossRef]
20. Irina, G.; Refaela, C.; Adi, B.; Avia, D.; Liron, H.; Chen, A.; Gad, S. Low Blood ALT Activity and High FRAIL Questionnaire Scores Correlate with Increased Mortality and with Each Other. A Prospective Study in the Internal Medicine Department. *J. Clin. Med.* **2018**, *7*, 386. [CrossRef]

21. Portal, D.; Hofstetter, L.; Eshed, I.; Dan-Lantsman, C.; Sella, T.; Urban, D.; Onn, A.; Bar, J.; Segal, G. L3 skeletal muscle index (L3SMI) is a surrogate marker of sarcopenia and frailty in non-small cell lung cancer patients. *Cancer Manag. Res.* **2019**, *11*, 2579–2588. [CrossRef]
22. Elinav, E.; Ben-Dov, I.Z.; Ackerman, E.; Kiderman, A.; Glikberg, F.; Shapira, Y.; Ackerman, Z. Correlation Between Serum Alanine Aminotransferase Activity and Age: An Inverted U Curve Pattern. *Off. J. Am. Coll. Gastroenterol. ACG* **2005**, *100*, 2201–2204. [CrossRef]
23. Restellini, S.; Chazouilleres, O.; Frossard, J.L. Hepatic manifestations of inflammatory bowel diseases. *Liver Int.* **2017**, *37*, 475–489. [CrossRef]
24. Mendes, F.D.; Levy, C.; Enders, F.B.; Loftus, E.V., Jr.; Angulo, P.; Lindor, K.D. Abnormal hepatic biochemistries in patients with inflammatory bowel disease. *Am. J. Gastroenterol.* **2007**, *102*, 344–350. [CrossRef]
25. Barendregt, J.; de Jong, M.; Haans, J.J.; van Hoek, B.; Hardwick, J.; Veenendaal, R.; van der Meulen, A.; Srivastava, N.; Stuyt, R.; Maljaars, J. Liver test abnormalities predict complicated disease behaviour in patients with newly diagnosed Crohn's disease. *Int. J. Colorectal Dis.* **2017**, *32*, 459–467. [CrossRef]
26. Cakir, M.; Sag, E.; Dogan, G.; Unal, F.; Kasirga, E. Clinical significance of low transaminase levels in children with inflammatory bowel disease. *World J. Pediatr.* **2019**, *15*, 143–147. [CrossRef]
27. Vadstrup, S. Subnormal alanine aminotransferase values in blood of patients with Crohn disease. *Scand. J. Gastroenterol.* **2004**, *39*, 554–556. [CrossRef] [PubMed]
28. Segev, A.; Itelman, E.; Avaky, C.; Negru, L.; Shenhav-Saltzman, G.; Grupper, A.; Wasserstrum, Y.; Segal, G. Low ALT Levels Associated with Poor Outcomes in 8700 Hospitalized Heart Failure Patients. *J. Clin. Med.* **2020**, *9*, 3185. [CrossRef] [PubMed]
29. Loftus, E.V., Jr.; Sandborn, W.J.; Lindor, K.D.; Larusso, N.F. Interactions between chronic liver disease and inflammatory bowel disease. *Inflamm. Bowel Dis.* **1997**, *3*, 288–302. [CrossRef] [PubMed]
30. Bargiggia, S.; Maconi, G.; Elli, M.; Molteni, P.; Ardizzone, S.; Parente, F.; Todaro, I.; Greco, S.; Manzionna, G.; Bianchi Porro, G. Sonographic prevalence of liver steatosis and biliary tract stones in patients with inflammatory bowel disease: Study of 511 subjects at a single center. *J. Clin. Gastroenterol.* **2003**, *36*, 417–420. [CrossRef] [PubMed]
31. Shelton, E.; Chaudrey, K.; Sauk, J.; Khalili, H.; Masia, R.; Nguyen, D.D.; Yajnik, V.; Ananthakrishnan, A.N. New onset idiosyncratic liver enzyme elevations with biological therapy in inflammatory bowel disease. *Aliment. Pharmacol. Ther.* **2015**, *41*, 972–979. [CrossRef]
32. Tobon, G.J.; Canas, C.; Jaller, J.J.; Restrepo, J.C.; Anaya, J.M. Serious liver disease induced by infliximab. *Clin. Rheumatol.* **2007**, *26*, 578–581. [CrossRef] [PubMed]
33. Fournier, M.R.; Klein, J.; Minuk, G.Y.; Bernstein, C.N. Changes in liver biochemistry during methotrexate use for inflammatory bowel disease. *Am. J. Gastroenterol.* **2010**, *105*, 1620–1626. [CrossRef]
34. Gisbert, J.P.; Gonzalez-Lama, Y.; Mate, J. Thiopurine-induced liver injury in patients with inflammatory bowel disease: A systematic review. *Am. J. Gastroenterol.* **2007**, *102*, 1518–1527. [CrossRef]
35. Bengoa, J.M.; Hanauer, S.B.; Sitrin, M.D.; Baker, A.L.; Rosenberg, I.H. Pattern and prognosis of liver function test abnormalities during parenteral nutrition in inflammatory bowel disease. *Hepatology* **1985**, *5*, 79–84. [CrossRef] [PubMed]
36. Yamamoto-Furusho, J.K.; Sanchez-Osorio, M.; Uribe, M. Prevalence and factors associated with the presence of abnormal function liver tests in patients with ulcerative colitis. *Ann. Hepatol.* **2010**, *9*, 397–401. [CrossRef] [PubMed]
37. Rasmussen, H.H.; Fallingborg, J.F.; Mortensen, P.B.; Vyberg, M.; Tage-Jensen, U.; Rasmussen, S.N. Hepatobiliary dysfunction and primary sclerosing cholangitis in patients with Crohn's disease. *Scand. J. Gastroenterol.* **1997**, *32*, 604–610. [CrossRef]
38. Yanai, H.; Goren, I.; Godny, L.; Maharshak, N.; Ron, Y.; Avni Biron, I.; Leibovitzh, H.; Banai Eran, H.; Aharoni Golan, M.; Rabinowitz, K.; et al. Early Indolent Course of Crohn's Disease in Newly Diagnosed Patients Is Not Rare and Possibly Predictable. *Clin. Gastroenterol. Hepatol.* **2021**, *19*, 1564–1572.e1565. [CrossRef]
39. Kogan, M.; Klempfner, R.; Lotan, D.; Wasserstrum, Y.; Goldenberg, I.; Segal, G. Low ALT blood levels are associated with lower baseline fitness amongst participants of a cardiac rehabilitation program. *J. Exerc. Sci. Fit.* **2018**, *16*, 1–4. [CrossRef]
40. Portal, D.; Melamed, G.; Segal, G.; Itelman, E. Sarcopenia as Manifested by L3SMI Is Associated with Increased Long-Term Mortality amongst Internal Medicine Patients—A Prospective Cohort Study. *J. Clin. Med.* **2022**, *11*, 3500. [CrossRef]
41. Gold, S.L.; Raman, M.; Sands, B.E.; Ungaro, R.; Sabino, J. Review article: Putting some muscle into sarcopenia—The pathogenesis, assessment and clinical impact of muscle loss in patients with inflammatory bowel disease. *Aliment. Pharmacol. Ther.* **2023**, *57*, 1216–1230. [CrossRef]
42. Ueland, P.M.; Ulvik, A.; Rios-Avila, L.; Midttun, Ø.; Gregory, J.F. Direct and functional biomarkers of vitamin B6 status. *Annu. Rev. Nutr.* **2015**, *35*, 33–70. [CrossRef]
43. Diehl, A.M.; Potter, J.; Boitnott, J.; Van Duyn, M.A.; Herlong, H.F.; Mezey, E. Relationship between pyridoxal 5′-phosphate deficiency and aminotransferase levels in alcoholic hepatitis. *Gastroenterology* **1984**, *86*, 632–636. [CrossRef] [PubMed]

44. Massironi, S.; Rossi, R.E.; Cavalcoli, F.A.; Della Valle, S.; Fraquelli, M.; Conte, D. Nutritional deficiencies in inflammatory bowel disease: Therapeutic approaches. *Clin. Nutr.* **2013**, *32*, 904–910. [CrossRef] [PubMed]
45. Wang, C.-S.; Wang, S.-T.; Chang, T.-T.; Yao, W.-J.; Chou, P. Smoking and alanine aminotransferase levels in hepatitis C virus infection: Implications for prevention of hepatitis C virus progression. *Arch. Intern. Med.* **2002**, *162*, 811–815. [CrossRef] [PubMed]

Journal of
Clinical Medicine

MDPI

Article

Reporting of Magnetic Resonance Enterography in Inflammatory Bowel Disease: Results of an Italian Survey

Cristiana Bonifacio [1,†], Arianna Dal Buono [2,*,†], Riccardo Levi [1,3], Roberto Gabbiadini [2], Christian Reca [1,2], Cristina Bezzio [2,3], Marco Francone [1,3], Alessandro Armuzzi [2,3] and Luca Balzarini [1]

1 Department of Radiology, Humanitas Research Hospital—IRCCS, Via Manzoni 56, Rozzano, 20089 Milan, Italy; cristiana.bonifacio@humanitas.it (C.B.); riccardo.levi@humanitas.it (R.L.); christian.reca@humanitas.it (C.R.); marco.francone@hunimed.eu (M.F.); luca.balzarini@humanitas.it (L.B.)
2 IBD Center, Humanitas Research Hospital—IRCCS, Via Manzoni 56, Rozzano, 20089 Milan, Italy; roberto.gabbiadini@humanitas.it (R.G.); cristina.bezzio@hunimed.eu (C.B.); alessandro.armuzzi@hunimed.eu (A.A.)
3 Department of Biomedical Sciences, Humanitas University, Pieve Emanuele, 20072 Milan, Italy
* Correspondence: arianna.dalbuono@humanitas.it
† These authors contributed equally to this work.

Abstract: Background/Objectives: Inflammatory bowel diseases (IBDs) are chronic disorders that require close monitoring with imaging techniques such as magnetic resonance enterography (MRE). Standardization of radiological reports is crucial for the optimal management of IBD. We surveyed Italian radiologists regarding their experiences with MRE examinations and reporting for IBD. **Methods:** All members of the Italian Society of Medical and Interventional Radiology (SIRM) were invited to complete an anonymous questionnaire in April 2023. Comparison tests between variables were assessed using the χ^2 test or Fisher exact test according to the least frequency group. Significance level was set for p-value < 0.05. **Results:** A total of 253 radiologists responded to the survey. Around 70% of the respondents declared personal clinical experience with IBD. Great agreement with the items included and described for both disease activity (i.e., intestinal wall thickness, presence of mucosal ulcers, presence of edema, mucous enhancement) and complications was reported. One-third of the respondents regularly used a structured MRE report. Centers with a high number of IBD patients per year (>1000) mostly used 3 T scanners or both 1.5 T and 3 T scanners ($p < 0.001$). The incorporation of scores of disease activity was associated with university and high-volume hospitals ($p < 0.001$). **Conclusions:** This survey highlighted the current routine practice and experience of MRE reports of IBD patients among Italian radiologists. We found deficiencies in the use of radiological scores in MRE reports and attendance at IBD multidisciplinary meetings.

Keywords: reporting; cross-sectional imaging; magnetic enterography; inflammatory bowel disease; survey

1. Introduction

Inflammatory bowel diseases (IBDs) are chronic, disabling, and incurable conditions of the gastrointestinal tract that exhibit a relapsing–remitting behavior [1]. The burden of IBDs is rising globally, and the prevalence in Europe and the United States is estimated at 1 in every 200–300 people [2].

Close monitoring and adequate assessment of response to therapy through objective measures are currently the backbone of managing IBDs [3,4]. Cross-sectional imaging methods, including intestinal ultrasound (IUS), magnetic resonance enterography (MRE), and computed tomography (CT), have been demonstrated as being highly accurate for the diagnosis and assessment of disease activity and severity, and for detecting complications in IBDs [5,6]. The pooled sensitivity and specificity of cross-sectional imaging are estimated to be >85% and >95%, respectively, with few differences among the techniques regarding disease extension, location, severity, and complications [7].

Several studies have demonstrated that the achievement of transmural healing, alongside with mucosal healing, is a complementary predictor of better long-term clinical outcomes in CD (i.e., lower risk of hospitalization, surgery, and/or corticosteroid use) [8–10]. Indeed, transmural healing, evaluated through MRI and defined as a bowel thickness <3 mm, without an increased T2 mural intensity or increased contrast enhancement on T1 sequences, was associated with reduced hospitalization rates, surgery, and treatment escalation over 5 years of follow-up in CD patients [8].

At present, the regular assessment of radiological response is recommended after therapy starts, with modification and/or escalation in IBD patients, especially in CD [4].

Recently, both gastroenterological and radiological societies have published guidelines that establish technical standards for cross-sectional imaging in IBD, define parameters, and indicate how to report the results [11–13]. Standardization of radiological reports is crucial for the optimal management of IBD in order to reliably guide therapeutic decision making. At present, there are no national guidelines regarding radiological monitoring in patients with IBD and the behavior of Italian Centers towards MRE in IBD patients is unknown. The aim of this study was to investigate technical and reporting standards in the use of MRE among Italian radiologists involved in the management of IBD patients. We evaluated radiologists' experiences with MRE examinations for IBD and with the reporting of MRE results by surveying members of the Italian Society of Medical and Interventional Radiology (SIRM).

2. Materials and Methods

To explore the application of MRE in the assessment of IBD patients by Italian radiologists, we developed an anonymous survey that was endorsed by SIRM. The questionnaire was developed using a dedicated software platform (Google forms, Google, Mountain View, CA, USA) and was anonymous.

2.1. Participants

In April 2023, a sample of SIRM members received an email invitation to complete the survey (n = 934). The survey remained available for 14 consecutive days, and participants could access it only once. A reminder was sent 4 days before the survey's closure. All completed questionnaires were included in the analysis.

2.2. Procedures

To estimate the time needed to complete the survey (approximately 6–8 min), we asked 10 colleagues to time themselves on a test run before opening the survey to SIRM members.

The survey comprised 21 multiple choice questions, of which 14 permitted only one answer and 7 permitted more than one. The questionnaire was administered in Italian, while an English translation is provided in Table 1.

Table 1. Questions and items included in the administered questionnaire.

Q1	Where do you work?	A.	Northern Italy
		B.	Center Italy
		C.	Southern Italy and islands
Q2	How old are you?	A.	<35 years
		B.	35–50 years
		C.	>50 years

Table 1. *Cont.*

Q3	What is your qualification?	A. Hospital doctor B. Resident C. Independent practitioner
Q4	In what type of facility do you work?	A. Public Hospital B. University Hospital C. Private Hospital/Clinic D. Non Hospital structure
Q5	How many patients with IBD are treated at your Center annually?	A. <100 B. 100–500 C. 500–1000 D. >1000
Q6	How many MRE are performed at your Center weekly (only for patients with IBD)?	A. ≤1 B. 2–3 C. 4–5 D. >5
Q7	Which magnetic field is used in your Center for enteric MRI?	A. 1.5 Tesla B. 3 Tesla C. 1.5 and 3 Tesla
Q8	Do you have experience in IBD?	A. Yes B. No
Q9	If yes, how many years have you been involved in IBD?	A. <5 years B. 5–10 years C. >10 years
Q10	Do you usually use a structured report for MRE of patients with IBD?	A. Yes B. Upon request C. Only for clinical trials D. No
Q11	Among general findings, what is included in your Center's reports for MRE of patients with IBD (multiple answers possible)?	A. Clinical indications B. Technical details C. Oral contrast volume D. IBD clinical characteristics E. None of the above
Q12	In the assessment of disease activity, which of the following parameters are included in your Center in the reports of MRE of patients with IBD (multiple answers possible)?	A. Presence of stenosis, fistulas or abscesses B. Mucosal enhancement C. Intestinal wall thickness D. Presence of edema E. Presence of mucosal ulcers
Q13	In the assessment of disease activity, what other findings are included in your Center in the reports of MRE of patients with IBD (multiple answers possible)?	A. Extra-intestinal characteristics (e.g., reactive lymphadenopathy, perivisceritis) B. Longitudinal extension of inflamed intestinal tract C. DWI characteristics D. Hyperenhancement E. Signs of sacroiliitis F. None of the above

Table 1. *Cont.*

Q14	Do you usually quantify numerically the wall thickness (in mm)?	A. Yes B. Upon request C. No
Q15	In the evaluation of stenosis, which of the following findings are included in your Center in the reports of MRE of patients with IBD (multiple answers possible)?	A. Location of stenosis B. Lengths of stenosis C. Presence of pre-stenotic dilation D. Number of intestinal stenoses E. Degree (diameter) of pre-stenotic dilation F. None of the above
Q16	In the evaluation of stenosis, which of the following findings are included in the reports of MRE of patients with IBD at your Center (multiple answers possible)?	A. Presence of adjacent fistulas/abscesses to the stenosis B. Presence of signs of active inflammation within the stenosis C. Relation to surgical anastomosis (if present) D. None of the above
Q17	In the evaluation of abscesses, which of the following findings are included in the reports of MRE of patients with IBD at your Center (multiple answers possible)?	A. Localization B. Dimensions (in mm or cm) C. Possible relations with fistula/s D. Possible relations with surgical anastomoses (if present) E. Morphology F. None of the above
Q18	Do you use scores in the assessment of IBD at your Center?	A. Yes, at least one B. Only upon gastroenterologist's request C. No
Q19	If yes, which scores are usually included (multiple possible)?	A. MaRIA score B. MaRIA simplified score C. MEGS score
Q20	How confident do you feel with MaRIA or MaRIAs?	A. Very confident B. Rather confident C. Non confident
Q21	Do you participate as a radiologist in multidisciplinary IBD meetings?	A. Always B. Only for complex cases and if invited by colleagues C. I'm interested, but I'm not involved D. I'm not interested E. Multidisciplinary IBD meetings is not present in my center

IBD: inflammatory bowel diseases; MRE: magnetic enterography; MaRIA: Magnetic Resonance Index of Activity; MEGS: magnetic resonance global score.

Overall, 10 questions inquired about the respondents' demographics (age, professional qualifications, experience in MRE for IBD) and work setting, whereas 11 questions focused on the use of MRE for IBD (i.e., machines and protocols) and the reporting of these results (i.e., items assessed and described in the radiological report for disease activity, severity, and complications) (Table 1).

Statistical analyses were performed on survey answers as categorical data. Data were described as absolute count and relative percentages. Comparison tests between variables were assessed using the χ^2 test or Fisher exact test according to the least frequency group. A significance level was set for p-value < 0.05.

3. Results

3.1. General Questions, Experience in IBD, Characteristics of the Centers

A total of 253 radiologists responded to the survey (response rate 21.7% of the invited), and 45.3% of respondents had an age between 35 and 50 years (n = 115). The study group comprised 191 radiologists (75.5%) and 62 radiology residents (24.5%). Just under half of respondents (n = 119; 47.1%) worked in a public hospital, while 92 (36.3%) worked at a university hospital and 42 (16.6%) worked at a private hospital or clinic. The respondents worked across Italy, and 188 (74.3%) claimed to have experience with IBD. Table 2 elucidates the main characteristics of the study population.

Table 2. Characteristics of the radiologists who responded to the questionnaire and of their work settings.

Characteristics		n = 253 n (%)
Age class		
	<35 years	79 (31.1)
	35–50 years	115 (45.3)
	>50 years	59 (23.6)
Professional qualification		
	Radiologist	191 (75.5)
	Hospital doctor	166 (86.9)
	Independent practitioner	25 (13.1)
	Radiology resident	62 (24.5)
Site of employment		
	Public hospital	119 (47.1)
	University hospital	92 (36.3)
	Private hospital or clinic	34 (13.4)
	Non-hospital structure	8 (3.2)
Geographic area of work		
	Northern Italy	113 (44.9)
	Central Italy	66 (26.0)
	Southern Italy or islands	74 (31.1)
Experience with IBD		
	Yes	188 (74.3)
	No	65 (25.7)
Duration of IBD experience, years		
	<5	68 (36.2)
	5–10	59 (31.4)
	>10	61 (32.4)
Hospital case load of patients with IBD, number per year		
	<100	97 (38.3)
	100–500	80 (31.6)
	500–1000	47 (18.6)
	>1000	29 (11.5)
Hospital case load of MRE examinations for IBD, number per week		
	≤1	74 (29.2)
	2–3	95 (37.6)
	4–5	35 (13.8)
	>5	49 (19.4)
Participation in multidisciplinary IBD meetings		
	Yes, always	25 (9.9)
	Mainly for complex cases and when invited by colleagues	29 (11.5)
	I'm interested, but I'm not involved	43 (17.0)
	I'm not interested in participating, although there is a multidisciplinary IBD meeting in my center	24 (9.5)
	No, because multidisciplinary IBD meetings are not held in my center	132 (52.1)

Table 2. *Cont.*

Characteristics	n = 253 n (%)
MRI scanner's magnetic field	
1.5 Tesla	189 (74.7)
3 Tesla	26 (10.3)
1.5 and 3 Tesla	38 (15.0)

MRI: magnetic resonance imaging; IBD: inflammatory bowel disease.

In terms of the participants' place of work, 97 respondents (38.3%) worked in a setting with an IBD case load below 100 patients/year, and 80 respondents (31.6%) reported a case load between 100 and 500 patients/year, whereas 76 respondents (30.1%) reported a case load above 500 patients/year. Regarding the clinical management and discussion of imaging findings, 121 respondents (47.8%) indicated having a multidisciplinary IBD meeting in their hospital, with a higher presence in university hospitals compared with public hospitals: 76.1% and 30.0%, respectively ($p < 0.001$).

MRE examinations were mostly performed on 1.5 T MRI scanners (n = 189, 74.7%), while small numbers of respondents indicated that they used both 1.5 and 3 T scanners (38/253, 15.0%) or only 3 T scanners (26/253, 10.3%). The use of 1.5 T and 3 T scanners was found to be different among Centers with a higher percentage of 1.5 T in public (87.5%) and non-hospital Centers (87.5%) ($p < 0.001$), whereas 3 T scanners were mostly used in private hospitals (23.5%) and university hospitals (12.0%) ($p < 0.001$). Notably, Centers with high numbers of patients with IBD per year (>1000) were mostly associated with 3 T scanners (17.2%) or both 1.5 T and 3 T scanners (48.3%) ($p < 0.001$).

Figure 1 summarizes the answers to questions regarding the assessment of disease activity and complications.

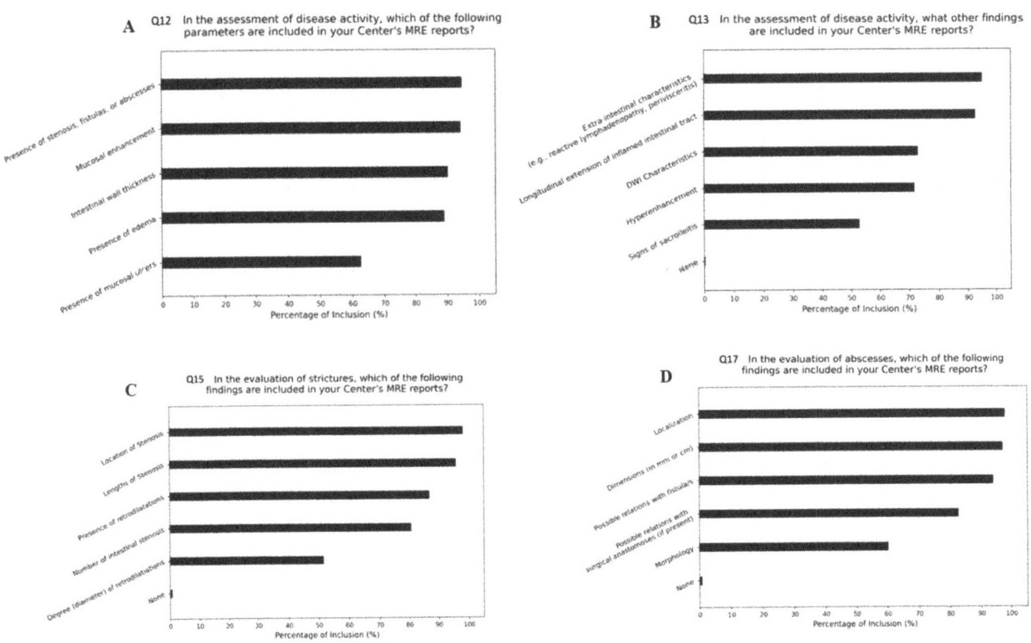

Figure 1. Details of answers to questions regarding assessment of disease activity and complications.

In Figure 1, the main items investigated through the questions are about disease activity and complications. In Q12 (panel A), the general features of transmural activity were asked to the participants (i.e., intestinal wall thickness, mucosal enhancement, mucosal ulcers and/or complications); Q13 (panel B) addressed adjunctive radiological features of active disease (i.e., extra-intestinal characteristics, concomitant sacro-ileitis); and Q15 and Q17 (panels C and D, respectively) specifically addressed items included for describing strictures and abscess/es.

3.2. Reporting Details

The second part of the questionnaire focused on MRE examinations and reports. When asked if the results of MRE examinations for patients with IBD were reported on a structured radiological report, only 77 respondents answered yes (30.4%). No significant association was found between the use of structured forms and the geographical area of Italy ($p = 0.553$), type of hospital ($p = 0.606$), or professional qualification ($p = 0.442$). Even fewer respondents indicated that they routinely include IBD clinical scores in the reports ($n = 26$, 10.3%) or include a score only when requested by a gastroenterologist ($n = 39$, 15.4%). The use of IBD activity scores was highest among respondents based in Northern Italy (76.9% vs. 23.1% for Central Italy, Southern Italy and islands, $p = 0.004$). It was also higher for radiology residents working at university hospitals (57.7% vs. 42.3% for radiologists, $p = 0.005$).

Concerning the evaluation of IBD activity (Figure 1A), half of respondents ($n = 138$, 54.5%) reported including all the following items: intestinal wall thickness, presence of mucosal ulcers, presence of edema, mucous enhancement. Moreover, almost all respondents include the presence of fistulas or abscesses ($n = 240$, 94.9%). Approximately one-third of the respondents ($n = 77$, 30.4%) include further descriptive items in the MRE report (Figure 1B), such as extra-intestinal features (i.e., reactive lymphadenopathy, periviscerititis), hyperenhancement, DWI features, the longitudinal extent of the inflamed intestinal tract and signs of sacro-ileitis.

In the evaluation of IBD-related stenosis (Figure 1C), more than 86.5% ($n = 219$) of the respondents include a numerical evaluation of wall thickness (in mm). More than one-third of the respondents ($n = 109$, 43.1%) consider it valuable to include the following items in the radiology report: the number of intestinal strictures, the location of the stricture(s), the length of the stricture(s), the presence and the degree (diameter) of pre-stenotic dilation. Moreover, 179 (70.7%) of the respondents found it relevant to report the following findings related to stenosis in the MRE report: the relationship to surgical anastomoses (if present), the presence of signs of active inflammation within the stricture, and the presence of fistulas/abscesses adjacent to the stricture.

Concerning the evaluation of abscesses (Figure 1D), 56.1% ($n = 142$) included all the following findings: location, dimensions (in mm or cm), morphology, and any relationship with fistula(s) and with surgical anastomoses (if any). The most frequently included feature in the report was the location of the abscess ($n = 249$, 98.4%).

3.3. Structured Report, Scores of Disease Activity, and Multidisciplinary Meetings

Overall, a structured MRE report was found to be used by a small percentage of respondents ($n = 83$, 32.8%). In more detail, 58 respondents (22.9% of the overall study population, 68.8% of users) said they use it on a daily basis, whereas the remaining 25 respondents use it only for clinical trials or upon gastroenterological request. Among the respondents, no differences were found in the use of a structured report in relation to geographical location ($p = 0.553$) (Figure 2), working qualification ($p = 0.442$), or type of Center ($p = 0.606$).

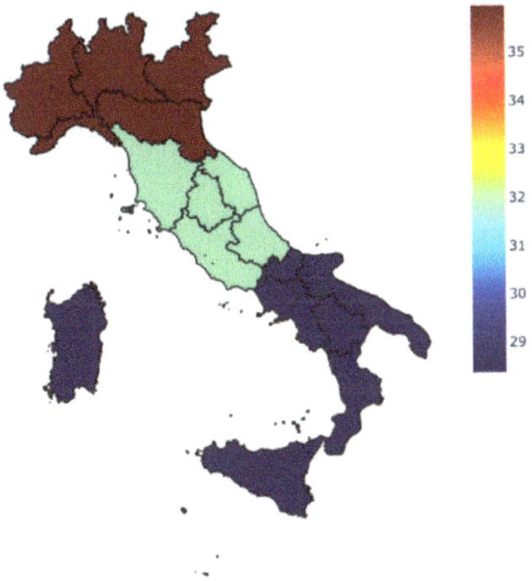

Figure 2. Percentage of usage of structured report for patients with IBD among geographical areas.

Regarding the adoption of scores in the MRE report, those sampled routinely include IBD clinical scores in reports ($n = 26$, 10.3%) in their daily practice: the use of IBD activity score/s in MRE reports is mainly adopted in the north of Italy (17.5%, $p = 0.004$), by radiology residents (25.4%, $p < 0.001$), and in university hospital (38.4%, $p < 0.001$) (Table 3).

Table 3. Statistical results for structured MRE report and disease activity scores.

	Adoption of Structured MRE Report	Adoption of Disease Activity Scores
Geographical Location	$\chi^2 = 1.20$, p-value = 0.55 [1]	$\chi^2 = 15.28$, p-value = 0.004 [1]
Responder's Age	$\chi^2 = 3.17$, p-value = 0.21 [1]	$\chi^2 = 15.70$, p-value = 0.003 [1]
Type of Hospital	p-value = 0.606 [2]	p-value = 0.005 [2]
Working Occupation	p-value = 0.442 [2]	p-value = 0.004 [2]

[1] Chi-squared test; [2] Fisher exact test.

The most adopted score is the simplified MaRIA score ($n = 12/65$, 46.2%), followed by the MaRIA score ($n = 18/65$, 27.7%) and MEGS ($n = 1/65$, 4%) (Table 3).

High confidence in MaRIA/sMaRIA score use was reported by only 8 respondents (30.7% of users, 3.1% of all respondents), and moderate confidence was reported by 53 respondents (81.5% of users, 20.9% of all respondents) (Table 3).

Multidisciplinary IBD meetings are accessible for 121 respondents (47.6%) (Table 2). Among those, 25 radiologists reported always participating (20.7%), 29 participate only for complex cases (24.0%), 43 are interested but not invited (35.5%), and 24 are not interested in participating (19.8%) (Table 2). Italian Centers in central regions (18,2%, $p = 0.014$), respondents between ages 35 and 50 years (13.0%, $p < 0.001$), and those working in university hospitals (18.5%, $p < 0.001$) were associated with higher participation in multidisciplinary IBD meetings.

4. Discussion

The increased availability and the accuracy of cross-sectional imaging in detecting complications, monitoring therapeutic response, and predicting long-term clinical outcomes place the radiologist at center stage in the management of IBD [14].

Our survey sought to highlight the current routine practice and experience with MRE reports for patients with IBD among Italian radiologists, highlighting high and low points. To the best of our knowledge, this is the first survey addressed to all members of a national Italian radiological society on this topic. This survey was mostly completed by radiologists with a declared personal expertise in IBD (>70% of the participants), thus representing a close picture of the daily clinical practice in this field.

An important result of the survey is the great agreement with the items included and described for both disease activity and complications (around 55% and 86–94% of agreement, respectively). This result lays the foundations for homogeneous and optimal MRE reporting among Italian radiologist with experience in IBD and can improve communication between different specialties. On the other hand, only 22.9% of the respondents use a structured reports in their daily practice, and most of them scarcely adopt radiological scores, with very low rates of confidence only concerning the MaRIA/sMaRIA scores. This is a relevant drawback, since it has been demonstrated that the MaRIA score is highly effective in detecting mucosal healing in CD [15,16], supporting its use as a therapeutic endpoint and maybe reducing the number of colonoscopies requested for monitoring patients. Calculating the MaRIA score can be time-consuming; however, the simplified MaRIA, which requires less time (sMaRIA: median 4.50 min vs. MaRIA: median 12.35 min), was thereafter developed to overcome this possible limitation [17,18] and can assess CD activity with a high correlation with the simple endoscopic score for CD (SES-CD) and excellent inter-rater reliability between expert and resident radiologists [6,19]. Accordingly, our survey showed that the most used score is the sMaRIA, and the adoption of scores was found to be most frequent among radiology residents (40.7%, $p = 0.005$), in university hospitals (38.0%, $p = 0.004$), and in hospitals with more than 1000 patients with IBD per year (55.2%, $p < 0.001$).

Another main issue of our study regards the involvement of radiologists in multidisciplinary IBD meetings, which appears to be higher in university hospitals compared with public hospitals (76.1% and 30.0%, respectively ($p < 0.001$)). This topic should be stressed and implemented in clinical practice as it seems that, similarly to oncology, multidisciplinary meetings can ameliorate the clinical management of IBD and represent a standard quality of care as expressed by the European Crohn's and Colitis Organisation and European Society of Radiology [20–22].

Consistently with previous data [23], MRE is performed with both 1.5 T and 3 T scanners, with a wider accessibility with 1.5 T. Few data are available on the performance differences between the two scanners in IBD, showing a slight superiority of 3 T as concerns the detection of mucosal ulcers [24]. In addition, 3 T displayed a shorter scan time. Therefore, if at one's disposal, 3 T is preferred in patients with ileo-colonic CD [24]. However, larger studies are warranted to better assess this issue.

Our study has some limitations. First, despite the declared experience with IBD of the participants, few highly specialized/third-level Centers were included (approximately 30% of high-volume IBD Centers [>500 patients treated yearly]). The members of the SIRM currently number approximately 12,000, and the participants in this survey are evidently radiologists with a specific interest in the field of IBD, with a possible associated selection bias. Secondly, few questions addressed technical aspects regarding MRE protocol. Finally, this survey did not separate pediatric from adult physicians, with possible mixed results.

Overall, this study helps to determine and understand the differences that exist in IBD diagnostic strategies between Italian Centers and radiologists, emphasizing common and widespread conduct, as well as areas for possible growth and improvement.

5. Conclusions

Our study helps provide an understanding of the current reporting standards among Italian radiologists specifically regarding MRE in patients with IBD. These data might improve radiology practices with respect to the incorporation of relevant items and descriptions to drive medical decisions more accurately, finally improving the outcomes of patients with IBD. According to our results, investing resources in dedicated educational and training programs in this field appears to be of evident importance. These findings can be used for better standardization of the reporting in MRE, specifically regarding the use of a structured report and the incorporation of MRE scores of disease activity, thus improving the quality of patients' care.

Author Contributions: Conceptualization, C.B. (Cristiana Bonifacio), A.D.B., R.G. and R.L.; methodology, R.L.; software, formal analysis, R.L.; data curation, A.D.B. and R.L.; writing—original draft preparation, C.B. (Cristina Bezzio), A.D.B., C.R. and R.L.; writing—review and editing, R.G., M.F., A.A. and L.B. All authors have read and agreed to the published version of the manuscript.

Funding: This work was partially supported by "Ricerca Corrente" funding from Italian Ministry of Health to IRCCS Humanitas Research Hospital.

Institutional Review Board Statement: Not applicable.

Informed Consent Statement: Not applicable.

Data Availability Statement: The datasets generated or analyzed during the study are available from the corresponding author on reasonable request.

Acknowledgments: The authors thank all participants to this survey. We acknowledge the Society of Medical and Interventional Radiology (SIRM) for their support in promoting the survey.

Conflicts of Interest: A. Armuzzi has received consulting fees from AbbVie, Allergan, Amgen, Arena, Biogen, Boehringer Ingelheim, Bristol-Myers Squibb, Celgene, Celltrion, Eli-Lilly, Ferring, Galapagos, Gilead, Janssen, MSD, Mylan, Pfizer, Protagonist Therapeutics, Roche, Samsung Bioepis, Sandoz, and Takeda; speaker's fees from AbbVie, Amgen, Arena, Biogen, Bristol-Myers Squibb, Eli-Lilly, Ferring, Galapagos, Gilead, Janssen, MSD, Novartis, Pfizer, Roche, Samsung Bioepis, Sandoz, Takeda, and Tigenix; and research support from Biogen, MSD, Takeda, and Pfizer. C Bezzio received lecture fees and served as a consultant for Takeda, MSD, Ferring, Abbvie, Galapagos, and Janssen. R. Gabbiadini has received speaker's fees from Pfizer and MSD. A. Dal Buono has received speaker's fees from AbbVie and Galapagos. C Bonifacio has served speaker's fees for Takeda and Janssen. M Francone has received speaker's fees from Bracco Suisse and Bayer Pharma. R Levi has received speaker's fees from Esaote. L Balzarini. C Reca declares no conflicts of interest.

References

1. Roda, G.; Chien Ng, S.; Kotze, P.G.; Argollo, M.; Panaccione, R.; Spinelli, A.; Kaser, A.; Peyrin-Biroulet, L.; Danese, S. Crohn's Disease. *Nat. Rev. Dis. Primers* **2020**, *6*, 22. [CrossRef] [PubMed]
2. Alatab, S.; Sepanlou, S.G.; Ikuta, K.; Vahedi, H.; Bisignano, C.; Safiri, S.; Sadeghi, A.; Nixon, M.R.; Abdoli, A.; Abolhassani, H.; et al. The Global, Regional, and National Burden of Inflammatory Bowel Disease in 195 Countries and Territories, 1990–2017: A Systematic Analysis for the Global Burden of Disease Study 2017. *Lancet Gastroenterol. Hepatol.* **2020**, *5*, 17–30. [CrossRef] [PubMed]
3. Torres, J.; Bonovas, S.; Doherty, G.; Kucharzik, T.; Gisbert, J.P.; Raine, T.; Adamina, M.; Armuzzi, A.; Bachmann, O.; Bager, P.; et al. ECCO Guidelines on Therapeutics in Crohn's Disease: Medical Treatment. *J. Crohn's Colitis* **2020**, *14*, 4–22. [CrossRef] [PubMed]
4. Turner, D.; Ricciuto, A.; Lewis, A.; D'Amico, F.; Dhaliwal, J.; Griffiths, A.M.; Bettenworth, D.; Sandborn, W.J.; Sands, B.E.; Reinisch, W.; et al. STRIDE-II: An Update on the Selecting Therapeutic Targets in Inflammatory Bowel Disease (STRIDE) Initiative of the International Organization for the Study of IBD (IOIBD): Determining Therapeutic Goals for Treat-to-Target Strategies in IBD. *Gastroenterology* **2021**, *160*, 1570–1583. [CrossRef] [PubMed]
5. Bettenworth, D.; Bokemeyer, A.; Baker, M.; Mao, R.; Parker, C.E.; Nguyen, T.; Ma, C.; Panés, J.; Rimola, J.; Fletcher, J.G.; et al. Assessment of Crohn's Disease-Associated Small Bowel Strictures and Fibrosis on Cross-Sectional Imaging: A Systematic Review. *Gut* **2019**, *68*, 1115–1126. [CrossRef] [PubMed]
6. Rimola, J.; Torres, J.; Kumar, S.; Taylor, S.A.; Kucharzik, T. Recent Advances in Clinical Practice: Advances in Cross-Sectional Imaging in Inflammatory Bowel Disease. *Gut* **2022**, *71*, 2587–2597. [CrossRef]
7. Panés, J.; Bouzas, R.; Chaparro, M.; García-Sánchez, V.; Gisbert, J.P.; Martínez De Guereñu, B.; Mendoza, J.L.; Paredes, J.M.; Quiroga, S.; Ripollés, T.; et al. Systematic Review: The Use of Ultrasonography, Computed Tomography and Magnetic Resonance Imaging for the Diagnosis, Assessment of Activity and Abdominal Complications of Crohn's Disease. *Aliment. Pharmacol. Ther.* **2011**, *34*, 125–145. [CrossRef]
8. Fernandes, S.R.; Serrazina, J.; Botto, I.A.; Leal, T.; Guimarães, A.; Garcia, J.L.; Rosa, I.; Prata, R.; Carvalho, D.; Neves, J.; et al. Transmural Remission Improves Clinical Outcomes up to 5 Years in Crohn's Disease. *United Eur. Gastroenterol. J.* **2023**, *11*, 51–59. [CrossRef]
9. Deepak, P.; Fletcher, J.G.; Fidler, J.L.; Barlow, J.M.; Sheedy, S.P.; Kolbe, A.B.; Harmsen, W.S.; Loftus, E.V.; Hansel, S.L.; Becker, B.D.; et al. Radiological Response Is Associated With Better Long-Term Outcomes and Is a Potential Treatment Target in Patients With Small Bowel Crohn's Disease. *Am. J. Gastroenterol.* **2016**, *111*, 997–1006. [CrossRef]

10. Castiglione, F.; Imperatore, N.; Testa, A.; De Palma, G.D.; Nardone, O.M.; Pellegrini, L.; Caporaso, N.; Rispo, A. One-Year Clinical Outcomes with Biologics in Crohn's Disease: Transmural Healing Compared with Mucosal or No Healing. *Aliment. Pharmacol. Ther.* **2019**, *49*, 1026–1039. [CrossRef]
11. Bruining, D.H.; Zimmermann, E.M.; Loftus, E.V.; Sandborn, W.J.; Sauer, C.G.; Strong, S.A.; Fletcher, J.G. Consensus Recommendations for Evaluation, Interpretation, and Utilization of Computed Tomography and Magnetic Resonance Enterography in Patients With Small Bowel Crohn's Disease. *Radiology* **2018**, *286*, 776–799. [CrossRef]
12. Maaser, C.; Sturm, A.; Vavricka, S.R.; Kucharzik, T.; Fiorino, G.; Annese, V.; Calabrese, E.; Baumgart, D.C.; Bettenworth, D.; Borralho Nunes, P.; et al. ECCO-ESGAR Guideline for Diagnostic Assessment in IBD Part 1: Initial Diagnosis, Monitoring of Known IBD, Detection of Complications. *J. Crohns Colitis* **2019**, *13*, 144–164. [CrossRef]
13. Sturm, A.; Maaser, C.; Calabrese, E.; Annese, V.; Fiorino, G.; Kucharzik, T.; Vavricka, S.R.; Verstockt, B.; Van Rheenen, P.; Tolan, D.; et al. ECCO-ESGAR Guideline for Diagnostic Assessment in IBD Part 2: IBD Scores and General Principles and Technical Aspects. *J. Crohns Colitis* **2019**, *13*, 273–284E. [CrossRef]
14. Deepak, P.; Axelrad, J.E.; Ananthakrishnan, A.N. The Role of the Radiologist in Determining Disease Severity in Inflammatory Bowel Diseases. *Gastrointest. Endosc. Clin. N. Am.* **2019**, *29*, 447–470. [CrossRef]
15. Buisson, A.; Pereira, B.; Goutte, M.; Reymond, M.; Allimant, C.; Obritin-Guilhen, H.; Bommelaer, G.; Hordonneau, C. Magnetic resonance index of activity (MaRIA) and Clermont score are highly and equally effective MRI indices in detecting mucosal healing in Crohn's disease. *Dig. Liver Dis.* **2017**, *49*, 1211–1217. [CrossRef]
16. Ordás, I.; Rimola, J.; Rodríguez, S.; Paredes, J.M.; Martínez-Pérez, M.J.; Blanc, E.; Arévalo, J.A.; Aduna, M.; Andreu, M.; Radosevic, A.; et al. Accuracy of Magnetic Resonance Enterography in Assessing Response to Therapy and Mucosal Healing in Patients with Crohn's Disease. *Gastroenterology* **2014**, *146*, 374–382.e1. [CrossRef]
17. Park, S.H.; Park, S.H. Simplified Magnetic Resonance Index of Activity for Crohn's Disease—Let's Try to Kick It Up a Notch. *Gastroenterology* **2020**, *158*, 281–282.e1. [CrossRef]
18. Williet, N.; Jardin, S.; Roblin, X. The Simplified Magnetic Resonance Index of Activity (MARIA) for Crohn's Disease Is Strongly Correlated with the MARIA and Clermont Score: An External Validation. *Gastroenterology* **2020**, *158*, 282–283. [CrossRef]
19. Roseira, J.; Ventosa, A.R.; de Sousa, H.T.; Brito, J. The New Simplified MARIA Score Applies beyond Clinical Trials: A Suitable Clinical Practice Tool for Crohn's Disease That Parallels a Simple Endoscopic Index and Fecal Calprotectin. *United Eur. Gastroenterol. J.* **2020**, *8*, 1208–1216. [CrossRef]
20. Ferman, M.; Lim, A.H.; Hossain, M.; Siow, G.W.; Andrews, J.M. Multidisciplinary Team Meetings Appear to Be Effective in Inflammatory Bowel Disease Management: An Audit of Process and Outcomes. *Intern. Med. J.* **2018**, *48*, 1102–1108. [CrossRef]
21. Fiorino, G.; Lytras, T.; Younge, L.; Fidalgo, C.; Coenen, S.; Chaparro, M.; Allocca, M.; Arnott, I.; Bossuyt, P.; Burisch, J.; et al. Quality of Care Standards in Inflammatory Bowel Diseases: A European Crohn's and Colitis Organisation [ECCO] Position Paper. *J. Crohn's Colitis* **2020**, *14*, 1037–1048. [CrossRef] [PubMed]
22. "Role of Radiology in a Multidisciplinary Approach to Patient Care": Summary of the ESR International Forum 2022 | Enhanced Reader. Available online: https://insightsimaging.springeropen.com/articles/10.1186/s13244-023-01377-x (accessed on 12 December 2023).
23. Gandhi, N.S.; Dillman, J.R.; Grand, D.J.; Huang, C.; Fletcher, J.G.; Al-Hawary, M.M.; Anupindi, S.A.; Baker, M.E.; Bruining, D.H.; Chatterji, M.; et al. Computed tomography and magnetic resonance enterography protocols and techniques: Survey of the Society of Abdominal Radiology Crohn's Disease Disease-Focused Panel. *Abdom. Radiol.* **2020**, *45*, 1011–1017. [CrossRef] [PubMed]
24. Fiorino, G.; Bonifacio, C.; Padrenostro, M.; Mrakic Sposta, F.; Spinelli, A.; Malesci, A.; Balzarini, L.; Peyrin-Biroulet, L.; Danese, S. Comparison Between 1.5 and 3.0 Tesla Magnetic Resonance Enterography for the Assessment of Disease Activity and Complications in Ileo-Colonic Crohn's Disease. *Dig. Dis. Sci.* **2013**, *58*, 3246–3255. [CrossRef]

Journal of
Clinical Medicine

MDPI

Article

Clinical, Radiological, and Surgical Risk Factors for Endoscopic Anastomotic Recurrence Following Surgery in Crohn's Disease

Laura Maria Minordi [1], Franco Sacchetti [2,*], Domenico Balzano [2], Rossella Maresca [3], Francesca Bice D'Angelo [1], Luigi Larosa [1], Davide Carano [1], Lucrezia Laterza [3], Daniela Pugliese [3,4], Paola Caprino [2], Angelo Eugenio Potenza [2], Franco Scaldaferri [3,4], Luigi Sofo [2] and Evis Sala [1]

1 UOC di Radioterapia Oncologica ed Ematologia Dipartimento di Diagnostica per Immagini, Fondazione Policlinico Universitario "A. Gemelli" IRCCS, 00168 Rome, Italy; lauramaria.minordi@policlinicogemelli.it (L.M.M.); francescabice.dangelo01@icatt.it (F.B.D.); luigi.larosa@policlinicogemelli.it (L.L.); davide.carano@guest.policlinicogemelli.it (D.C.); evis.sala@policlinicogemelli.it (E.S.)
2 UOC di Chirurgia Addominale, Dipartimento di Scienze Mediche e Chirurgiche, Fondazione Policlinico Universitario "A. Gemelli" IRCCS, 00168 Rome, Italy; domenico.balzano01@icatt.it (D.B.); paola.caprino@policlinicogemelli.it (P.C.); angeloeugenio.potenza@policlinicogemelli.it (A.E.P.); luigi.sofo@policlinicogemelli.it (L.S.)
3 UOS Malattie Infiammatorie Croniche Intestinali, Centro Malattie Apparato Digerente (CeMAD), Dipartimento di Scienze Mediche e Chirurgiche, Fondazione Policlinico Universitario "A. Gemelli" IRCCS, 00168 Rome, Italy; rossella.maresca12@gmail.com (R.M.); lucrezia.laterza@policlinicogemelli.it (L.L.); daniela.pugliese@policlinicogemelli.it (D.P.); franco.scaldaferri@policlinicogemelli.it (F.S.)
4 Dipartimento di Medicina e Chirurgia Traslazionale, Università Cattolica del Sacro Cuore, 00168 Rome, Italy
* Correspondence: franco.sacchetti@policlinicogemelli.it

Abstract: Objective: This study investigated the radiological, clinical, and surgical factors linked to the risk of endoscopic recurrence following ileocolic resection for Crohn's disease. **Materials and Methods:** We conducted a retrospective analysis of data from all patients who underwent primary ileocecal resection for Crohn's disease in a single colorectal unit between 2004 and 2020. We analyzed the potential risk factors subdivided by the clinical, radiological, and surgical factors associated with morphological recurrence, as detected by endoscopy within 2 years after surgery. Cox regression was employed to ascertain the risk factors associated with such recurrence. **Results:** In total, 63 patients were included, and 24 (38%) had endoscopic recurrence. The age of the patient at the time of surgery was identified as a significant clinical factor associated with the risk of recurrence (HR: 1.04; p = 0.003), indicating that the probability of recurrence increases by 1% as the surgical age increases each year. The radiological factors associated with an increased risk of recurrence included localization in the distal ileum (HR: 3.526; p = 0.015), the number of pathological small-bowel segments affected by the disease (HR: 1.15; p = 0.004), and the total length of the pathological intestinal segment (HR: 1.002; p = 0.014). The presence of granulomas (HR: 6.003; p = 0.004) and the length of the resected bowel (HR: 1.01; p = 0.003) were surgical factors associated with a higher risk of recurrence. **Conclusions:** This study delineated several clinical, radiological, and surgical factors that serve as predictors for the endoscopic recurrence of Crohn's disease after surgery.

Keywords: Crohn's disease; postoperative recurrence; endoscopic recurrence; radiological recurrence

1. Introduction

Up to 80% of patients with Crohn's disease (CD) undergo surgery during their lifetime, despite improvements in medical therapy with the introduction of new drugs [1]. Moreover, there has been important progress in surgery, with a tendency to carry out more limited surgical demolitions and/or stricture-plastic [2].

The pre-surgical evaluation of patients with CD is complex and requires a multidisciplinary approach with gastroenterologists, surgeons, and radiologists. Moreover, once the surgery has been performed, the clinical course of the patient is variable, with frequent postoperative relapses or recurrence, which may require a new surgery [3]. According to ECCO 2016 [4], the term "relapse" refers to the appearance of symptoms in a patient in clinical remission, either spontaneously or after medical therapy, and this must be confirmed by laboratory tests, radiological tests, or endoscopy. The term "recurrence" must be used to indicate the appearance of lesions after surgical therapy, and it is divided into morphological and clinical recurrence. Clinical recurrence consists of the appearance of symptoms in a patient undergoing surgery with complete resection of macroscopic disease. Morphological recurrence consists of the appearance of new lesions after complete resection of macroscopic disease and usually affects the terminal ileum before the anastomosis. Morphological recurrence is identified via endoscopy, radiology, or a new surgery.

In the literature, there are some studies that have evaluated the predictive risk factors of recurrence on the basis of clinical and laboratory parameters [5], while the role of imaging has not been thoroughly investigated [6], or it has been evaluated only in clinical studies [7]. The identification of patients with a high risk of recurrence is important in order to plan the correct therapeutic strategy after surgery.

The aim of this study was to evaluate the radiological factors that can predict the onset of endoscopic recurrence after surgery in association with clinical and surgical factors. The secondary objective was the evaluation of the survival time to the onset of recurrence after surgery.

2. Materials and Methods

2.1. Study Population and Data Source

We performed a monocentric retrospective study of a cohort of patients with known Crohn's disease, which was submitted and approved by our Ethics Committee.

In the surgery department, electronic patient records were interrogated to identify patients who had undergone ileocolic resection for the first time between January 2014 and December 2020. Patients with a postoperative diagnosis of ulcerative colitis or unclassified inflammatory disease, previous surgical intestinal resection, postoperative diagnosis of tuberculosis, and histological evidence of invasive malignancy were excluded from this study. Patients of <18 years were also excluded. The diagnosis of Crohn's disease was confirmed upon review of the medical records based on standard clinical, radiological, endoscopic, and histological reports.

For each patient, data were extracted from their medical records in the gastroenterology department to include demographic information, the Crohn's disease clinical setting, operative and histological data, and medication history, while radiological exams (CT enterography, abdomen CT, and MR enterography) were evaluated in the radiological department.

All patients had either an abdomen CT or MR enterography performed within 6 months before surgery and underwent endoscopy within 2 years after the surgery.

The CT and MR enterography were independently evaluated by 3 radiologists with at least 10 years of abdominal radiology experience.

According to ECCO 2016 [4], we stated morphological recurrence in case of new CD lesions after complete resection of macroscopic disease, detected by endoscopy within 2 years.

In this study, the risk factors were divided into three groups: clinical, radiological, and surgical factors.

2.2. Clinical Evaluation

The clinical potential risk factors for the development of postoperative recurrence evaluated in this study were (1) age at the moment of diagnosis; (2) age at the moment of surgery; (3) gender; (4) the duration of the disease; (5) perianal disease; (6) a habit of smoking; (7) the presence and type of extra-intestinal manifestations; and (8) the type of medical therapy performed before surgical resection.

2.3. Technique and Radiological Evaluation

The radiological examinations performed on the patients within 6 months before surgery were evaluated. In the presence of multiple studies, the examination closest to the surgery was considered.

Both the CT and MR-E exams were performed according to standardized protocols used in our department [8,9].

In particular, the CT enterography (CT-E) exams were performed after injection of iodinated contrast medium and acquired 75 s after intravenous injection of 100–130 mL of iodinated contrast agent, administered in two consecutive boluses, the first bolus at a rate of 1.5 mL/sec (comprising 1/3 of the total amount of iodinated contrast agent given to the patient), and the second bolus at a rate of 3 mL/second (covering the remaining 2/3 of the total amount of iodinated contrast agent given to the patient).

The MR enterography (MR-E) exams were performed before and after intravenous administration of paramagnetic contrast medium using the following sequences: single-shot T2-weighted and balanced steady-state free precession (bSSFP), and T2-weighted fat-suppressed, multiphase 3D T1-weighted fat-suppressed post-contrast images. Diffusion-weighted imaging (with values of 0–800 s/mm^2) sequences were performed but not evaluated in this study. Enhanced sequences were performed in the arterial, venous, and tardive phases.

In both the CT-E and MR-E, all patients had drunk a polyethylene glycol solution (1.5–2 L) in the 30 min preceding the examination. An anticholinergic was always administered in the MR-E exams, while it was optional in the CT-E exams, so it was not infused in all patients.

Abdomen CT was performed before and after injection of iodinated contrast medium and acquired 75 s after intravenous injection of 100–130 mL of iodinated contrast agent.

The following data were reported in an Excel sheet (Table 1):

1. Type of radiological examination (CTE; MR-E, abdomen CT);
2. Site of pathology;
3. Number of small-bowel pathological loops;
4. Characteristics of small-bowel pathological loops;

Length of each small-bowel pathological loop.

The measurement of the extent was performed in both CT and MRI, using vessel analysis software. The CT or MR images were reconstructed with post-processing "multiplanar reformatting" (MPR), and a specific software (Vue PACS Carestream V12) was applied to create a virtual image that permitted us to have a tubular vision of the small-bowel loops (Figure 1) [10]. This applied to the sum of inflammation in the discontinuous loops. The length of each pathological loop and the sum of the lengths of the pathological segments were calculated in patients with more than one small-bowel pathological loop.

Based on the signs described above, at the end of the radiological evaluation, a radiological judgment was expressed on the type of disease: active inflammatory, fistulizing, or fibrostenotic. In particular, the fistulizing subtype was identified in the presence of fistulas, sinus tracts, or abscesses.

Table 1. Radiological findings evaluated in CT/MR-E.

Type of Radiological Examination	MR Enterography or Abdomen CT or CT Enterography
Site of pathological loops	Proximal jejunum, distal jejunum, proximal ileum, distal ileum, last ileal loop, appendix, ascending colon, transverse colon, descending colon, sigmoid colon, and rectum
Number of small-bowel pathological loops	Counting as pathological any segment with radiological signs of CD separated from another lesion by a normal intestinal loop

Table 1. *Cont.*

Type of Radiological Examination	MR Enterography or Abdomen CT or CT Enterography
Characteristics of small-bowel pathological loops	• Mural thickening: a wall thickness of more than 3 mm; • Mucosal ulcers: deep depressions in the mucosal surface; • Bowel wall enhancement: stratified in the active inflammatory subtype (intense enhancement of the mucosa and serosa and low signal intensity in the submucosa) or homogeneous in the fibrostenotic subtype; • Halo fatty sign: the presence of fatty signals in the submucosa; • Engorgement of the vasa recta: hyperemia of the near mesentery; • Stenosis: upstream dilatation with a loop caliber greater than 2 cm; • Fibrofatty proliferation: excess of mesenteric fat; • Sinus tracts: wall defects that extend outside the intestinal wall but have no connection to an epithelialized structure, such as adjacent organs or skin; • Fistulas: communication with a near structure, e.g., entero-enteric, entero-colic, entero-cutaneous, and entero-vesicular fistulas; • Abscesses: capsulated fluid collection near pathological loop, which could contain air; • Lymph node enlargement: a short diameter of greater than 1 cm; • Others: involvement of other structures, such as the colon, appendix, genital organs, etc.; • In patients studied by MRI: bowel wall edema (a hyperintense signal in the wall compared with the skeletal muscle in T2-weighted sequences) and diffusion restriction in DWI (diffusion weighted imaging) sequences.
Length of each small-bowel pathological loop	• In the presence of more than one pathological loop: the loop with greater extension; • In the presence of more than one loop affected by pathology: the sum of the extension of the intestinal loops in which these segments are evident.
Type of disease	• Active inflammatory; • Fistulizing; • Fibrostenotic.

2.4. Surgical and Postoperative Evaluation

In an Excel sheet, we reported the type of surgery (ileocecal resection, ileocolic resection, or small-bowel resection); traditional (LPT) or laparoscopic surgery; emergency or elective surgery; the length of the intestinal segment removed (cm); the presence of granulomas in the specimen; histological signs of Crohn's disease in the resection margins; the type of anastomosis (stapled anastomosis or hand-sewn anastomosis); and ileostomy/colostomy.

In an Excel sheet, we reported postoperative complications. The Clavien–Dindo system was used to evaluate the grade of postsurgical complications [11].

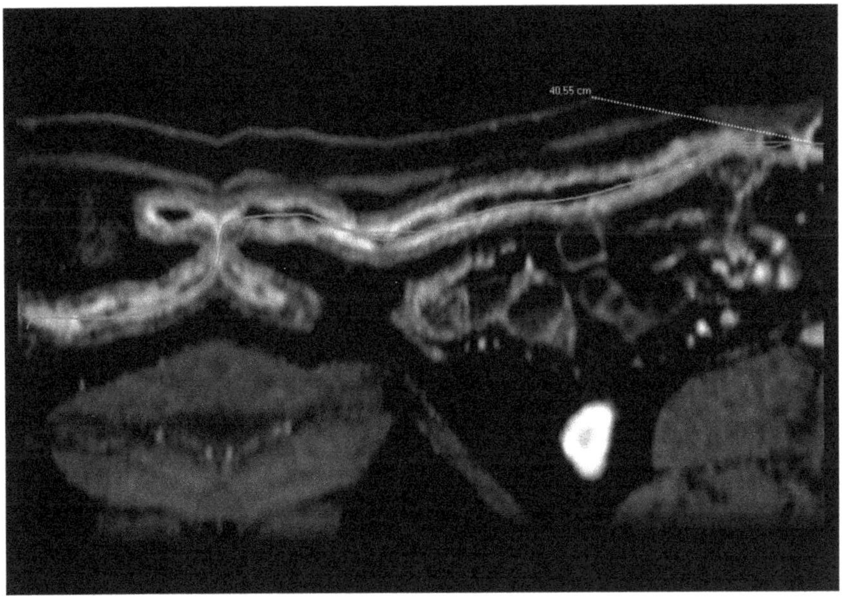

Figure 1. Post-processing reconstruction of the images enabled us to generate a linear view of the small bowel, allowing for the measurement of its length.

2.5. Statistical Analysis

The clinical and demographic characteristics of the enrolled sample are shown with the descriptive statistics. Particularly, the quantitative variables are represented as means ± standard deviation (SD) or medians (IQR), as appropriate, according to the results of the Shapiro–Wilk test.

The qualitative variables are described in terms of absolute and percentage frequencies. The chi-squared and/or Fisher's exact test were used to compare the categorical variables. Student's *t*-tests and the Mann–Whitney test were used to compare the quantitative unpaired data, as appropriate.

Kaplan–Meier plots and log-rank tests were used to estimate and compare two or more survival curves. Cox proportional hazard regression models were applied to the estimated hazard ratios (HRs) and the effects of the predictor factors upon survival for their prognostic relevance. A *p*-value of <0.05 was considered statistically significant. The statistical analysis was assessed using the R software, version 4.4.0 (R Core Team (2024)).

3. Results

3.1. Baseline Characteristics

Two hundred and twenty-nine patients were identified for this study. Of these, 109 were excluded because they did not have radiological imaging within 6 months before surgery. Of the remaining 120, 57 patients were excluded because they had not had endoscopic exams in the two years following surgery or were lost to follow-up.

Of the remaining 63 patients who met all the criteria, 35 (55%) patients were evaluated by MR-E, 13 (21%) by CT-E, and 15 (24%) by abdomen CT.

All patients underwent endoscopy in the two years following surgery. Endoscopic recurrence of the disease was found in 24 patients (38%).

3.2. Clinical Evaluation

The clinical factors are described in Tables 2 and 3, particularly the following:

(a) Age at diagnosis and at the time of surgery: the mean age was 32 years at the time of diagnosis (range: 10–69 years ±16.1) and 40 years at the time of surgery (range: 18–70 ±15.4 years).
(b) Gender: 35 males (56%) and 28 females (44%).
(c) Duration: the duration of the disease ranged from 0.5 to 46 years, with a mean of 8.4 years (±9.2 years).
(d) Perianal disease: perianal disease was present in 4 (6%) patients.
(e) A habit of smoking was present in 11 (17%) patients.

Extra-intestinal disease was present in 12 (9%) patients.

Age at the time of surgery was the only statistically significant factor (HR: 1.04; CI 1.01–1.06; $p = 0.003$) (Table 4).

In other words, the probability of having a recurrence increased by 1% for every year of increase in age. The other clinical factors were not statistically significant factors. In particular, age at diagnosis and the type of medical therapy were not statistically significant factors (Table 4).

Table 2. Demographic characteristics of patients.

	Minimum (Years)	Maximum (Years)	Mean (Years)	Standard Deviation
Age at diagnosis	10.7	69	31.9	16.1
Age at the moment of surgery	18	70	39.9	15.4
Duration of the disease	0.5	46	8.4	9.2

Table 3. Clinical factors and medical treatment of patients.

	Number of Patients	Percentage (%)
Male	35	55.6
Female	28	44.4
Smoking habit	11	17.5
Extra-intestinal manifestations:	12	9
Dermatological	2	3.2
Rheumatological	10	15.9
Perianal disease	4	6.3
Medical therapy:		
- Anti-TNF [a]	11	17.5
- Anti-IL23 [b]	2	3.2
- Anti-integrin	5	7.9
- Immunosuppressive drugs	5	7.9
- Budesonide	12	19.7
- Systemic corticosteroids	2	3.2
- 5-ASA [c]	14	23

[a] Anti-tumor necrosis factor; [b] anti-interleukin 23; [c] 5-acetylsalicylic acid.

Table 4. Statistical descriptive results of enrolled sample.

	HR (95% IC, *p*-Value)
Clinical factors:	
- Age at surgery (for each increment of one year)	1.04 (1.01–1.06, $p = 0.003$)
- Age at diagnosis	1.02 (0.99–1.04, $p = 0.135$)
- Gender	0.80 (1.24–0.34, $p = 0.601$)
- Duration of disease	1.07 (1.02–1.12, $p = 0.051$)
- Perianal disease	NA
- Habit of smoking:	
No	1.67 (0.63–4.36, $p = 0.295$)
Yes	3.08 (0.86–11.04, $p = 0.083$)
- Extra-intestinal manifestations	1.05 (0.41–2.67, $p = 0.905$)
- Anti-TNF [a]	0.91 (0.31–2.63, $p = 0.860$)
- Anti-IL22 [b]	1.51 (0.19–11.35, $p = 0.691$)
- Anti-integrin	0.96 (0.22–4.21, $p = 0.962$)
- Immunosuppressive drugs	1.14 (0.25–5.02, $p = 0.866$)
- Budesonide	1.08 (0.27–4.27, $p = 0.905$)
- Systemic corticosteroids	0.76 (0.09–5.92, $p = 0.796$)
- 5-ASA [c]	1.46 (0.48–4.38, $p = 0.499$)
Radiological factors:	
- Small-bowel thickening	0.96 (0.85–1.09, $p = 0.525$)
- Mucosal ulcers	1.12 (0.50–2.52, $p = 0.771$)
- Stratified CE	NA
- Halo fatty sign	NA
- Engorgement of vasa recta	0.44 (0.05–3.29, $p = 0.425$)
- Stenosis (lumen diameter)	0.78 (0.56–1.08, $p = 0.137$)
- Caliber of upstream loop	1.02 (1.00–1.04, $p = 0.088$)
- Sinus tracts	0.701 (0.31–1.63, $p = 0.418$)
- Fistulas	0.807 (0.35–1.82, $p = 0.609$)
- Abscesses	0.71 (0.24–2.08, $p = 0.529$)
- Lymph nodes	2.34 (0.54–9.98, $p = 0.251$)
- Localization in distal ileum	3.52 (1.19–9.03, $p = 0.015$)
- Number of small-bowel pathological loops	1.15 (1.05–1.27, $p = 0.004$)
- Length of small-bowel pathological loops	1.001 (0.99–1.004, $p = 0.452$)

Table 4. *Cont.*

	HR (95% IC, *p*-Value)
- Sum of small-bowel pathological loops	1.002 (1.00–1.54, $p = 0.014$)
- MRI hyperintensity	NA
- MRI restriction	NA
Surgical factors:	
- Laparotomic surgery	2.17 (0.96–4.86, $p = 0.061$)
- Length of resected intestine	1.01 (1.00–1.02, $p = 0.003$)
- Presence of granulomas	6.00 (1.05–1.27, $p = 0.004$)
- Histological involvement of resection margins	0.77 (0.32–1.78, $p = 0.536$)
- Hand-sewn anastomosis	6.67 (0.89–5.02, $p = 0.033$)
Postoperative evaluation:	
- Complications	0.54 (0.21–1.38, $p = 0.204$)

[a] Anti-tumor necrosis factor; [b] anti-interleukin 23; [c] 5-acetylsalicylic acid.

3.3. Radiological Evaluation

The radiological exams identified 115 small-bowel loops affected by pathology. For each patient, the number of pathological small loops varied from 1 to 20 (medium: 3).

Table 5 shows the frequency distribution of the number of segments in our study.

Table 5. Localizations of pathological intestinal loops in CT-E and MR-E.

	Number of Patients	Percentage (%)
Proximal jejunum	1	1.6
Distal jejunum	5	7.9
Proximal ileum	6	9.5
Distal ileum	41	65.1
Last ileal loop	62	98.4
Involvement of other intestinal loops:		
Appendix	16	25.4
Ascending colon	11	17.5
Transverse colon	3	4.8
Distal colon	2	3.2
Sigma	6	9.5
Rectum	3	4.8

The most frequent localizations were the last ileal loop (62 segments (98%)) and the distal ileum (41 segments (65%)). Even if the radiological evaluation was aimed at studying only the small intestine, we reported each colonic localization appreciable with the method, identifying 41 colonic segments affected by pathology. For each patient, the number of colonic localizations varied from zero to four (medium: one).

Concerning the radiological findings, small-bowel wall thickening was present in all patients, stenosis in 60 (95%), and intestinal dilatation in 32 (51%).

In Table 6, the values of the wall thickening, lumen diameter, and pre-stenotic loop caliber in all patients are reported.

Table 6. CT/MRI small-bowel pathological loops.

	Minimum	Maximum	Mean	Standard Deviation
Wall thickening (mm)	5	25	10.8	2.9
Lumen diameter (mm)	1	7	2.6	1.3
Pre-stenotic loop caliber (mm)	13	95	28.5	13.7

In Table 7, the frequency values of the radiological signs found in this study are reported. In particular, fistulas were found in 27 patients (48%) and sinus tracts in 23 (36%). In six patients, sinus tracts were present without associated fistulas.

Table 7. MR-E, CT-E, and CT findings (35 MR-E, 15 CT, and 13 E-CT).

	Number of Patients	Percentage (%)
Mural thickening	63	100
Mucosal ulcers	27	42.9
Stratified CE	63	100
Halo fatty sign	3	4.8
Engorgement of vasa recta	59	93.7
Stenosis	60	95.2
Pre-stenotic dilatation	32	50.8
Fibrofatty proliferation	8	12.7
Sinus tracts	23	36.5
Enterocutaneous fistulas	5	7.9
Entero-enteric fistulas	25	39.7
Abscesses	15	23.8
LFN	54	85.7
Occlusion	8	12.7
MRI hyperintensity	35	97.2
MRI DWI restriction	30	85.7

In patients who underwent MR-E (35 patients), an increased intramural T2 signal was found in all patients (100%) and restricted diffusion in DWI in 30 (86%) (Table 6).

Table 8 reports the length of each small-bowel pathological loop. The sum of the pathological segments is reported for patients with more than one small-bowel pathological loop.

Table 8. Extension of small-bowel disease in CT and MR exams.

	Minimum	Maximum	Mean	Standard Deviation
Extension of each pathological loop (mm)	20	600	186.1	120.4
Sum of the length of pathological loops (mm)	20	881	258.9	167.5

On the basis of the signs described above, active inflammatory disease was found in 26 (41%) patients, fistulizing in 33 (52%) patients, and fibrostenotic in 4 (6%) patients.

As complications, occlusion was present in 8 (13%) patients. None of the patients reported perforation or bleeding.

Localization in the distal ileum (HR: 3.526; $p = 0.015$; 1.19–9.03) and the number of pathological small-bowel loops (HR: 1.15; 1.05–1.27; $p = 0.004$) were statistically significant radiological factors (Table 3). In other words, patients who had localization in the distal ileum were 3.5 times more likely to develop recurrence than patients who did not have localization in the distal ileum (Figure 2), while the probability of recurrence increased by 1% for each increase in the number of small-bowel loops.

In patients with localization in the distal ileum, the median time from ileocolic resection to clinical postoperative recurrence was 12.5 months.

The sum of small-bowel pathological loops was also a statistically significant factor (HR. 1.002; IC: 1.00–1.54; $p = 0.014$). In other words, the probability of having a recurrence increased by 1% for every increase in cm. The other radiological factors were not statistically significant factors (Table 3).

3.4. Surgical Evaluation

Ileocecal resection was performed in 48 (76%) of patients, and the laparoscopic technique was used for 46 patients (73%). The other surgical factors are described in Table 9. The length of the resected small bowel had a minimum of 3 cm, a maximum of 175 cm, and a mean of 40.7 cm.

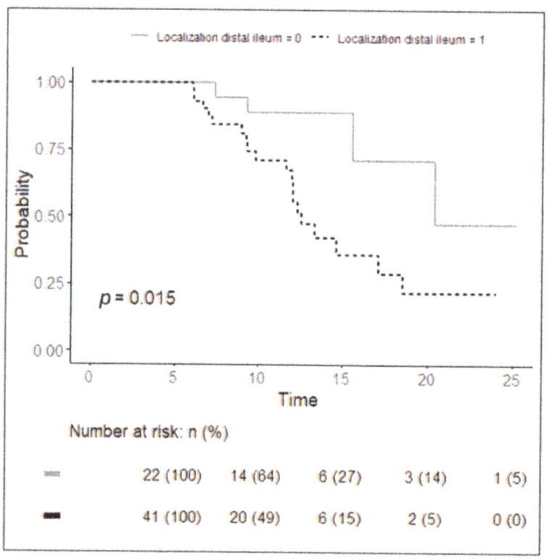

Figure 2. Kaplan–Meier curves of probability to have a recurrence in patients with radiological distal ileum localization (dotted black line) and patients who did not have radiological localization in the distal ileum (continuous grey line).

Table 9. Surgical potential risk factors for postoperative recurrence.

	Number of Patients	Percentage (%)
Type of surgical resection:		
Ileocecal resection	48	76.2
Ileocolic resection	14	22.2
Right hemicolectomy	1	1.6
Laparoscopic surgery	46	73
Emergency surgery	1	1.6
Histological involvement of resection margins	23	36.5

Table 9. *Cont.*

	Number of Patients	Percentage (%)
Type of anastomosis:		
Stapled anastomosis	11	17.5
Hand-sewn anastomosis	52	82.5
Presence of granulomas in the specimen	4	26.7
Transfusions	2	3.2
Ileostomy/colostomy	4	6.3

The length of the resected intestine (HR: 1.01; 1.00–1.02; $p = 0.003$) was a statistically significant factor. In other words, the probability of recurrence increased by 1% for each cm of increase in the length (Table 4). The presence of granulomas (HR: 6.003; IC: 1.05–1.27; $p = 0.004$ (Figure 3)) and hand-sewn anastomosis (HR: 6.67; 0.89–5.02; $p = 0.033$) were also statistically significant factors (Table 4). This means that the probability of recurrence was six times more likely to be in the presence of granulomas and almost seven times more likely to be in the case of hand-sewn anastomosis.

In patients with hand-sewn anastomosis, the median time from ileocolic resection to clinical postoperative recurrence was 14.6 months, while it was 13.4 months in patients with granulomas.

The other surgical factors were not statistically significant factors (Table 4).

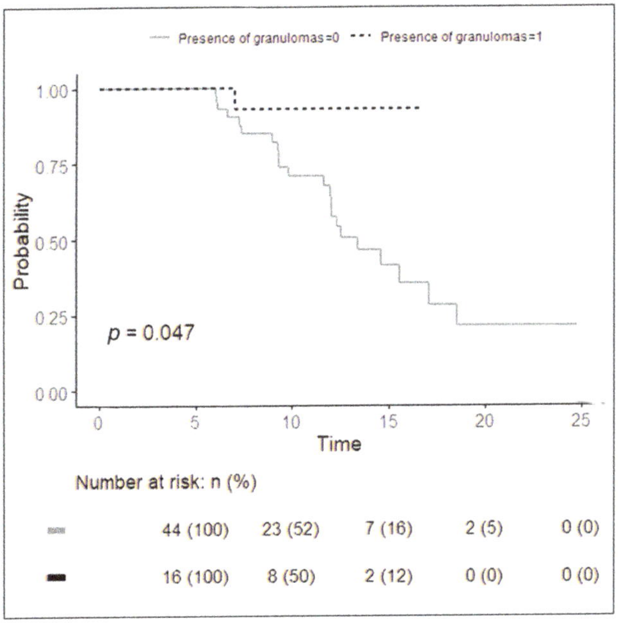

Figure 3. Kaplan–Meier curves of probability to have a recurrence in patients with the presence of granulomas in the specimens (dotted black line) and patients without the presence of granulomas (continuous grey line).

3.5. *Postsurgical Evaluation*

After surgery, 22 (35%) patients had complications (Table 10). The most frequent complication was melena/rectorrhagia in 9 (14%) patients

Table 10. Postsurgical complications and related Clavien–Dindo score.

	Number of Patients	Percentage (%)
Postoperative complications:	22	35
Anastomotic dehiscence	2	3
Sepsis	1	1
Fever (>37.5°)	9	9
Intra-abdominal fluid collection	3	5
Urinary tract infection	3	5
Anemization	5	8
Melena/rectorrhagia	9	14
Vomiting	1	1
High stomal output	1	1
Bladder globe	1	1
Hypoadrenal crisis	1	1
Resumption of parenteral nutrition	1	1
Delay of canalization	0	0
Clavien–Dindo grade:		
0	41	65
1	12	19
2	7	11
3a	1	2
3b	2	3

The presence of complications was not a statistically significant factor for recurrence (Table 4).

4. Discussion

4.1. *Definition of Recurrence*

In the literature, scientific papers are not homogeneous regarding the method of evaluation and identification of postoperative recurrence. In 2014, Li et al. [6] evaluated patients with endoscopic recurrence. In 2015, De Cruz, P. et al. [12] evaluated patients with clinical relapse, defined as the recurrence of Crohn's disease symptoms leading to hospitalization or therapeutic modifications. In 2021, Navaratne et al. [7] distinguished between clinical relapse and symptomatic relapse: clinical relapse was defined as the recurrence of Crohn's disease symptoms leading to hospitalization or therapeutic modifications, according to De Cruz [12], while postoperative relapse was defined as symptomatic when clinical recurrence was confirmed by the presence of recurrence in endoscopic and/or radiological examinations. In 2021, in a paper by Otzgur et al. [13], recurrence was evaluated based on the Crohn's Disease Activity Index or endoscopic findings. In 2016, the ECCO guidelines [4] standardized the terminology to be used in the definition of postoperative recurrence. According to the ECCO guidelines, we chose to evaluate patients with morphological recurrence identified by endoscopy within 2 years before surgery, with the aim of verifying the roles of clinical, surgical, and radiological factors in postoperative recurrence.

4.2. *Clinical Factor*

In 2015, Fornaro et al. [14] published a clinical narrative review and analyzed the roles of different factors in the occurrence of postoperative recurrence in patients surgically treated for CD. The paper aimed to determine which of these factors had been proven in the literature to have a predictive role. The authors underlined the discordant results reported in the literature for most of the clinical factors, even if some of them seemed to be correlated with a greater risk of recurrence. In particular, smoking was reported to be the most statistically significant among the clinical factors. On the contrary, in our study, smoking was not a statistically significant factor.

In 2021, in a study by Navaratne et al. [7], a univariate analysis of the Montreal classification A1 indicated that a Crohn's disease diagnosis age of <17 years appeared to be associated with an increased risk of symptomatic anastomotic postoperative recurrence. In our study, age at diagnosis was not a statistically significant factor. On the contrary, we found age at the time of surgery (HR: 1.04; CI: 1.01–1.06; $p = 0.003$) to be the only statistically significant clinical factor. To the best of our knowledge, this factor has not been evaluated in previous studies.

The other clinical factors were not statistically significant.

4.3. Radiological Factors

In our study, localization in the distal ileum was a statistically significant radiological factor ($p = 0.015$; HR: 3.526; 1.19–9.03). This means that patients who have localization in the distal ileum in radiological exams are more likely to develop recurrence than patients who do not have localization in the distal ileum. In patients with localization in the distal ileum, the median time from ileocolic resection to clinical postoperative recurrence was 12.5 months. Colic localization was not a statistically significant factor. However, in the literature, not all authors agree with the importance of intestinal localization. In fact, for some authors, colic localization seems to be associated with a lower recurrence rate than jejunal and ileal disease [15], while for others [16], localization of the disease in the colon is a predictive factor for recurrence.

In the literature, mesenteric hypertrophy is described in some studies as an indicator of a complicated course of Crohn's disease [6,17]. Li et al. [6] used computed tomography to measure the subcutaneous fat area and visceral fat area (VFA) and defined the mesenteric fat index (MFI) as the ratio of the VFA to the subcutaneous fat area. The authors found that a high VFA value is predictive of postoperative recurrence of Crohn's disease, so it plays a clinical role in optimizing prophylaxis for each patient. Navaratne et al. [7] evaluated the mesenteric fat index and the presence of fibrofatty proliferation in CT/MRI examinations carried out before surgery, and no association was found between the visceral fat area (VFA) or mesenteric fat index (MFI) and postoperative recurrence. In our study, we evaluated the presence of fibrofatty proliferation, and we found it not to be a statistically significant factor in predicting recurrence.

Finally, a significant radiological factor was the number of pathological small-bowel loops affected by pathology (HR: 1.15; 1.05–1.27; $p = 0.004$). To the best of our knowledge, this factor has not been evaluated in previous studies.

4.4. Surgical Evaluation

In "The Second European Evidence-Based Consensus on the Diagnosis and the Management of Crohn's Disease: Special Situations" [16], a penetrating behavior of the disease, extensive small-bowel resection, and prior intestinal surgery were also predictive factors for postoperative recurrence. In our study, we evaluated patients who underwent surgery for the first time; therefore, we were not able to make any judgments regarding this factor, and the presence of penetrating disease was not a statistically significant factor.

Concerning disease extension, Navaratne et al. [7] evaluated the extension of disease based on the extent of macroscopic disease seen at surgery and the resection length and found gastrointestinal involvement of >30 cm to be a statistically significant factor, while Fornaro [14] reported a length of intestinal disease of >100 cm to be a statistically significant factor. In our study, the length of intestinal disease was assessed both in radiological studies and surgical specimens. While the length of small-bowel pathological loops in radiological exams was not a statistically significant factor, we found both the sum of small-bowel pathological loops in radiological exams and the length of the resected intestine measured intraoperatively to be statistically significant. In particular, we found a correlation between the probability of recurrence and the grade of length increase. To the best of our knowledge, this correlation has not been verified in previous studies.

Finally, in our study, the presence of granulomas and hand-sewn anastomosis were statistically significant factors. In patients with granulomas, the median time from ileocolic resection to clinical postoperative recurrence was 13.4 months. However, the literature data regarding the impact on postoperative recurrence of the presence of granulomas in the resected specimen are contradictory. Some authors reported an association with a higher incidence of recurrence [18,19], while others reported a lower recurrence rate [20,21].

The result of an increased risk of recurrence in the case of hand-sewn anastomosis is a controversial fact that requires further investigation. In our opinion, although statistical significance was reached in our study, the result was influenced by the non-homogeneity of the numbers in the two groups (mechanical and hand-sewn anastomoses) and by the fact that, often, in our center, the decision to perform a mechanical anastomosis is influenced by the intraoperative characteristics, and, in the most difficult cases (fistulizing disease, abscesses, and extensive resections), a manual anastomosis is, generally, opted for.

The other surgical factors were not statistically significant factors.

4.5. Postsurgical Evaluation

The presence of complications was also not a statistically significant factor for recurrence.

In our study, we evaluated the risk of recurrence within two years of surgery and excluded patients who had already undergone surgery. On the contrary, Khoury et al. [5] evaluated the risk factors associated with early disease recurrence with the need for re-surgery and found that the risk factors for early disease recurrence were the presence of stenotic and penetrating disease (stricturing: odds ratio (OR)—12.1; penetrating: OR—9.9 (rather than non-stricturing and non-penetrating)) and the development of postoperative complications in a previous surgery.

4.6. Limitations

Our work presents several limitations that must be taken into consideration.

First and foremost, this was a retrospective study, and the validity of our conclusions is naturally influenced by this study's design. Additionally, the postoperative recurrence of Crohn's disease can be significantly affected by the postoperative pharmacological therapy and the timing of its initiation. Unfortunately, the data we had only provided partial information regarding the postoperative therapy taken by the patients in our study, which is why we chose not to include these data in our analysis. Certainly, this information could be incorporated into the design of a larger prospective study in the future.

5. Conclusions

Our study identified clinical, surgical, and radiological factors that could predict disease recurrence after intestinal resection for Crohn's disease. Younger patients with disease localization in the distal ileum, extensive radiological involvement of small-bowel loops, and specific histopathological features, such as granulomas and longer resected segments, represent a high-risk group for recurrence. Identifying these factors preoperatively allows for the possibility of more aggressive therapeutic interventions post-surgery, including, for example, the early introduction of immunosuppressive or biological agents, which may mitigate the risk of recurrence and improve long-term outcomes. These results not only offer valuable insights into patient-specific recurrence risks but also set the stage for future prospective studies aimed at optimizing postoperative management and improving the quality of life of patients with Crohn's disease. By refining our ability to predict recurrence, we can move closer to more personalized, precision-based treatment paradigms that address both the immediate postoperative period and long-term disease control.

Author Contributions: Conceptualization, L.M.M.; methodology, L.M.M., F.S. (Franco Sacchetti), D.P. and F.S. (Franco Scaldaferri); formal analysis D.B., R.M. and F.B.D.; investigation D.B., F.S. (Franco Sachetti), R.M., L.L. (Luigi Larosa), D.C., L.L. (Lucrezia Laterza), D.P., P.C., A.E.P. and F.S. (Franco Scaldaferri); data curation D.B. and R.M.; writing—original draft preparation, L.M.M., D.B. and F.S. (Franco Sachetti); writing—review and editing, L.M.M., D.B. and F.S. (Franco Sacchetti); supervision, L.L. (Luigi Larosa), L.L. (Lucrezia Laterza), P.C., A.E.P., L.S. and F.S. All authors have read and agreed to the published version of the manuscript.

Funding: This research received no external funding.

Institutional Review Board Statement: This study was conducted in accordance with the Declaration of Helsinki and approved by the Ethics Committee of Università Cattolica del Sacro Cuore, Rome (protocol 0016123/22 on 12 May 2022).

Informed Consent Statement: Informed consent was obtained from all subjects involved in this study.

Data Availability Statement: The raw data supporting the conclusions of this article will be made available by the authors upon request.

Conflicts of Interest: The authors declare no conflicts of interest.

References

1. Poggioli, G.; Pierangeli, F.; Laureti, S.; Ugolini, F.; Poggioli, G.; Pierangeli, F.; Laureti, S.; Ugolini, F. Indication and type of surgery in Crohn's disease. *Aliment. Pharmacol. Ther.* **2002**, *16* (Suppl. S4), 59–64. [CrossRef] [PubMed]
2. McLeod, R.S. Surgery for Inflammatory Bowel Diseases. *Dig. Dis.* **2003**, *21*, 168–179. [CrossRef] [PubMed]
3. Rutgeerts, P.; Geboes, K.; Vantrappen, G.; Beyls, J.; Kerremans, R.; Hiele, M. Predictability of the postoperative course of Crohn's disease. *Gastroenterology* **1990**, *99*, 956–963. [CrossRef] [PubMed]
4. Gomollón, F.; Dignass, A.; Annese, V.; Tilg, H.; Van Assche, G.; Lindsay, J.O.; Peyrin-Biroulet, L.; Cullen, G.J.; Daperno, M.; Kucharzik, T.; et al. 3rd European Evidence-based Consensus on the Diagnosis and Management of Crohn's Disease 2016: Part 1: Diagnosis and Medical Management. *J. Crohn's Colitis* **2017**, *11*, 3–25. [CrossRef] [PubMed]
5. Khoury, W.; Strong, S.A.; Fazio, V.W.; Kiran, R.P. Factors Associated with Operative Recurrence Early After Resection for Crohn's Disease. *J. Gastrointest. Surg.* **2011**, *15*, 1354–1360. [CrossRef]
6. Li, Y.; Zhu, W.; Gong, J.; Zhang, W.; Gu, L.; Guo, Z.; Cao, L.; Shen, B.; Li, N.; Li, J. Visceral fat area is associated with a high risk for early postoperative recurrence in Crohn's disease. *Color. Dis.* **2015**, *17*, 225–234. [CrossRef] [PubMed]
7. Navaratne, L.; Hurndall, K.; Richardson, D.M.; Stephenson, R.; Power, N.; Gillott, H.; Sánchez, S.R.; Khodatars, K.; Chan, C.L.H. Risk factors for symptomatic anastomotic postoperative recurrence following ileo-colic resection in Crohn's disease. *Color. Dis.* **2021**, *23*, 1184–1192. [CrossRef]
8. Minordi, L.M.; Larosa, L.; Bevere, A.; D'angelo, F.B.; Pierro, A.; Cilla, S.; Del Ciello, A.; Scaldaferri, F.; Barbaro, B. Imaging of Strictures in Crohn's Disease. *Life* **2023**, *13*, 2283. [CrossRef] [PubMed]
9. Minordi, L.M.; Bevere, A.; Papa, A.; Larosa, L.; Manfredi, R. CT and MRI Evaluations in Crohn's Complications: A Guide for the Radiologist. *Acad. Radiol.* **2022**, *29*, 1206–1227. [CrossRef]
10. Minordi, L.M.; Larosa, L.; Brizi, M.G.; Armuzi, A.; Manfredi, R. Length of the healthy and pathological small intestine in patients with Crohn's disease: Calculations using computed tomography and magnetic resonance enterography. *Diagn. Interv. Radiol.* **2023**, *29*, 24–28. [CrossRef]
11. Dindo, D.; Demartines, N.; Clavien, P.-A. Classification of Surgical Complications. *Ann. Surg.* **2004**, *240*, 205–213. [CrossRef] [PubMed]
12. De Cruz, P.; Kamm, M.A.; Hamilton, A.L.; Ritchie, K.J.; Krejany, E.O.; Gorelik, A.; Liew, D.; Prideaux, L.; Lawrance, I.C.; Andrews, J.M.; et al. Crohn's disease management after intestinal resection: A randomised trial. *Lancet* **2015**, *385*, 1406–1417. [CrossRef] [PubMed]
13. Ozgur, I.; Kulle, C.B.; Buyuk, M.; Ormeci, A.; Akyuz, F.; Balik, E.; Bulut, T.; Keskin, M. What are the predictors for recurrence of Crohn's disease after surgery? *Medicine* **2021**, *100*, e25340. [CrossRef] [PubMed]
14. Fornaro, R.; Caratto, E.; Caratto, M.; Fornaro, F.; Caristo, G.; Frascio, M.; Sticchi, C. Post-operative recurrence in Crohn's disease. Critical analysis of potential risk factors. An update. *Surgeon* **2015**, *13*, 330–347. [CrossRef]
15. Rutgeerts, P. Strategies in the prevention of post-operative recurrence in Crohn's disease. *Best Pract. Res. Clin. Gastroenterol.* **2003**, *17*, 63–73. [CrossRef]
16. Eugene, C. The second European evidence-based Consensus on the diagnosis and management of Crohn's disease. *Clin. Res. Hepatol. Gastroenterol.* **2011**, *35*, 257–259. [CrossRef]
17. Anseline, P.F.; Wlodarczyk, J.; Murugasu, R. Presence of granulomas is associated with recurrence after surgery for Crohn's disease: Experience of a surgical unit. *Br. J. Surg.* **1997**, *84*, 78–82. [CrossRef]
18. Malireddy, K.; Larson, D.W.; Sandborn, W.J.; Loftus, E.V.; Faubion, W.A.; Pardi, D.S.; Qin, R.; Gullerud, R.E.; Cima, R.R.; Wolff, B.; et al. Recurrence and impact of postoperative prophylaxis in laparoscopically treated primary ileocolic Crohn disease. *Arch. Surg.* **2010**, *145*, 42–47. [CrossRef]
19. Simillis, C.; Jacovides, M.; Reese, G.E.; Yamamoto, T.; Tekkis, P.P. Meta-analysis of the Role of Granulomas in the Recurrence of Crohn Disease. *Dis. Colon Rectum* **2010**, *53*, 177–185. [CrossRef]
20. Chambers, T.J.; Morson, B.C. The granuloma in Crohn's disease. *Gut* **1979**, *20*, 269–274. [CrossRef]
21. Glass, R.E.; Baker, W.N. Role of the granuloma in recurrent Crohn's disease. *Gut* **1976**, *17*, 75–77. [CrossRef]

MDPI AG
Grosspeteranlage 5
4052 Basel
Switzerland
Tel.: +41 61 683 77 34

Journal of Clinical Medicine Editorial Office
E-mail: jcm@mdpi.com
www.mdpi.com/journal/jcm